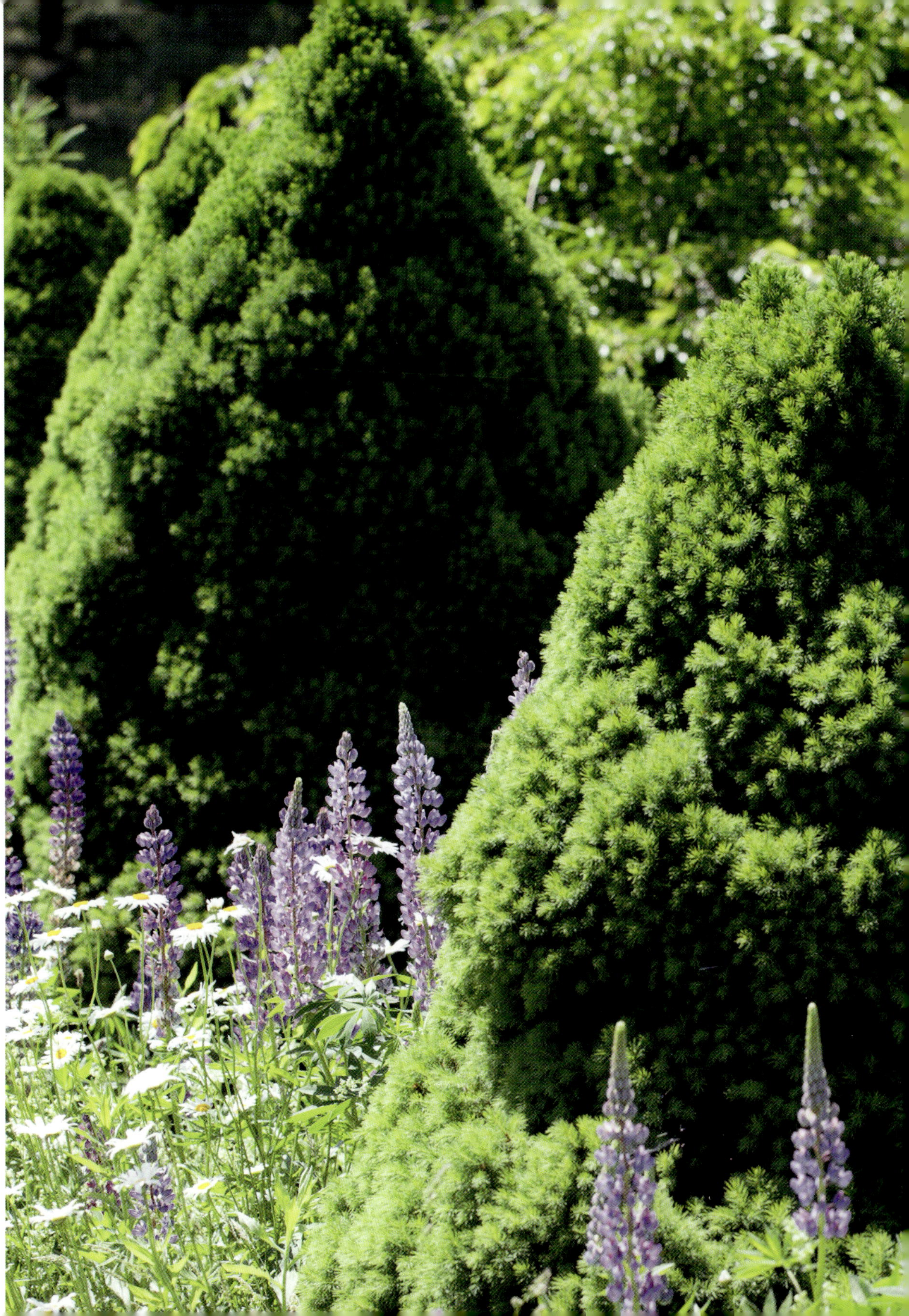

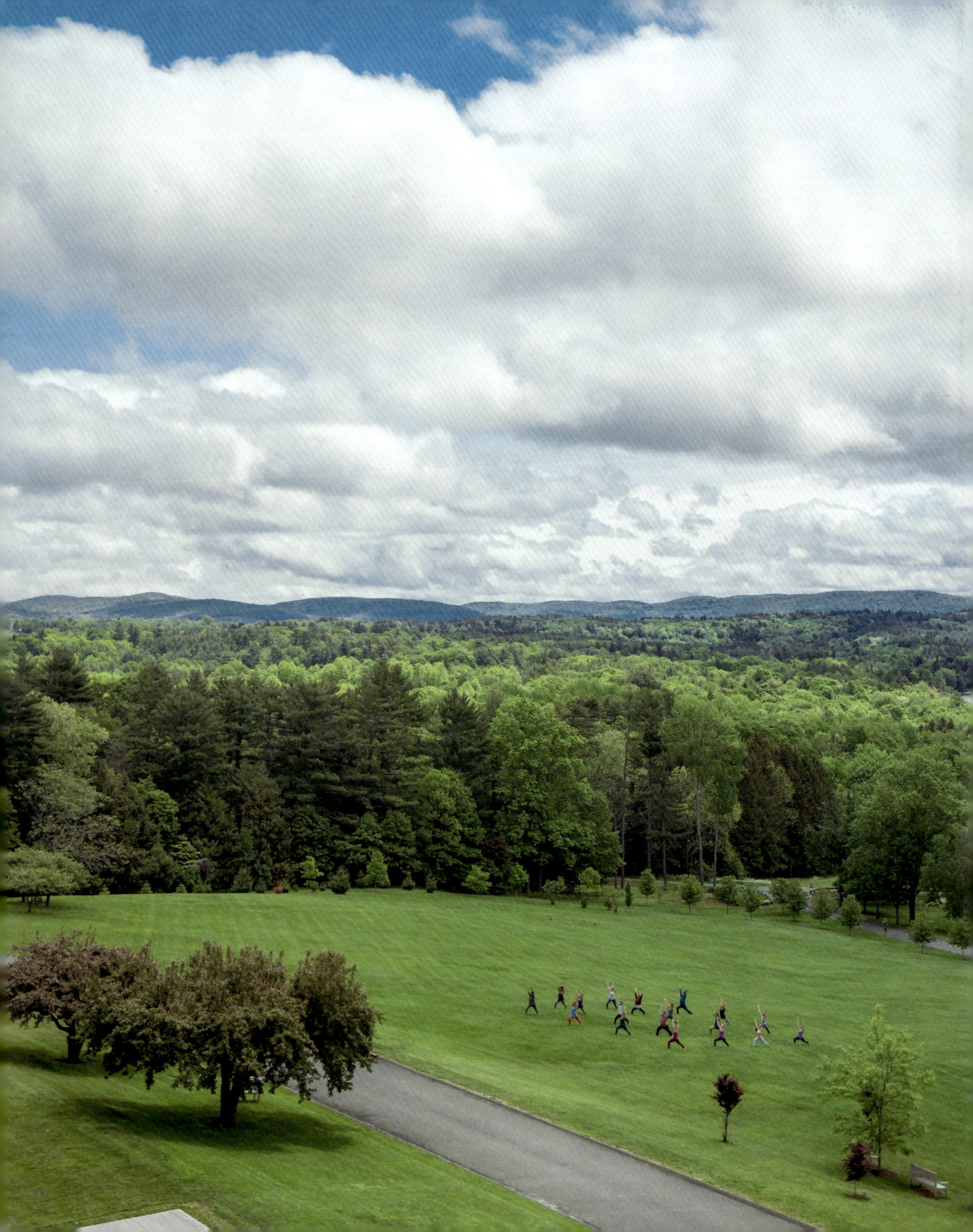

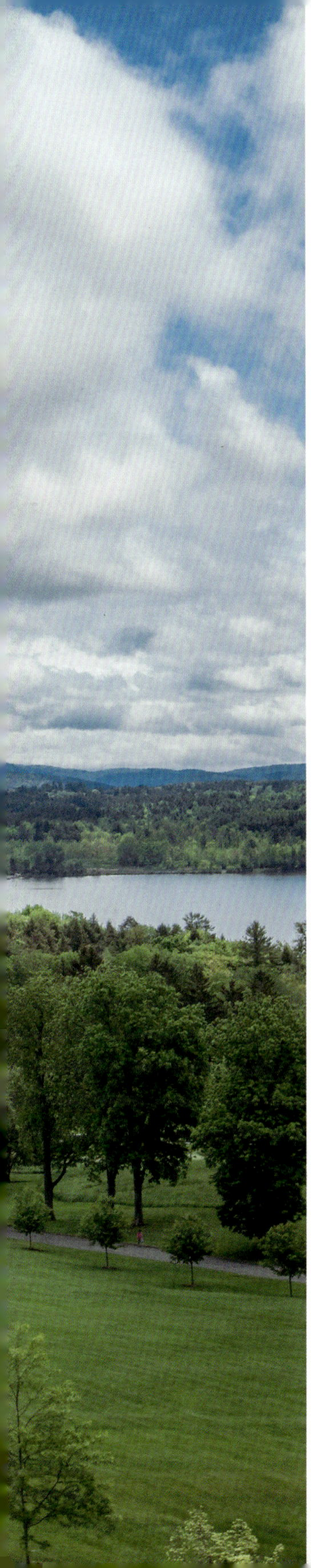

THE KRIPALU KITCHEN

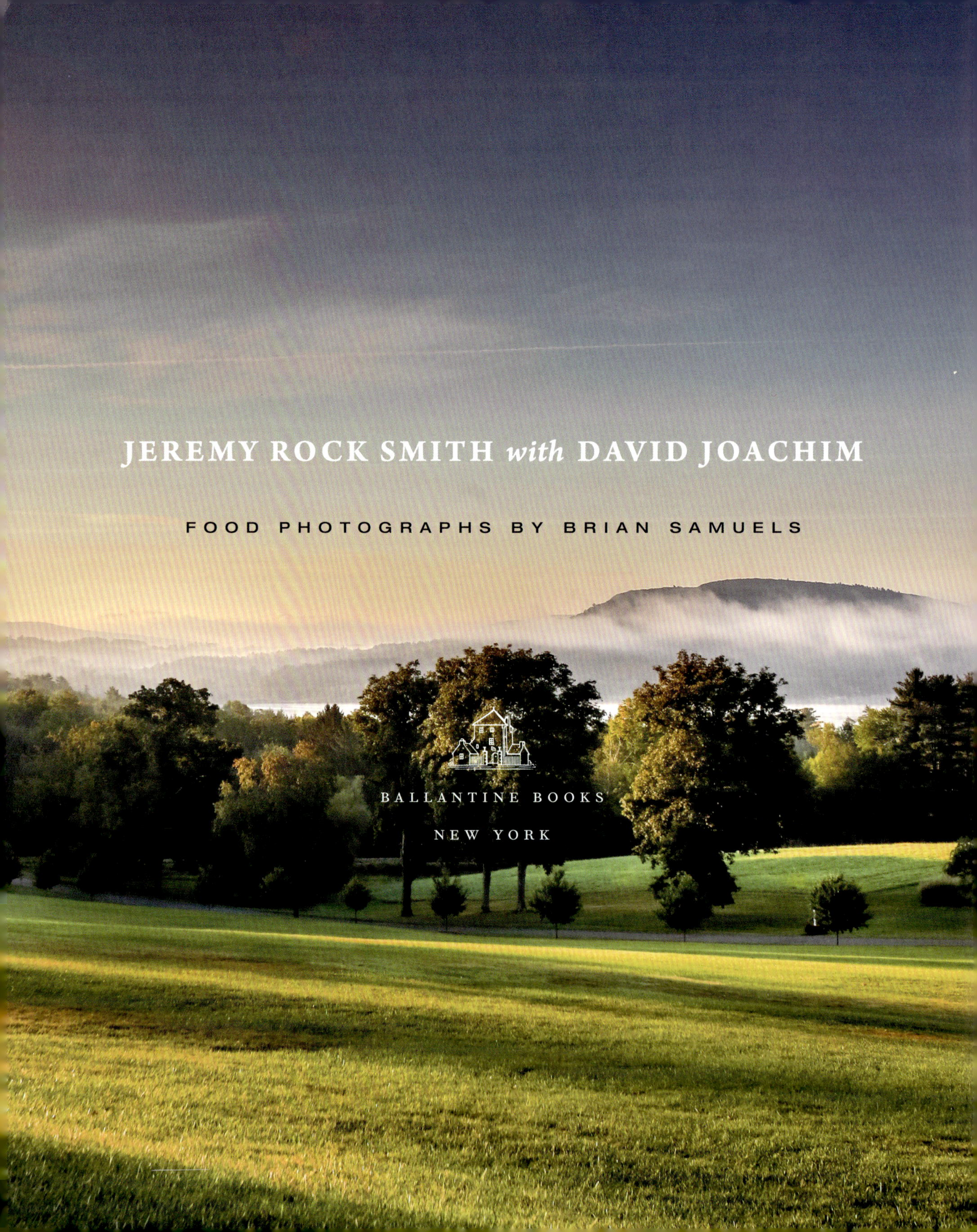

JEREMY ROCK SMITH *with* DAVID JOACHIM

FOOD PHOTOGRAPHS BY BRIAN SAMUELS

BALLANTINE BOOKS

NEW YORK

THE KRIPALU KITCHEN

NOURISHING FOOD *for* BODY AND SOUL

125
REVITALIZING RECIPES
FROM THE
POPULAR WELLNESS
RETREAT

Published in the United States by Ballantine Books,
an imprint of Random House, a division of
Penguin Random House LLC, New York.

BALLANTINE and the HOUSE colophon are registered
trademarks of Penguin Random House LLC.

Food photography by Brian Samuels
Landscape photography courtesy the Kripalu Center for Yoga & Health

LIBRARY OF CONGRESS CATALOGING-IN-PUBLICATION DATA

NAMES: Rock Smith, Jeremy, author. | Joachim, David, author.
TITLE: The Kripalu kitchen: nourishing food for body and soul
115 revitalizing recipes from the popular wellness retreat /
Jeremy Rock Smith with David Joachim; food photographs by Brian Samuels.
DESCRIPTION: New York: Ballantine Books, 2019. | Includes bibliographical references and index.
IDENTIFIERS: LCCN 2018051676 (print) | LCCN 2018051745 (ebook) |
ISBN 9781984817303 (ebook) | ISBN 9780525620815 (hardcover: alk. paper)
Subjects: LCSH: Cooking (Natural foods) | Nutrition. | LCGFT: Cookbooks.
CLASSIFICATION: LCC TX741 (ebook) | LCC TX741 .S62 2019 (print) |
DDC 641.3/02—dc23
LC record available at https://lccn.loc.gov/2018051676

Printed in China on acid-free paper

randomhousebooks.com

123456789

First Edition

Book design by Barbara M. Bachman

To Swami Kripalu

for spreading the love

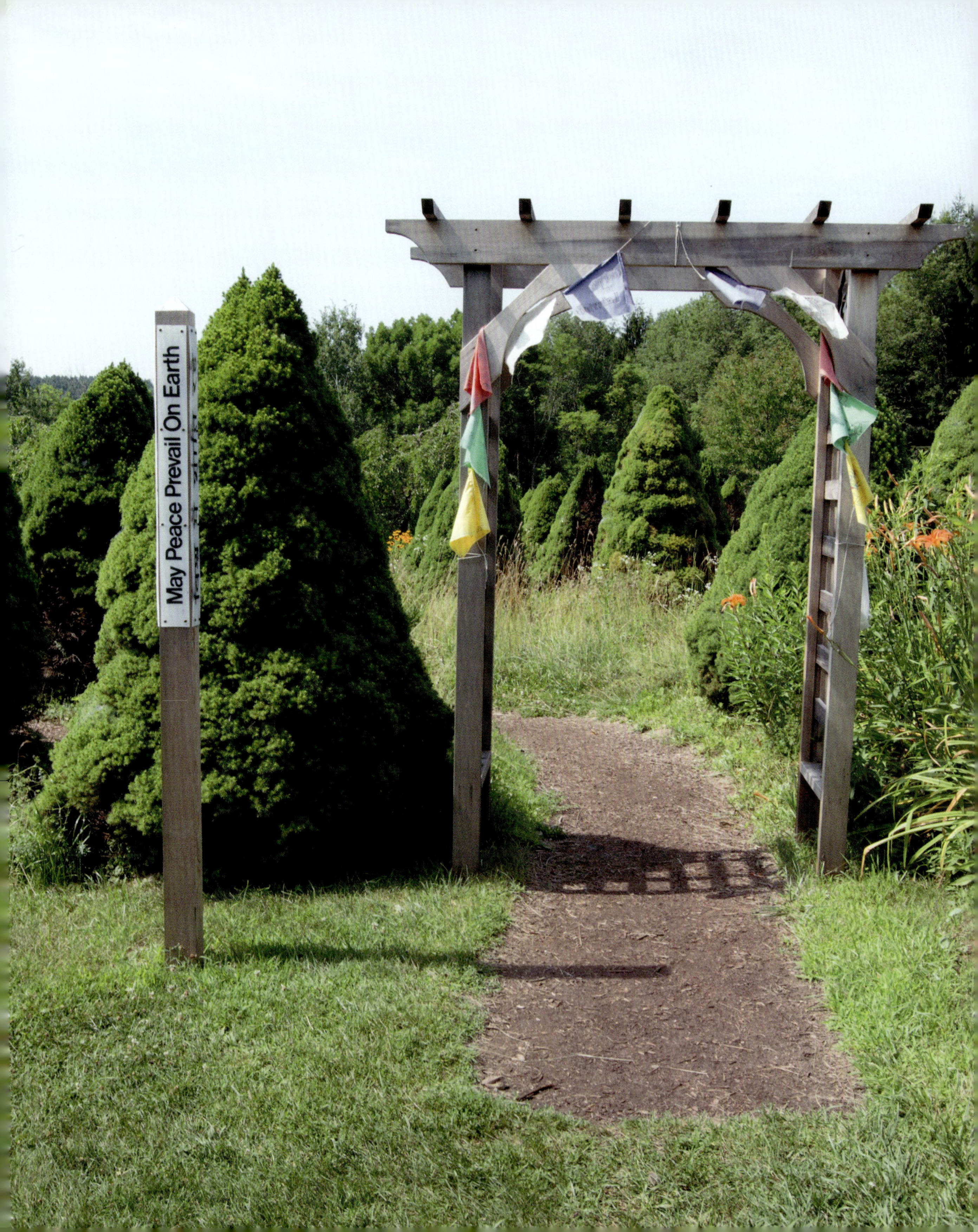
May Peace Prevail On Earth

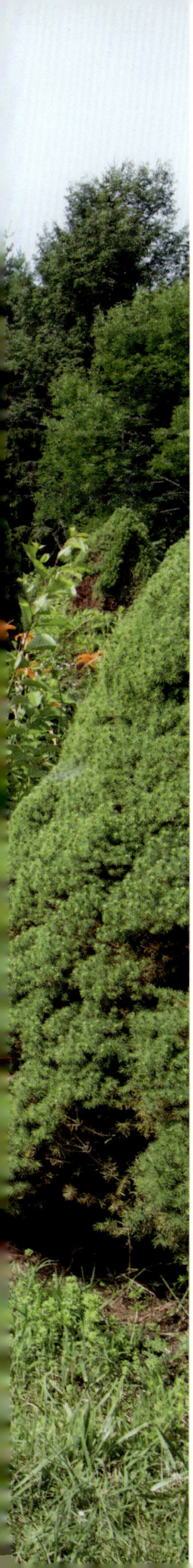

CONTENTS

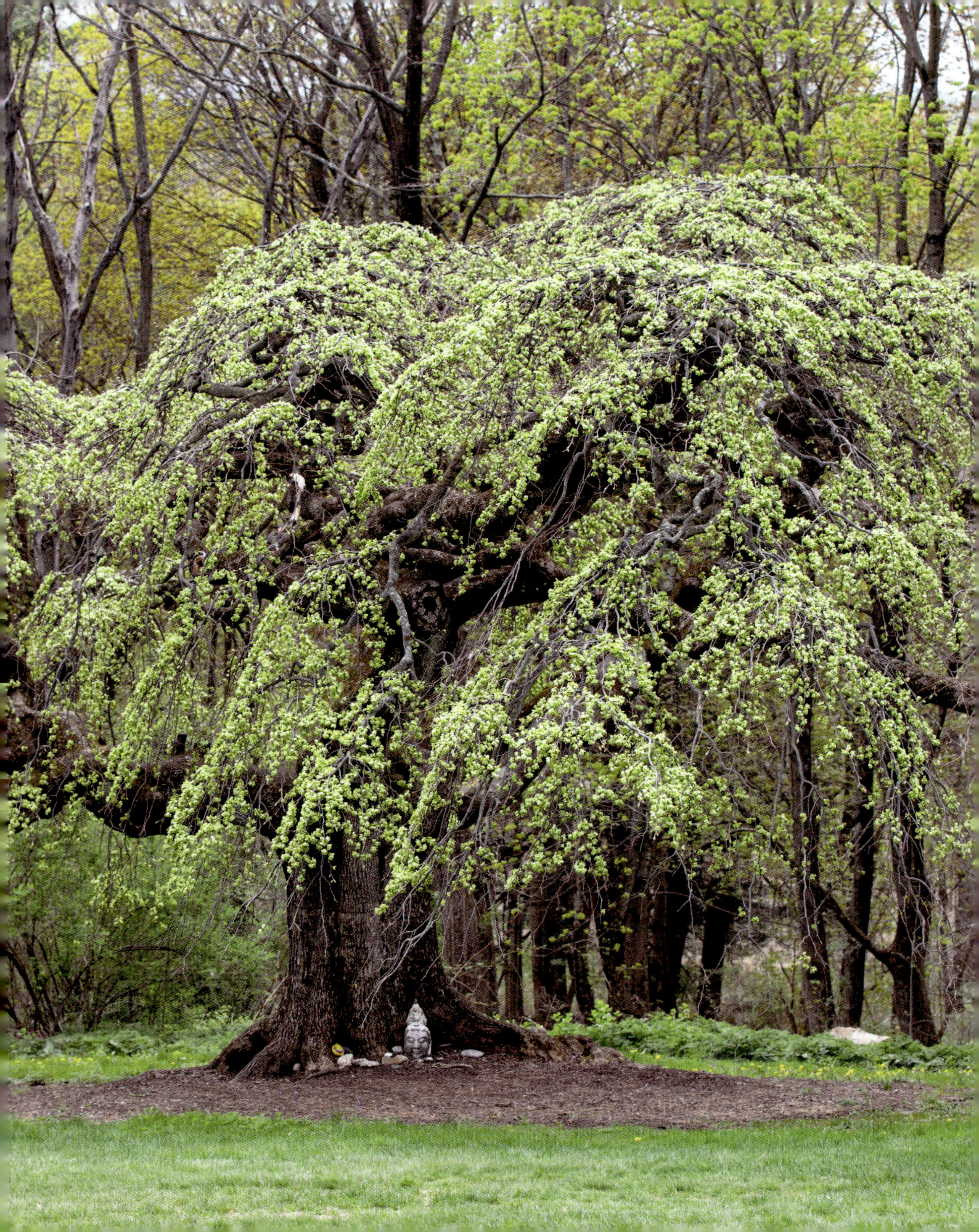

RECIPE LIST

BREAKFAST

MUFFINS, SCONES, AND BREADS

SOUPS

SALADS AND SANDWICHES

BASICS FROM THE BUDDHA BAR

MAIN DISHES

VEGETABLES AND GRAINS

SOMETHING SWEET

JUICES, TEAS, AND TONICS

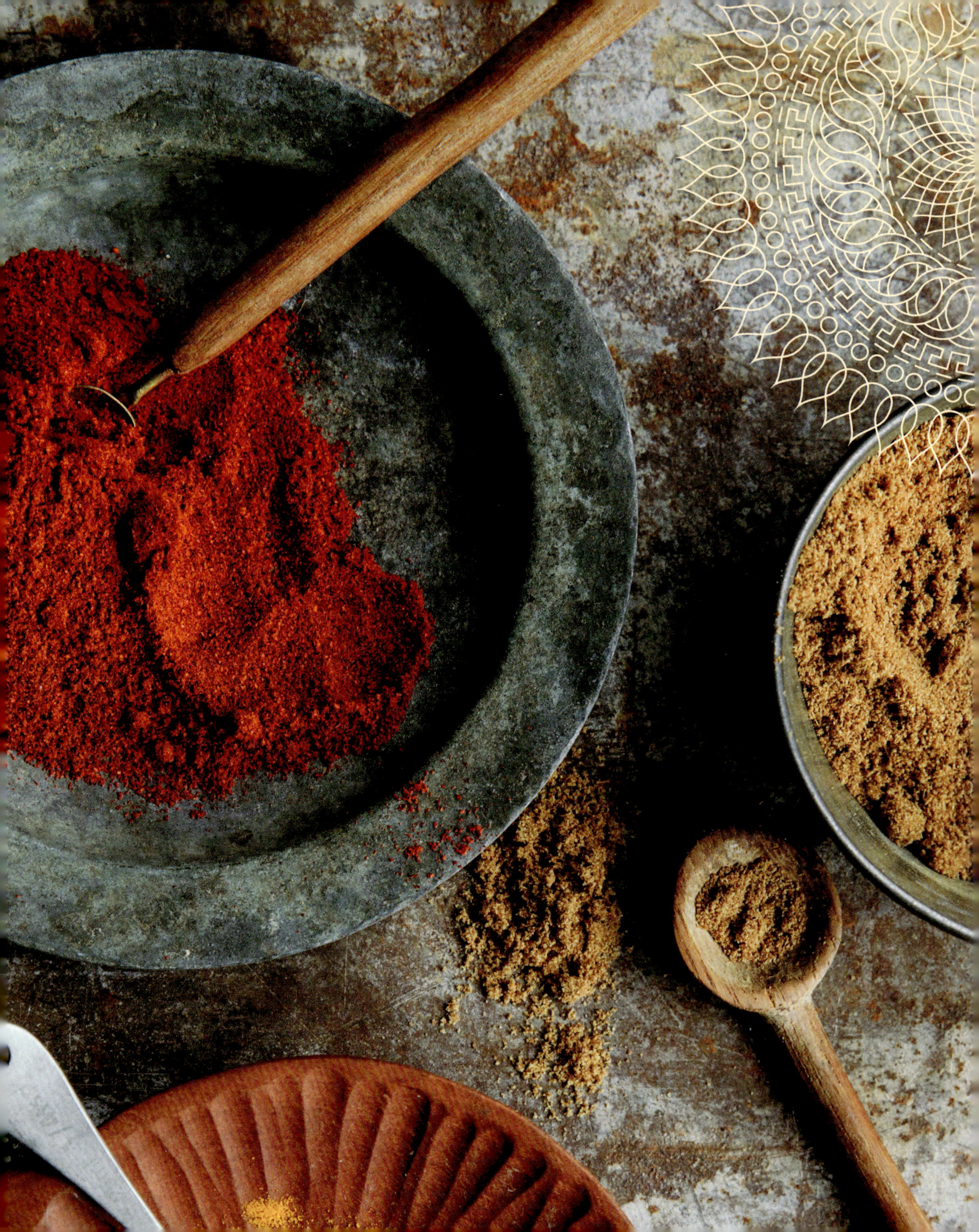

INTRODUCTION

WELCOME TO THE KRIPALU KITCHEN

Have you noticed that almost every small town in America has at least one yoga studio? In bigger cities, you find dozens. According to recent research from the Yoga Alliance and the *Yoga Journal*, more than 36 million Americans maintain some kind of yoga practice. Why? Because it feels good! More and more studies are verifying the health benefits of yoga, such as reducing stress, lowering blood pressure, improving heart health, fighting inflammation, reducing chronic pain, and improving mental health.

More people are also hiking, paddling, and taking up activities like tai chi. Along with the increasing popularity of these physical activities, demand for healing foods such as turmeric and ginger has also skyrocketed in recent years. Again, you can chalk it up to scientific research confirming the health benefits of these time-honored curative ingredients. Plus, they taste great!

Yoga, tai chi, paddling, turmeric, and ginger are all part of the larger American movement toward healthy living—from the foods we eat to the activities we enjoy. They are also key elements of the healthy lifestyle practiced at the Kripalu Center for Yoga & Health, North America's largest yoga-based healing and education center. This cookbook captures everything we do at Kripalu. It provides dozens of holistic wellness strategies and 125 deeply satisfying recipes with variations that create many more options, all of which can help you get healthy and stay healthy.

Kripalu has been teaching holistic living skills for more than forty years and attracts nearly fifty thousand guests every year. Our nonprofit facilities sit on more than three hundred acres in the picturesque Berkshire Hills of Western Massachusetts, and we offer approximately a thousand unique wellness programs a year. We also serve more than twelve hundred nourishing meals to guests every single day. In fact, the Kripalu Kitchen daily meals are one of the highest-ranked experiences among guests, aside from the beautiful grounds.

This cookbook brings the satisfaction and healing power of Kripalu's most popular foods to your table. It also provides a personalized approach to nutrition, including an introduction to the ancient practice of Ayurvedic healing, useful tips for mindful eating, a variety of delicious cross-cultural recipes, and menus for various dietary preferences ranging from vegan and vegetarian to gluten-free, grain-free, dairy-free, and sugar-free. No matter how busy you are, we encourage you to incorporate more healthy foods into your current lifestyle, so we also offer dozens of six-ingredient and thirty-minute recipes.

Over the years, the food we've prepared in the Kripalu Kitchen has woven together the wisdom of ancient healing practices, modern nutritional science, and both classic and contemporary culinary techniques. This cookbook features a wide range of recipes, including international twists on popular favorites such as Coconut French Toast with Thai Ginger Maple Syrup (page 62); healthy versions of quick and satisfying meals like Mushroom Cheesesteaks (page 203) and Linguine with Pumpkin Sage "Alfredo" and Kale Pesto (page 192); and restorative preparations such as Morning Broth (page 279) and Cucumber, Kale, Ginger, and Apple Juice (page 292).

Our cuisine needs to please anywhere from two hundred to six hundred individual palates a day, so these recipes come with simple adaptations for special diets, allowing you to serve a single dish such as Sautéed Barramundi with Harissa, Toasted Almonds, and Honey (page 212) to vegans and vegetarians as well as omnivores by replacing all or part of the fish with plant-based proteins such as tofu. About 80 percent of the recipes are naturally vegetarian and the other 20 percent come with easy vegan and vegetarian options. Many of our guests eat gluten-free, so we also include recipes for our most tried-and-true baked goods, such as Gluten-Free Salted Double Chocolate Chip Cookies (page 253), Gluten-Free

Whole-Grain Vegan Brownies (page 261), and Gluten-Free Vegan Swami Kripalu Birthday Cake (page 273).

But this is not just a cookbook. At Kripalu, our mission is to empower you to realize your full potential through the transformative wisdom of yoga, a union of mind and body. A critical part of any unified health practice is a nutritious diet, and this book helps you find the optimal diet for you. We include a simple test to determine your personal nutrition profile, and explain which foods are best for you to eat. To help you achieve and maintain your ideal health, every recipe in this book is marked as balancing or imbalancing for your personal constitution.

This concept of personal nutrition and personal choice is central to everything we do in the Kripalu Kitchen. We believe that each person has a unique path to health, and our goal is to gently guide you along that path. Let's get started!

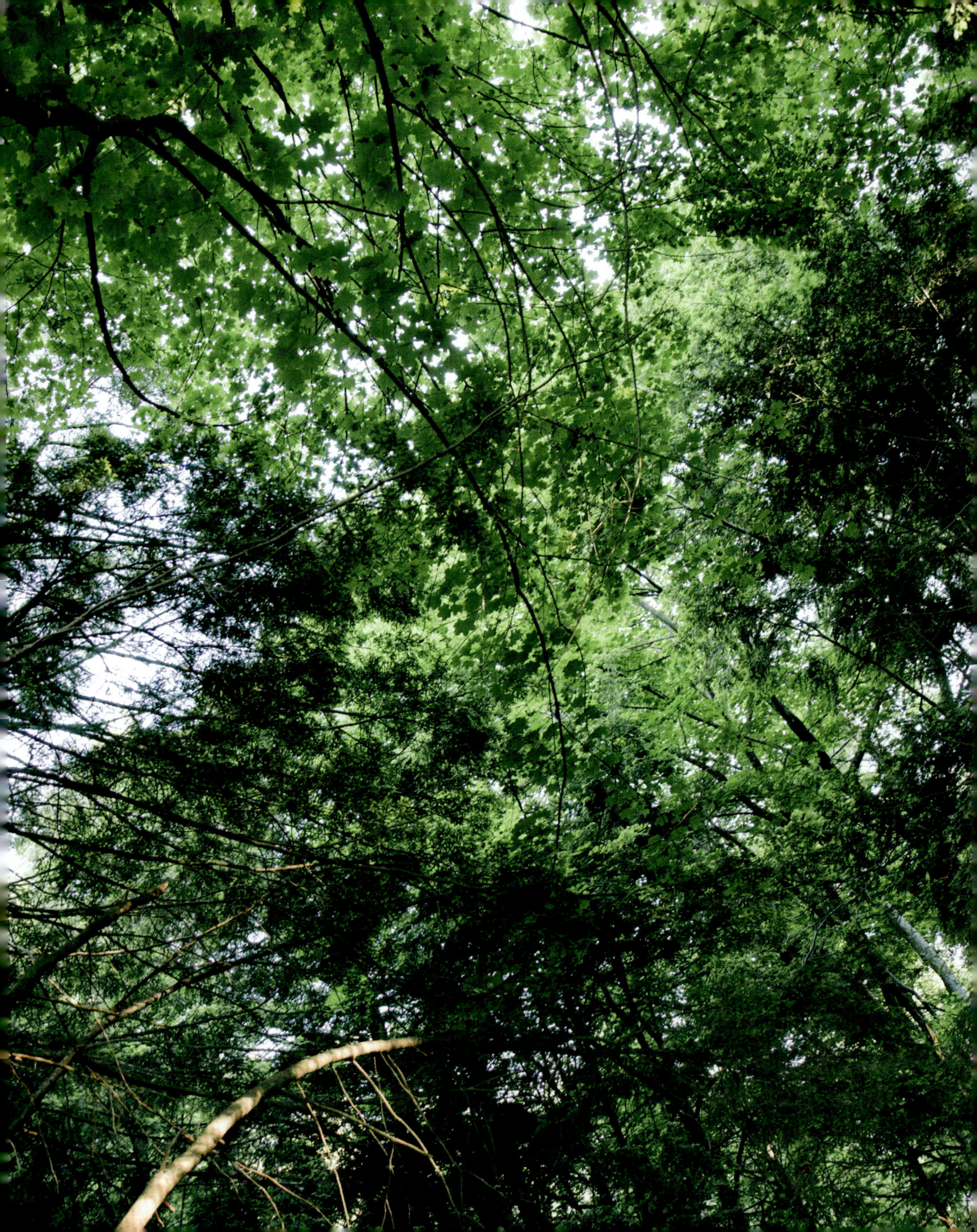

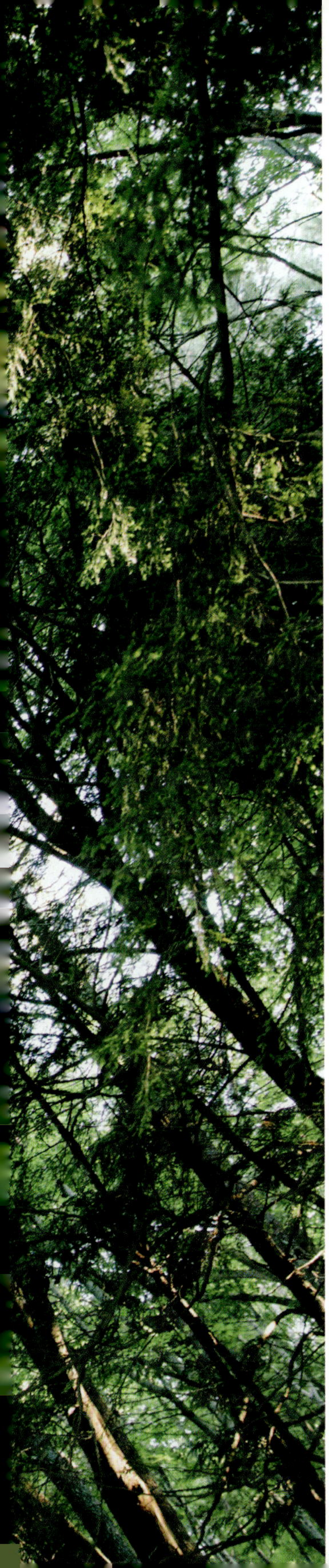

THE KRIPALU KITCHEN

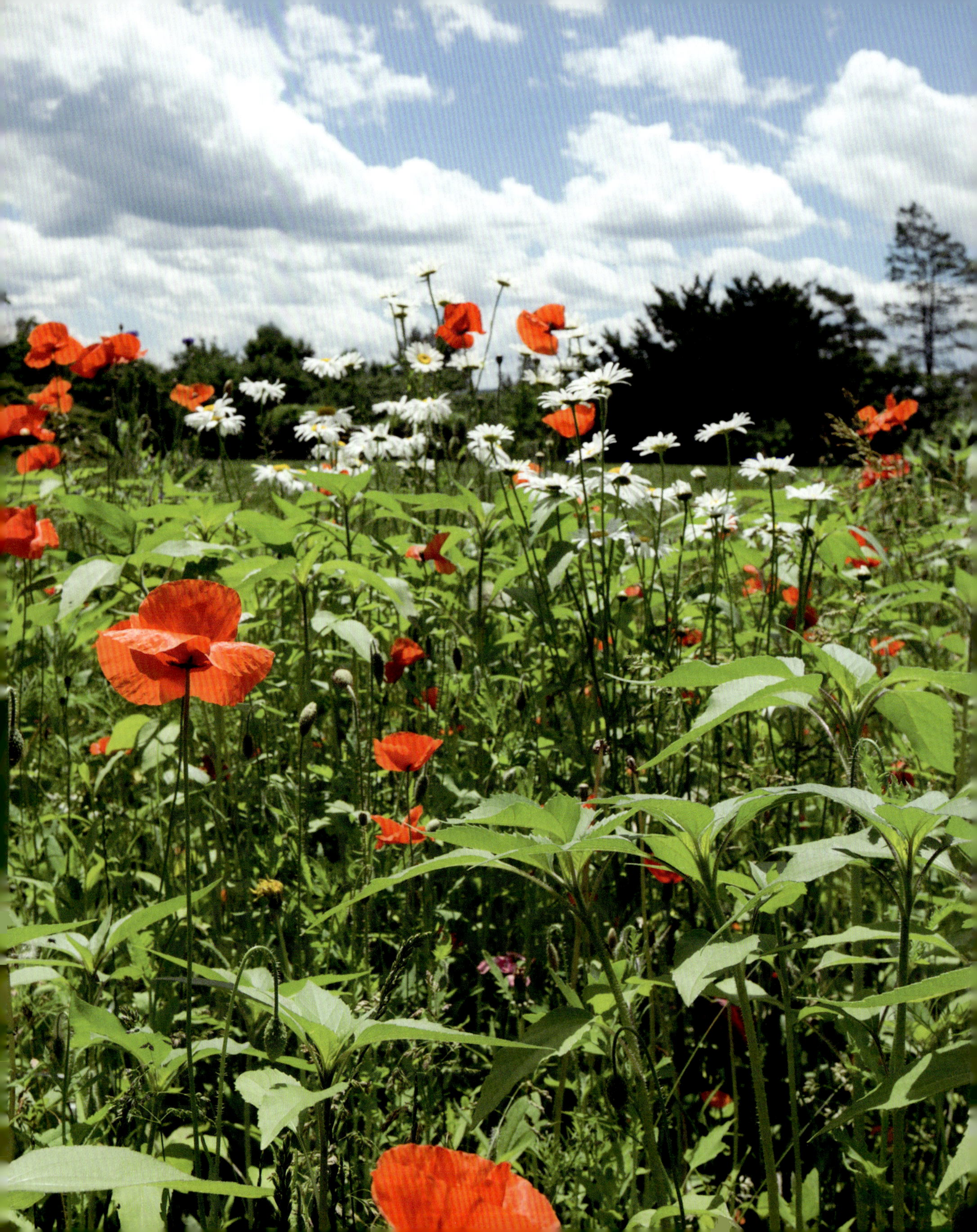

PERSONAL NUTRITION

WHEN AN ELEPHANT AND AN ANT DECIDE WHAT IS MODERATION, THEIR PORTIONS WILL BE DIFFERENT.

—SWAMI KRIPALU

At Kripalu, we are committed to helping our guests transform their health by deepening their understanding of food and nourishment. Our nutrition philosophy combines current scientific research with the wisdom of the yogic tradition, which views food as a source of *prana*, or life force. All of our dietary recommendations are geared toward increasing energy and vitality, improving digestion, boosting metabolism, and, if you have one, enhancing your yoga practice. We support a diversity of dietary choices but have one recommendation that applies to everyone: eat the highest-quality food possible. In the Kripalu Kitchen, that means enjoying the freshest, most nutritious, least-processed foods, and buying food locally, seasonally, and organic whenever possible. To help you bring balance to your food choices, we encourage what we call compassionate self-observation, a gradual process of accepting one's behavior without judgment and allowing transformation to occur naturally. Food is powerful medicine, and wise choices can improve not only your personal health but also the health of your environment, relationships, and community.

EAST MEETS WEST NUTRITION

What constitutes a "healthy diet" is a hotly debated topic. The truth is that there is no single way of eating that will always be healthy for every person, at every stage of life, around the globe. We all have slightly different dietary needs, depending on whether we are trying to lose weight, gain weight, boost immunity, reduce inflammation, or prevent disease. However, there are general patterns of eating that can be considered healthy for everyone. One of the world's most widely studied eating patterns has come to be known as the Mediterranean diet. This way of eating emphasizes plenty of vegetables, fruits, and other plant-based foods. These foods are often prepared with olive oil but are otherwise minimally processed. In this diet, whole grains and legumes (beans and peas) are favored along with moderate amounts of fish, poultry, and dairy products. Red meat and sweets are kept to a minimum.

Among the many diets out there, the Mediterranean diet has some of the most valid and reliable science backing up its healthfulness. Meta-analyses of several long-term studies have shown that this whole-food, plant-based eating pattern may help lower the risks of various major illnesses, including heart disease (the leading cause of death in the United States), cancer, diabetes, and Alzheimer's disease.

In many ways, the Mediterranean diet mirrors the eating patterns that have long been espoused by health practitioners in India. For thousands of years, these practitioners have emphasized eating whole, minimally processed plant foods as part of a general approach to health known as Ayurveda. Ayurvedic healers recommend enjoying these foods in season and in moderation. Yet, they go one step further. Ayurvedic practitioners advocate a personalized diet optimized for your particular health needs. In this way, Ayurvedic eating patterns are applicable to various modern dietary preferences ranging from vegetarian and vegan to low-carb, high-protein, gluten-free, grain-free, dairy-free, and sugar-free.

CORE PRINCIPLES OF AYURVEDA

Originating more than five thousand years ago in India, Ayurveda is the oldest continuously practiced healthcare system in the world. *Ayurveda* translates to the "science of life" and takes a holistic view of health. A key concept in Ayurvedic medicine is the universal connectedness of individuals to each other, to their environment, and to the universe itself. Ayurveda sees your optimal diet in the context of your body, mind, senses, and spirit, including factors such as your age, activity level, lifestyle, emotional state, and even the weather around you at any particular time.

While many contemporary medical practices focus solely on treating disease, Ayurveda also focuses on *preventing* disease. From the Ayurvedic perspective, being healthy is more than just the absence of disease: healthy people radiate vigor and vitality. The key to restoring your good health is regaining balance and moderation in both diet and lifestyle.

The soaring rates of stress-induced illness among Americans coupled with conflicting nutritional advice has led many Americans to revisit the ancient healing methods of Ayurveda. Now that medical professionals around the world have acknowledged diet and lifestyle as key components of disease prevention and health maintenance, the teachings of Ayurveda have found renewed importance. In fact, American interest in Ayurveda has grown so strong that the U.S. National Institutes of Health has devoted substantial resources to studying its effectiveness, sponsoring clinical trials on various Ayurvedic practices ranging from yoga to anxiety treatments.

KNOW THYSELF

While Ayurvedic practitioners advise everyone to eat whole, minimally processed foods in season and in moderation, the details of personal recommendations are based on each person's unique "constitution." Ayurvedic texts describe how human beings are made up of the same elements as everything else in the universe. Yet, as individual human beings, each of us has a distinct mix of elements that compose our unique self.

Ayurveda identifies five essential elements of the universe: ether, air, fire, water, and earth. Ether is considered to be the element of space; air the element of movement; fire the element of transformation; water the element of cohesion; and earth the element of structure. These elements come together in three basic combinations that Ayurveda calls *vata*, *pitta*, and *kapha*. *Vata* is a combination of ether and air, and it has distinctive qualities, including dryness, lightness, coldness, mobility, and subtlety. *Pitta* is a combination of fire and water; its distinctive qualities are oily, sharp/penetrating, hot, and spreading (dispersing). *Kapha* combines earth and water, and its qualities are heavy, dull, stable, cool, and sticky. These basic combinations of the elements are known as *doshas*. Together, the three doshas constitute your body and mind, and determine your overall health and growth. The doshas can be thought of as mind-body types. While Ayurvedic texts describe how the

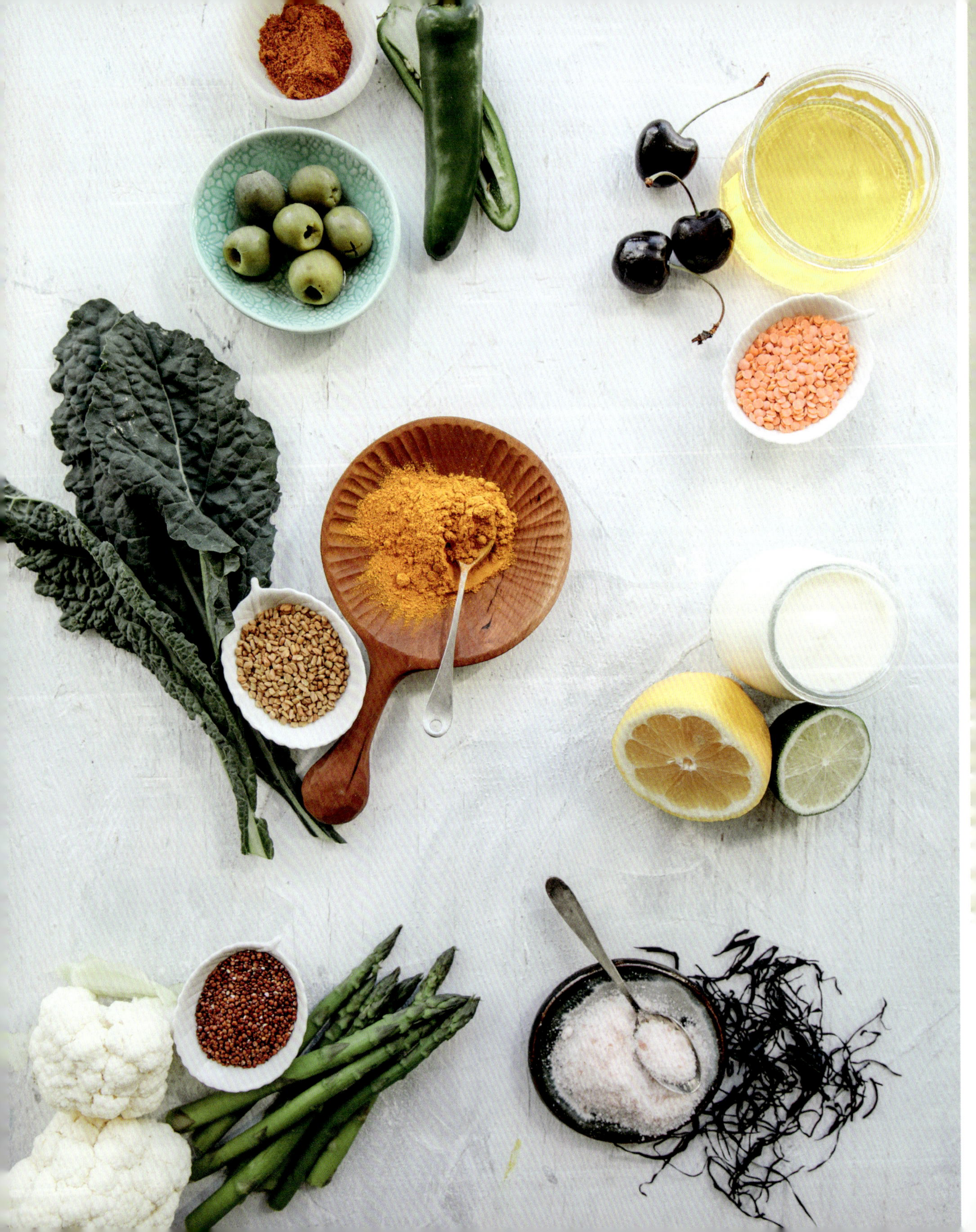

three doshas fluctuate in each person according to factors like the time of day, the time of year, and your stage of life, everyone has his or her own unique combination of doshas or personal constitution. The goal of Ayurvedic dietary recommendations is to bring all three of your doshas into harmony and balance.

WHAT'S MY PERSONAL CONSTITUTION?

Ayurveda identifies three basic mind-body types—*vata*, *pitta*, and *kapha*—called *doshas*. Your personal constitution is a unique mix of these mind-body types and their characteristics. To determine your personal constitution, answer the questions below (what is your body frame, weight, etc.) and circle one answer per category. Add the number of circles in each column and record the numbers at the bottom. The highest score indicates your dominant dosha, and lower scores indicate secondary doshas. Once you know your personal constitution, you can choose foods and meals that improve your personal health. Every recipe in this book is tagged as balancing (reducing) or imbalancing (increasing) for your dominant dosha.

	VATA	PITTA	KAPHA
Body frame	Thin, tall, or short	Medium	Heavy, broad
Weight	Hard to gain, easy to lose	Easy to gain, easy to lose	Easy to gain, hard to lose
Skin	Cool and dry, dark/sallow	Warm and moist, freckles, sunburns easily	Cool and moist, fair, oily, thick
Hair	Dry, frizzy, thin, dark	Fine, straight, premature graying or balding	Oily, wavy, thick
Eyes	Small, brown, gray, violet, unusual color	Almond-shaped, bright, intense gaze, green, hazel	Big, round, dark, blue, thick eyelashes
Appetite	Irregular (sometimes very hungry, sometimes skips meals)	Intense (gets irritated when hungry)	Consistent (sometimes skips breakfast, otherwise good appetite)
Evacuation	Constipated, dry stools, irregular, small quantity	Soft stools, regular, large quantity	Slow, thick stools, regular, moderate quantity

	VATA	PITTA	KAPHA
Sweat	Scanty	Profuse	Moderate
Temperament	Energetic, creative, enthusiastic, perceptive, fearful, indecisive, nervous, scattered	Intelligent, witty, goal-oriented, competitive, driven, critical	Reliable, grounded, calm, stable, greedy, stubborn, lack of motivation
Memory	Learns quickly, forgets quickly	Learns quickly, forgets slowly	Learns slowly, forgets slowly
Speech	Erratic, talkative, high-pitched, fast, peppy	Articulate, decisive, organized, clear, sharp	Slow, melodious, low tones, deep voice, booming voice
Climate	Prefers hot and humid, dislikes dryness and cold	Prefers cool temps, dislikes heat and humidity	Prefers warm and dry, dislikes humidity and dampness
Activity	Active, social, energized, restless	Competitive, intense	Calm, slow, likes leisure activity
Routines	Likes variety, dislikes routine	Likes planning and organizing	Works well with routine
Total			

THE SIX TASTES OF FOOD

Ayurvedic texts explain how different foods affect the doshas in different ways. For example, very hot and pungent spices aggravate pitta, while cold and light foods such as salads calm it down. This ability to affect the doshas is the underlying basis for your personalized dietary recommendations.

According to Ayurveda, the six basic tastes in food are sweet, sour, salty, pungent, bitter, and astringent. Most foods are sweet, sour, or salty—flavors considered building, grounding, and nourishing. Spices tend to be pungent, bitter, or astringent—flavors considered cleansing as well as supportive for digesting heavier foods. Here's a quick look at each taste and the foods that contain them.

SWEET: Includes grains, dairy, meats, fruits, and vegetables.

SOUR: Includes citrus fruits, yogurt, and fermented foods like pickles and kimchi.

SALTY: Includes salt, seaweed, and tamari.

PUNGENT: Includes garlic, onions, ginger, and hot peppers.

BITTER: Includes kale, collard greens, spinach, chard, broccoli, black tea, and turmeric.

ASTRINGENT: Includes legumes (beans and peas), sprouts, and pomegranates.

Ayurveda recommends balancing all six tastes at every meal. A balance of the six tastes promotes optimal digestion, metabolism, assimilation, and elimination. Balanced meals also help to curb your appetite and minimize cravings. Depending on your dominant dosha, your personal approach to nutrition will entail emphasizing or de-emphasizing certain foods. Here's how the tastes affect the different doshas and what time of year is best to favor foods containing those tastes.

SWEET: Reduces vata. Reduces pitta. Increases kapha. Favor in winter and summer.

SOUR: Reduces vata. Increases pitta. Increases kapha. Favor in winter.

SALTY: Reduces vata. Increases pitta. Increases kapha. Favor in winter.

PUNGENT: Increases vata. Increases pitta. Reduces kapha. Favor in spring.

BITTER: Increases vata. Reduces pitta. Reduces kapha. Favor in spring and summer.

ASTRINGENT: Increases vata. Reduces pitta. Reduces kapha. Favor in spring and summer.

When we create new dishes at Kripalu, the six tastes guide our choices. We strive to balance all six tastes in individual dishes as well as in composed meals. We often separate meals into their component parts, such as vegetables, proteins, sauces, and dressings, so that guests can build a meal better suited to their personal constitution. The recipes in this book often include several options so that you can adapt the food to your personal constitution at home.

VATA, PITTA, AND KAPHA LABELING

The recipes in this book are labeled to help you choose meals that optimize your personal health. Once you know your personal constitution and dominant dosha (see page 7), you can choose foods that reduce your dominant dosha and increase your secondary doshas. Some dishes may be "tridoshic," or balancing for all three doshas. The overall goal is to bring all three doshas into balance through what you eat. Here's a quick look at each label, what it means, and when to favor these foods.

↓V—Reduces vata. These foods are warming, grounding, and/or moistening. They are recommended to help reduce gas, bloating, and constipation; relieve dry skin and eyes; and reduce stress, nervousness, overstimulation, or insomnia. Favor these foods in the winter.

↑V—Increases vata. These foods are drying, lightening, stimulating, and/or cooling. They are not recommended if you are experiencing bloating, constipation, dryness, or stress. Minimize these foods in the winter.

↓P—Reduces pitta. These foods are cooling, refreshing, and/or anti-inflammatory. They are recommended to help relieve heartburn, skin inflammations/irritations, red and/or burning eyes, excessive body heat, and mental agitation. Favor these foods in the summer.

↑P—Increases pitta. These foods are heating, stimulating, acidic, and/or oily. They are not recommended if you are experiencing excessive heat, heartburn, or mental agitation. Minimize these foods in the summer.

↓K—Reduces kapha. These foods are warming, lightening, stimulating, and/or cleansing. They are recommended to help relieve sluggishness, water retention, slow digestion, low appetite, foggy thinking, lack of motivation, and feeling stuck. Favor these foods in the spring.

↑K—Increases kapha. These foods are heavy, rich, dense, sticky, and/or oily. They are not recommended if you are experiencing excessive heaviness or slow digestion. Minimize these foods in the spring.

= These foods neither increase nor reduce the doshas. Enjoy them in moderation in any season.

FOODS THAT ALLEVIATE CHRONIC INFLAMMATION

Many of the foods in traditional Ayurvedic meals help to reduce inflammation in the body. Inflammation is actually one of the body's healing responses. When you sustain an injury that gets bruised such as a knock on your elbow, the body sends white blood cells to the area to heal it. Inflammation is also your body's response when protecting you from harmful bacteria and viruses. On its own, inflammation is not a bad thing. But when inflammation continues over a period of weeks, months, or years, it can lead to more serious illness. In fact, low-level, chronic inflammation has been shown to play a critical role in most degenerative diseases, including heart disease, cancer, diabetes, and Alzheimer's.

Foods high in antioxidants, including most vegetables, fruits, and other plant foods, help to reduce inflammation. According to Ayurveda, these antioxidant-rich plant foods should form the basis of our diets, and consuming these foods may help explain why Ayurvedic eating patterns help to improve health and prevent disease. Spices also play a critical role in Ayurvedic cooking, and two in particular have been shown to contain effective anti-inflammatory compounds. Turmeric contains the compound *curcumin*, and several studies have shown that this compound can reduce low-level, chronic inflammation. According to meta-analyses from the U.S. National Institutes of Health (NIH), the anti-inflammatory properties of turmeric may even help reduce the symptoms of rheumatoid arthritis. Ginger, which contains the anti-inflammatory compound *gingerol*, is another spice used frequently in Ayurvedic cooking. NIH reviews show that ginger may help to minimize chronic inflammation and reduce the risks of associated degenerative diseases such as cancer and heart disease.

Ayurvedic cooking makes frequent use of turmeric, ginger, and other spices because most spices have multiple health benefits—as well as great flavor! For instance, ginger—both fresh and powdered—is not only anti-inflammatory; it also helps to reduce bloating and alleviate numerous digestive issues. Ayurvedic practitioners consider balanced digestion to be the cornerstone of good health, as explained in the next chapter (starting on page 15), so ginger is a key spice in Ayurvedic cooking. Try sautéing some minced fresh ginger along with the vegetables in your next stir-fry, or enjoy ginger in dishes such as Vegan Ginger Scones (page 80) and Coconut French Toast with Thai Ginger Maple Syrup (page 62). Ground turmeric can also be incorporated into simple dishes like scrambled eggs and roasted vegetables. Or stir it into Ojas Milk (page 285) to make Kripalu's version of the healing drink known as "golden milk."

According to Ayurveda, strong digestion and overall good health rely, in part, on skillfully choosing appropriate foods at each meal. Once you have determined your personal constitution, experiment with the recipes in this book to help you shift into a more balanced relationship with food and with your body. Eating mindfully can help you find the foods that increase your energy and vitality the most. Keep in mind that your personal constitution may change based on your stage of life, emotional well-being, environment, physical health, and activity level. If necessary, revisit the questions under "What's My Personal Constitution?" (page 7) to reconfirm your dominant and secondary doshas. Then choose the foods and recipes that best improve your health. You will likely find that these recipes also taste the most satisfying to you. This is the Ayurvedic art of personalized eating and cooking.

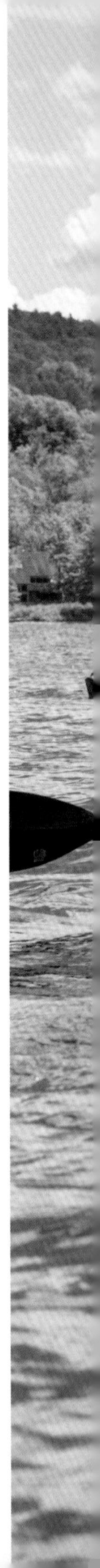

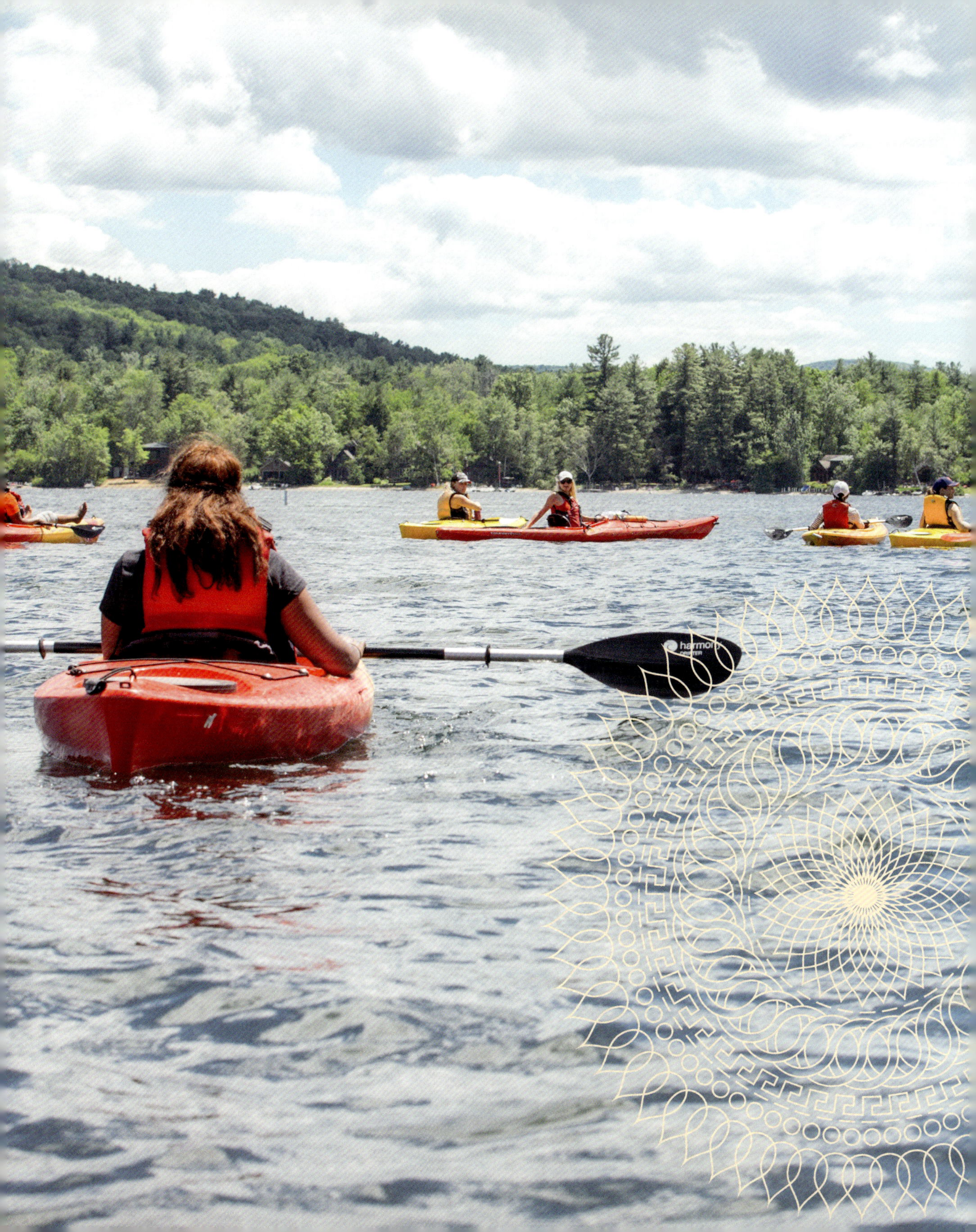

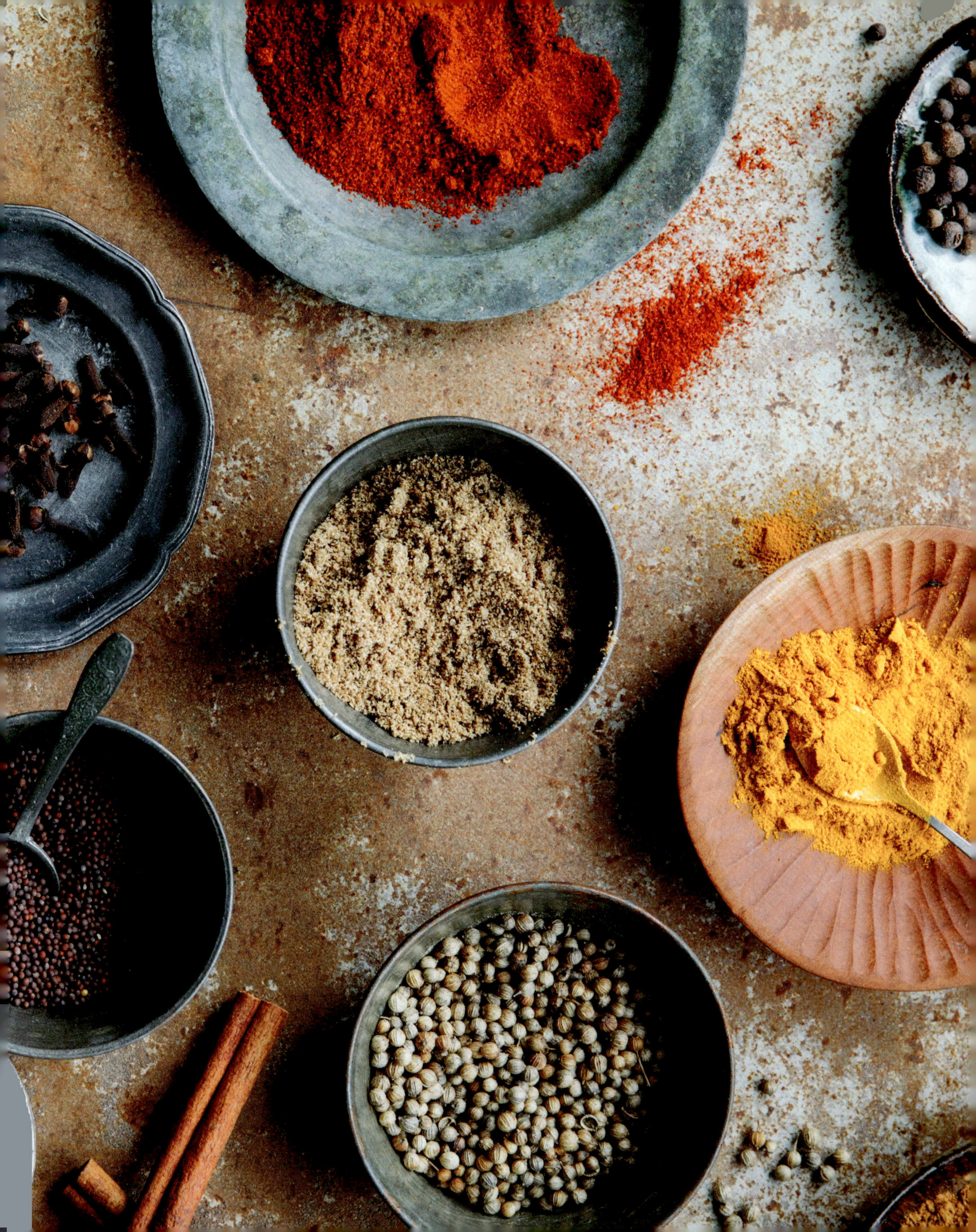

MINDFUL EATING

THE HIGHEST SPIRITUAL PRACTICE IS SELF-OBSERVATION WITHOUT JUDGMENT.

—SWAMI KRIPALU

Have you ever been watching TV and munching on popcorn when suddenly you look down and find that the entire bowl of popcorn is gone? This scenario epitomizes the concept of "mindless eating." You repeatedly bring food to your mouth and consume it but don't fully taste it or comprehend how much food you are eating because your attention is focused elsewhere.

Mindful eating is the exact opposite: it is being fully present when you eat, knowing full well what you are eating and how much, and savoring every mouthful. Eating mindfully is a central tenet of the ancient Indian healing practices known as Ayurveda. In a nutshell, it means eating moderately, eating in season, and taking time to enjoy your meals. Mindful eating can help you reduce stress, improve digestion, curb overeating, manage your weight, and give you a greater sense of well-being. Most important, it can make food a greater source of pleasure!

EAT WITH THE RHYTHMS OF NATURE

As a holistic health approach, Ayurveda emphasizes living in harmony with natural rhythms. When you stray from the basic patterns of nature, unhealthy imbalances begin to appear in your body. Mindful eating, in part, means consuming food in accordance with the daily and seasonal changes in your environment. From an Ayurvedic perspective, you are essentially a microcosm of the larger universe, and when the sun is at its highest in the sky, it also feels the hottest to your body. The Ayurvedic word for fire is *agni*; it applies to both the energy of the sun and your own internal energy. Both the sun's fire and your internal digestive fire are at their strongest in the middle of the day. The goal is to keep agni balanced, which means feeding it more when it is burning strong, and feeding it less when your digestive fire is low. Hence the Ayurvedic recommendation to make lunch your big meal of the day when you can.

Conversely, it's best to enjoy lighter meals in the evenings. It also helps to eat dinner at least two hours before going to bed. At night when you sleep, your digestive fire is at its lowest point. If you eat a big dinner or try to sleep too soon after eating, your meal may not be fully digested, which can lead to imbalances such as heartburn, bloating, irritable bowel syndrome, and interrupted sleep.

This principle of eating with the sun may help to explain why the Mediterranean diet is so healthy. It may not be simply due to *what* food is eaten (mostly plant-based food) but *how* and *when* that food is eaten. In the Mediterranean, as with the recommendations of the Ayurvedic diet, lunch is the main meal of the day.

In today's working world, the idea of eating your largest meal at lunch may seem impossible. But do your best. If you work in an office during the week, at least shut down the computer, find a quiet place, and take the time to enjoy your meal without getting distracted. Then, when you are home on the weekends, take full advantage of eating with the sun: enjoy leisurely midday meals.

EAT SEASONAL AND LOCAL FOODS

Eating with nature's rhythms also means eating seasonally. What your body needs most is whatever food is ready for harvest at any particular time of year. In the heat of summer, we naturally reach for cooling foods such as cucumbers and juicy fruit like peaches and melons, and we eat lighter meals overall. In the colder months, it's the opposite: our appetites instinctively increase to help build up our inner warmth. We eat a bit more food overall in the winter and focus on richer dishes, heartier grains such as oatmeal, root vegetables like sweet potatoes, and hot soups and stews.

It's easy to eat seasonally *and* healthfully in the summer because so many nutrient-rich plants thrive in that season. Farm-fresh lettuces and greens are everywhere, and salads are always an option. In the winter, however, it may seem more difficult to eat healthfully because there are fewer vegetables overall. But most of us have not fully explored the wide variety of delicious winter squashes such as delicata, cruciferous vegetables like cauliflower, and winter greens like collards. There is also an entire class of winter vegetables that many people overlook: sea greens. Seaweeds like kombu, dulse, wakame, and arame are traditionally harvested in the winter and provide your body with a wealth of beneficial minerals. They lend a satisfying, savory flavor to a variety of winter soups and stews. Try to incorporate sea greens into your meals in addition to classic winter greens such as kale. If you are new to cooking with sea greens, try Morning Broth (page 279) or Tofu in Tamari Ginger Broth (page 158), both of which get umami flavor from kombu. You could also try Arame and Tempeh (page 160).

Think local, too. Ayurveda reminds us that we are merely reflections of our local environment. Eating in harmony with nature's rhythms means eating the food that grows closest to you. If you eat food grown on the other side of the globe, you are eating the food of a different environment. Shop at your local farmer's market. Join a community-supported agriculture group (CSA) or farm share. Buying locally produced food also makes it easier to eat in season because whatever is growing locally is naturally what's in season. This "eat local" principle explains why pure maple syrup is the preferred sweetener at Kripalu: it is produced right outside our doors in the Berkshire Hills of Massachusetts.

SEASONAL FOOD GUIDE

In U.S. supermarkets, you can get most fresh fruits and vegetables year-round. But strawberries shipped to your market in January will never be as delicious as local strawberries picked in late May or June. They also won't have to be shipped from as far away. Get in the habit of choosing vegetables and fruits that are at peak ripeness during any particular season in your locality. In North America in the spring, focus on foods like asparagus and potatoes. Go for corn and tomatoes in the summer, pumpkins and mushrooms in the fall, and broccoli and kale in winter. Here's when various other foods are in season.

SEASON	VEGETABLES	FRUITS
Spring	Artichokes, asparagus, avocados, beets, broccoli, carrots, celery, dandelion greens, endive, green beans, parsnips, potatoes, radishes, rutabagas, scallions, spinach, watercress, wax beans	Bananas, grapefruit, oranges, pineapples, rhubarb, strawberries
Summer	Asparagus, beets, broccoli, cabbage, carrots, cauliflower, celery, chard, chicory, corn, cucumbers, dandelion greens, eggplant, green beans, lettuces, lima beans, mustard greens, okra, onions, parsnips, peas, peppers, potatoes, radishes, scallions, spinach, summer squash, tomatoes, turnips, wax beans	Apricots, bananas, blackberries, blueberries, cantaloupe, cherries, grapes, honeydew melon, lemons, limes, peaches, pineapples, raspberries, rhubarb, strawberries, watermelon
Fall	Beets, broccoli, Brussels sprouts, cabbage, carrots, cauliflower, celery, chard, corn, cucumbers, eggplant, endive, escarole, lettuces, lima beans, mushrooms, onions, parsnips, peas, peppers, potatoes, pumpkins, radishes, rutabagas, sweet potatoes, tomatoes, turnips, winter squash	Apples, cantaloupe, dates, dried berries, figs, grapes, pears, plums, pomegranates, raisins
Winter	Broccoli, Brussels sprouts, carrots, cauliflower, celery, collard greens, endive, kale, parsnips, potatoes, rutabagas, sweet potatoes, turnips, winter squash	Dates, dried berries, grapefruit, oranges, pomegranates, raisins, tangerines

EAT IN MODERATION

Mindful eating is not only a matter of *when* you eat but *how much*. In Ayurveda, this concept is called *mitahar*, which literally means "the moderate taking of food." Mitahar can be defined as taking only the amount of food necessary to keep your body alert and functioning efficiently. If you overeat, you make your body work harder to metabolize the excess food.

Eating in moderation has proven metabolic benefits. It can reduce oxidative stress and improve digestion, leading to better overall health. If you remain keenly aware of your body and its needs, mitahar can be summed up as follows: When you are hungry, eat. When you're not, don't. Regular mealtimes can help to regulate your appetite as well, so try to eat breakfast, lunch, and dinner at similar times every day.

It takes some careful consideration to practice mitahar, especially when we are surrounded by "hyper-palatable" foods. Hyper-palatable food products are designed to make us hungrier. The sugar in candy makes us want more. The salt in potato chips drives us to keep eating them. The fat in ice cream makes us eat the whole tub. But the food itself may offer our bodies very little in the form of sustained nourishment. It leaves us feeling hungry. After all, the manufacturers of these hyper-palatable food products are not in the business of nourishing us. They are in the business of selling more food. And they are succeeding. Junk food makes it very difficult to eat in moderation.

The key is to pay close attention to your hunger cues. Are you actually hungry, or are you really just thirsty? Or are you eating to provide comfort from some kind of stress? If you are stress eating, is there something else you could do to relieve stress? Perhaps meditation, yoga, or some physical activity? And if you are truly hungry, is the food you are eating really satisfying that hunger? Or is it only providing a quick flavor fix? Try to reach for whole foods that are minimally processed to offer your body more sustained satisfaction.

Keep in mind that mitahar does not necessarily mean eating a small quantity of food. Your dietary needs change according to things like the time of day, the time of year, your personal constitution (see page 7), and your activity level. If you practice vigorous vinyasa yoga, are very athletic, or do frequent physical labor, your nutritional needs will be very different from someone who is a more meditative yogi, a more sedentary person, or a nine-to-five office worker. More active people need more calories. Those who work their bodies harder also need more protein to rebuild their muscles. Or, let's say your activity level varies from day to day. On active days, your appetite will naturally increase, and you should heed those hunger cues by eating a bit more. When you are less active, your appetite and metabolism slow down, so you should eat less. The essence of mitahar is remaining fully aware of your body and paying attention to what it needs and does not need at any particular time. Then, you can provide yourself with just the right amount of food—no more, no less.

Mitahar is not only good dietary practice. It is also an essential part of yoga. Eating only what your body needs can transform your yoga, empowering you to discover new sources of energy and allowing you to reach your full potential. Mitahar is also considered one of the foundations of spiritual progress. Full awareness of yourself and your dietary needs connects you more deeply to the world around you and the role that you play in it. But it takes practice. We all know that it's best to eat in moderation. Doing so is another matter entirely. When you begin, you may find it challenging. Take it slow. Instead of going cold turkey, make gradual dietary changes that you are more likely to stick with. Over time, practicing mitahar will help you steadily shift into a more balanced and healthy pattern of eating.

TAKE TIME TO ENJOY YOUR MEALS

Mindful eating also encourages us to focus on the food itself. Try not to eat on the run or while multitasking. In today's fast-paced culture, it is common to eat while standing up, in the car, in front of the computer, watching television, and talking on the phone. Distracted eating may seem benign, but it is the opposite of mindful eating. Over time, distracted eating can impede your digestion and lead to imbalances that deteriorate your health. Try to focus on the food when you eat. Avoid taking meals when you are upset, angry, or arguing. If you are entering mealtime from a stressful situation or environment, take a few moments to relax before sitting down. Then, put yourself in a calm, seated, and settled environment, and direct your attention to the food itself. It doesn't matter whether you eat for ten minutes or one hour: during meals, you should be engaged in the act of eating.

Observe the colors and shapes of everything on the plate or in the bowl. Use your nose to inhale the food's alluring aromas. Give thanks to those who grew, harvested, and prepared the meal. Enjoy the food at a moderate pace, and put down the fork occasionally so you can chew each bite thoroughly. As you eat, open all of your senses: fully experience the tastes, the textures, the temperatures, and even the sounds. Sip warm or room-temperature water throughout the meal to ease digestion. After eating, relax for a few minutes. Maybe take a walk to stimulate your circulation. And allow at least a few hours between meals to encourage complete digestion.

These mindful practices of eating in season, eating in harmony with nature's rhythms, and eating moderately and slowly are intended to improve your overall digestive health. Remember: your digestive fire, or *agni*, is merely a reflection of the sun, the fire in the sky. Mindful eating promotes balanced digestion, and a strong digestive system helps give you sustained energy through the day.

The essence of mindful eating is recognizing and respecting the critical role that food plays in your body's health. Food provides the basic building blocks for all life, and the food you eat has the power to improve or impair your health. To optimize your health, get to know yourself and feed your body the best possible food that you can. It helps to prepare your own food instead of relying on fast food, packaged foods, and restaurant meals. Learning how to cook even a few whole-food, plant-based meals can go a long way toward healing illness, revitalizing your body, and nourishing your soul.

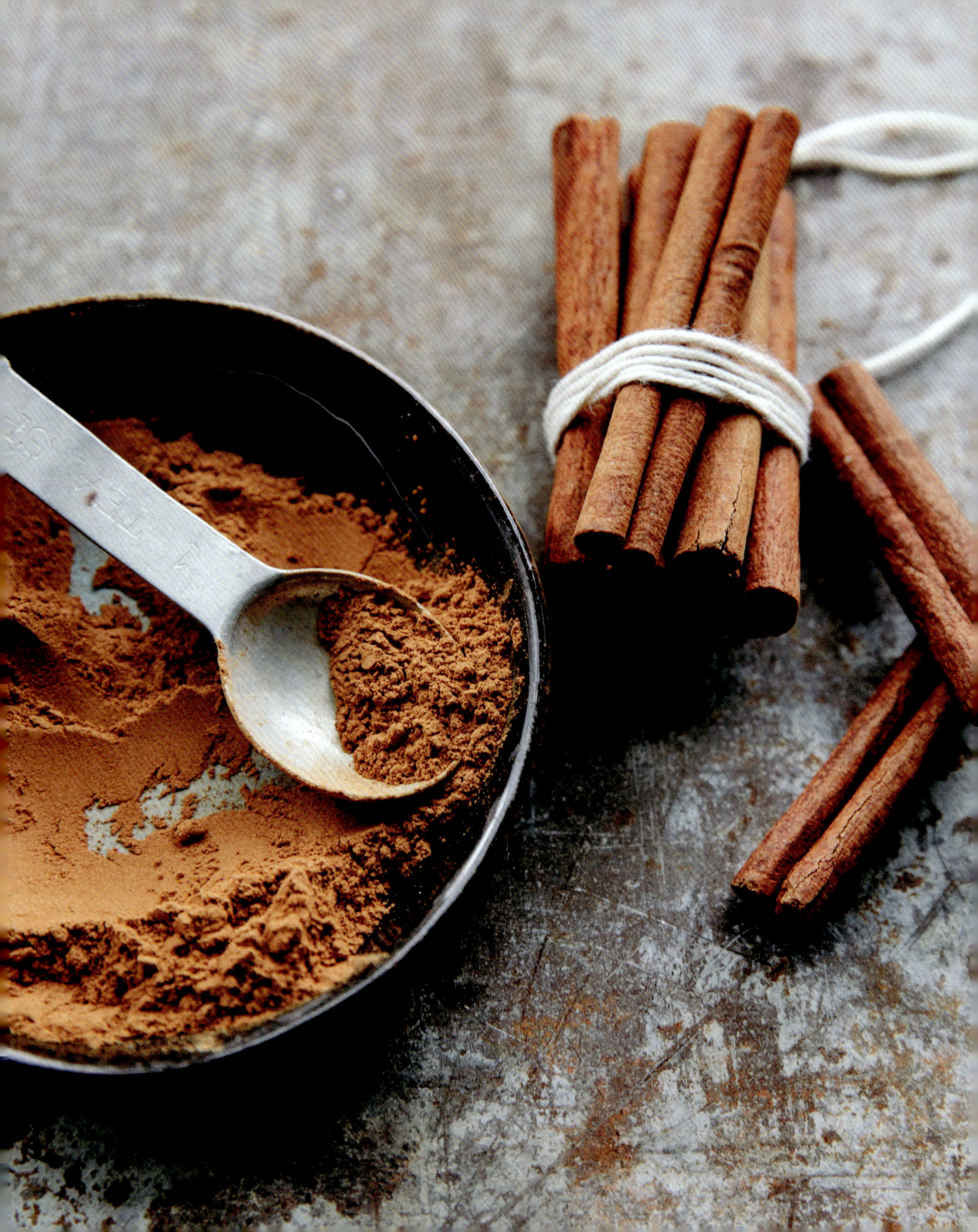

KRIPALU KITCHEN AT HOME

SERVE WITH A FULL HEART. WHEN YOU MAKE OTHERS HAPPY, YOU MAKE YOURSELF HAPPY.

—SWAMI KRIPALU

In the Kripalu dining room, we serve about twelve hundred healthy meals a day. Over the decades, we have learned how to streamline our shopping, planning, kitchen prep, and cooking to appeal to a broad range of tastes and dietary needs. Whether preparing meals for a large group or just one or two at home, the truth is that serving healthy food every day does not have to be an arduous task. A little planning, a few key cooking techniques, and some basic equipment like a well-balanced chef's knife make it easier. Our other strategies are outlined below.

Just remember to chill. As with yoga, cooking is a practice, and mistakes are part of the process. If something doesn't work out like you hoped and you end up ordering takeout, you can always try again the next day. Do your best to work within the guidelines that follow, but don't worry if you have to compromise on something: your whole diet isn't going to crash. Just continue to approach cooking with your full attention, and the quality of your food will continue to improve. That's when cooking becomes truly joyful and rewarding.

SHOP SMART

Cooking your own meals is one of the best things you can do to improve your health. Most of the extra calories, fat, sodium, and carbs in our diets come not from home-cooked meals but from restaurant meals and packaged foods. Cook your own meals, and you can control what goes into them and how big the portions will be. The first step: shop for those foods you want to eat more often—and avoid buying what you don't want to eat. Surround yourself with healthy food and that is what you will end up eating. Buy the highest-quality food that you can, and consider it an investment in your health. Here's what to look for.

Choose whole foods. Try to buy food in its most natural state. That way, you get the most nutrients and the most flavor. Buy whole fruits and vegetables; whole grains like farro, quinoa, and brown rice; whole-wheat flour and other whole-grain flours such as oat flour; and dried beans and lentils. Go for a whole head of garlic instead of jarred minced garlic. Your food will taste better and you'll get more nutrients from the fresh garlic. The fact is that food processing of any kind, even just grinding whole spices into ground spices, begins to erode nutrients and flavor. Put extra emphasis on whole fresh vegetables and fruits. The recipes in this book provide dozens of ways to enjoy fresh produce. And if you don't feel like making a recipe, just eat the vegetables or fruits raw. Eat a raw carrot, or munch on a red bell pepper (they both taste sweet). When you eat whole and minimally processed foods, you will begin to notice a difference in your health.

Buy local when you can. Many Ayurvedic practices are intended to bring your body into balance with its environment. Buying locally grown food supports that goal. Buying local also reduces your environmental impact because your food does not have to be shipped long distances, which uses more of the earth's valuable resources. Shop at your local farmer's market, and you'll find a variety of colorful vegetables, fruits, baked goods, honey, and other products that have been grown, harvested, and prepared within a few miles of where you live.

Buy organic when you can. Back in 2000, the U.S. Department of Agriculture set standards for certified "USDA Organic" foods. These foods must be grown and produced without any synthetic pesticides, chemical fertilizers, or GMOs (genetically modified organisms). Organic meat, egg, and dairy products cannot include growth hormones or antibiotics, and livestock are required to have year-round grazing access and non-GMO feed. To be certified as USDA Organic, farms must also prove that they have been free of these prohibited substances for three years prior to certification. When we eat organic food, these potentially harmful substances don't end up in our bodies or in our environment, including our water supplies. Keep in mind that some farms may not be "certified" organic but may still produce food using organic methods. Federal organic certification is expensive, and some small farms simply use common sense, often going beyond the federal organic standards to ensure the health of their farms, their food, and their customers. When in doubt, ask the farmer how his or her farming methods compare to the national organic standards.

Eat seasonal. Here's another plus for farmer's market shopping: the food is always in season. If it's not at the farmer's market, it's not in season. If you find yourself eyeing the ears of sweet corn at the supermarket in wintertime, remember that corn is not in season until the summer. To find out what vegetables and fruits are in season throughout the year in North America, see the chart on page 18. At any given time of year, try to eat in harmony with your environment by choosing food that is in season.

Use a delivery service. Many farmers and markets now work with local delivery services that aggregate items from different farms. These services bring fresh, local, seasonal, and often organic food right to your doorstep. To simplify the process of buying local, seasonal food, ask around at your local market or search online for farmer's market delivery services in your area.

Frozen vegetables and fruits are fine. If you can't find good fresh produce, buy it frozen so you are stocked when you want that produce most. Frozen vegetables and fruits are nutritious and convenient. Keep some peas and carrots in the freezer and you'll be able to make Vegetable Biryani (page 246) at a moment's notice. Frozen corn kernels come in handy, as do frozen berries, cubed mango, and sliced peaches.

Some canned foods are okay. In winter, skip the pale supermarket tomatoes. They tend to be low in flavor and nutrients and have earned a ton of frequent flyer miles. Go for canned tomatoes instead. In fact, canned tomatoes are higher in heart-healthy lycopene than fresh tomatoes. Similarly, canned beans work in place of dried beans in a pinch. Plenty of other healthy foods like coconut milk and pumpkin puree also come in cans.

Avoid the marketing labels. Just keep in mind that the healthiest foods don't have labels. Very few foods in the produce aisle, which are the foods you should eat most, have labels that scream "Low Fat! Gluten-Free! Healthy!" Shop mostly for fresh, whole foods that don't have fancy packages and advertising slogans. For the packaged foods you do buy, look at the ingredient list. The fewer ingredients, the better.

HEALTHY INGREDIENT NOTES

Most of the recipes in this book use basic ingredients like fresh vegetables and fruits. We also use some international ingredients like tamari, tahini, and chili paste. Many of these ingredients are explained in the recipes themselves, where substitutions are offered. Here are some details on other ingredients used throughout the book.

Beans. Chickpeas, black beans, cannellini beans, and various lentils such as red and brown are good basic ingredients to keep in your pantry. For emergencies, keep some canned beans on hand. Preferably, though, stock dried beans and soak them overnight to reduce cooking time. We usually cook our dried beans over low heat with a strip of kombu seaweed. The kombu adds savory umami flavor and some iodine, which helps to regulate the body's metabolism. Kombu also helps to break down beans as they cook, so the beans are easier for our bodies to digest. When buying canned beans, look for brands that include kombu, such as Eden. Either way, it's a good idea to rinse canned beans to reduce the sodium content.

Breads. Naturally leavened sourdough breads are best. Look for those made with whole-grain flour and/or sprouted grain flour. These breads provide beneficial minerals and fiber, which helps to slow the absorption of the carbohydrates and avoid sharp spikes in your blood sugar.

Canned fish. If you eat fish, keep some cans on hand for quick meals. Canned wild salmon, sardines, and anchovies are high in heart-healthy omega-3 fatty acids.

Chicken. If you eat chicken, buy organic and, whenever possible, local. You'll avoid the hormones, antibiotics, and pesticides often found in commercially raised birds. Organic chicken is fed organic feed and tends to taste better, too.

Dried fruit. Sweet and nutritious, dried fruit is perfect for snacking and adding to salads and rice or grain dishes. Keep some raisins, dates, currants, dried cranberries, and dried cherries in your pantry. They have a very long shelf life.

Eggs. We use large eggs and always buy organic. We go through a huge volume of eggs every week, so we use the national brand Pete & Gerry's because we can get them in the large quantities we need. Any brand of organic eggs will do, or buy local eggs from an organic farm.

Fish. Seafood presents a minefield of choices. Generally, wild-caught fish makes a better choice than farm raised. The fish we serve at Kripalu is always wild caught and sustainably harvested. It comes from a conscientious local purveyor who sources directly from Boston, Massachusetts. To make wise fish choices in your area, consult the Monterey Bay Aquarium's Seafood Watch guide at seafoodwatch.org. Choosing the fish listed there and buying from a reputable fishmonger will help to ensure the long-term health and vitality of our oceans.

Flours. In addition to all-purpose flour, keep some whole-grain flours on hand, such as whole-wheat flour, oat flour, cornmeal, buckwheat flour, and whole-wheat pastry flour (for more tender quick breads). The term "stone-ground" indicates a whole-grain flour because stone mills grind the whole grain. Whole-grain flours are higher in fiber and beneficial nutrients. If you eat gluten-free, various flours such as oat flour, tapioca flour, rice flour, and coconut flour help to create satisfying gluten-free baked goods. Look for these flours from local farmers and mills or from nationally distributed brands like Bob's Red Mill. We have spent decades experimenting with gluten-free flours and perfecting our recipes for baked goods like Gluten-Free Blackberry Chocolate Chip Muffins (page 77), Gluten-Free Whole-Grain Vegan Brownies (page 261), Gluten-Free Vegan Carrot Cake (page 270), and Gluten-Free Pizza Dough (page 91). Consult the recipes for the specific flours used in each.

Ghee. The preferred fat of traditional Indian and Ayurvedic cooking, ghee is similar to clarified butter but not exactly the same thing. Ghee is cooked longer to evaporate more moisture, and in the process, the milk solids turn golden brown. The browned solids are then strained out, leaving behind a satisfying toasted flavor. Ghee is a lactose-free butterfat with a higher smoke point than butter, meaning it won't burn as fast as butter. You can buy it or make it yourself. It is our preferred fat and can be kept at room temperature or in the refrigerator. Olive oil and coconut oil are both suitable substitutes, but they don't impart the same nutty taste as ghee.

Grains. We serve brown rice, basmati rice, quinoa, and millet almost daily. Other whole grains to keep in your pantry include whole oats, farro, amaranth, barley, bulgur, and buckwheat. Whole grains make for very satisfying meals and provide a wealth of antioxidants, fiber, vitamins, and minerals that can help reduce your risk of heart disease, stroke, cancer, and diabetes. Keep a variety of whole grains on hand and eat them often.

Herbs. Among dried herbs, oregano and thyme top the list. Most other delicate herbs are best kept fresh, including basil, cilantro, mint, and flat-leaf parsley. If you can, keep an herb garden—even on your windowsill—so you can reap the flavor and health benefits of fresh herbs whenever you cook.

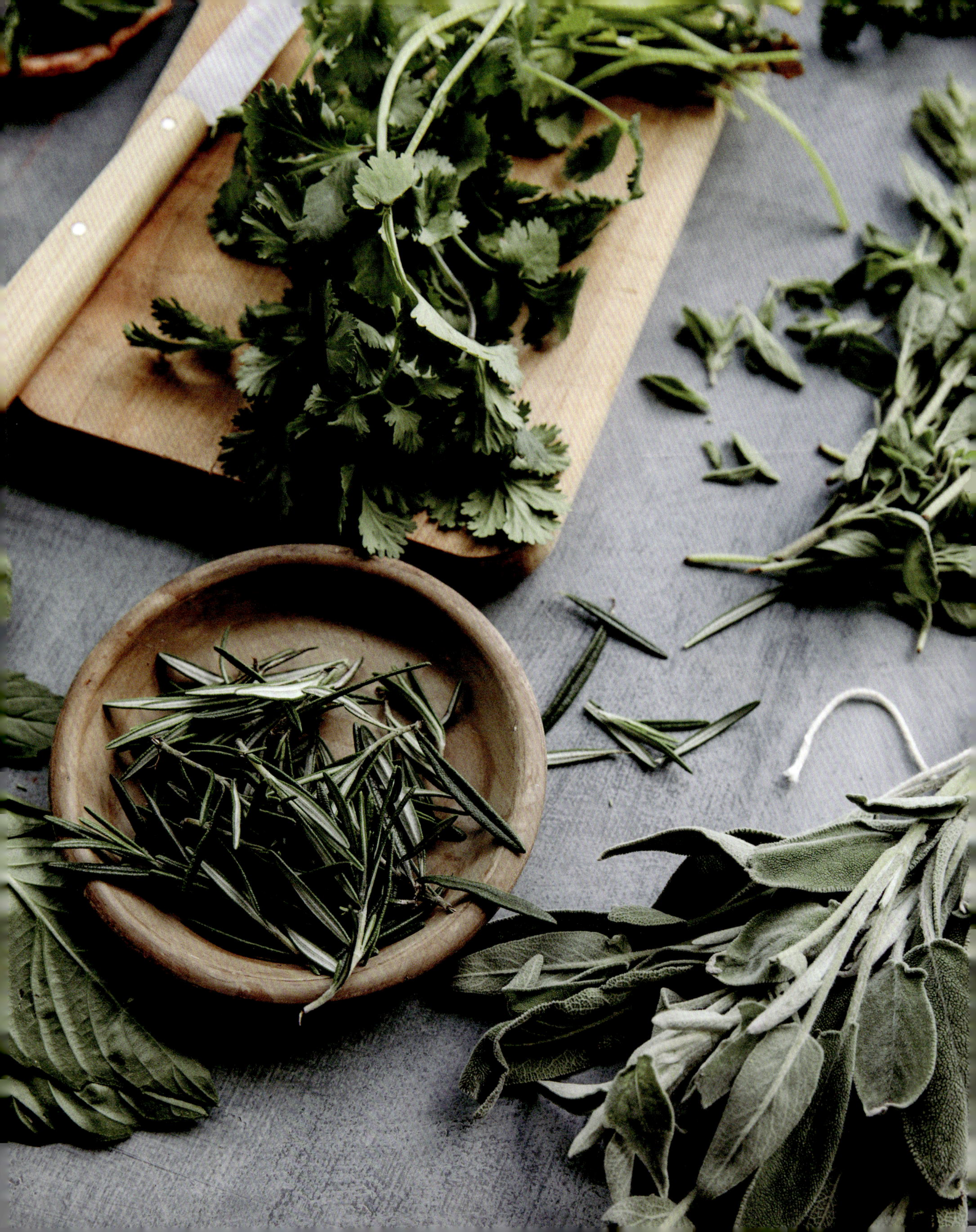

Hot sauce. At Kripalu, we use Cholula hot sauce, but Crystal hot sauce or Tabasco make suitable substitutes.

Milk. We get our milk from High Lawn Farm, a local farm that raises Jersey cows on grass. The milk has a rich taste and a wealth of nutrients from the fertile grasses eaten by the cows. If you can't find milk from grass-fed cows, go for organic milk. As with organic chicken, it's worth the extra money to ensure that your milk is free of potentially harmful hormones, antibiotics, and synthetic pesticides.

Nondairy milks. If you eat dairy-free, keep some unsweetened soy milk, rice milk, or almond milk on hand for cooking. Everyone has his or her favorite. Even if you like dairy milk, you'll love the taste of coconut milk in dishes such as Coconut French Toast with Thai Ginger Maple Syrup (page 62). When buying coconut milk for cooking, look for pure, 100 percent full-fat coconut milk sold in cans. You could also use reduced-fat ("lite") canned coconut milk if you prefer, but avoid using the coconut beverages sold in aseptic or refrigerated cartons. These coconut beverages often include gums and other ingredients that could negatively affect the recipe.

Nutritional yeast. Often used in vegan cookery, nutritional yeast is deactivated yeast with a yellow color and savory taste reminiscent of cheese. It's also high in B vitamins. Look for nutritional yeast in health food stores such as Whole Foods Market. We use it in a few vegan dishes such as Chickpea of the Sea (page 126) and Gluten-Free Vegan Gravy (page 130).

Nuts and nut butters. Great for snacking, nuts provide protein, good fats, and beneficial minerals. It's a good idea to keep a variety of nuts in your pantry, including walnuts, almonds, pecans, cashews, pistachios, and peanuts. Almond butter, cashew butter, and peanut butter also come in handy for dishes like Ginger Almond Broccoli Salad (page 133) and Gluten-Free Chocolate Peanut Butter Bars (page 258).

Oil. At Kripalu, we use a variety of oils, including extra-virgin olive oil, toasted sesame oil, grapeseed oil, coconut oil, and sunflower oil. For all-purpose sautéing, we use olive oil or sunflower oil. We also keep olive oil in spray bottles for greasing baking sheets. For high-heat searing, go for grapeseed oil, which has a higher smoke point and a neutral taste. Grapeseed oil is available in many markets now. For salad, drizzling, and low-temperature cooking, we recommend organic, cold-pressed, extra-virgin olive oil. And if you're looking for vegan "lard," use coconut oil. I call it "jungle lard" because it has a light tropical flavor. It also has a great mouthfeel. Coconut oil is solid at room temperature and liquid over 76°F or so. Some companies sell coconut oil that is mixed with other oils. Look for 100% pure, unrefined, cold-pressed, organic coconut oil from brands such as Spectrum. When recipes call for melted coconut oil, you may be able to put it on a sunny windowsill to liquefy it.

Onions. We mostly use common yellow (Spanish) onions. Sometimes we use red onions for color, milder-tasting white onions, or sweet onions such as Vidalia. Recipes specify these onions when necessary.

Pasta. Keep your pantry stocked with a variety of long strand pastas such as spaghetti or linguine and short pastas such as penne or rotini. They make it easy to whip up a quick, nutritious meal that features whatever vegetables and protein foods you happen to have in the kitchen, such as Farfalle with Asparagus, Mushrooms, and Creamed Leeks (page 196). If you prefer gluten-free options, look for pasta made from rice, corn, quinoa, or a blend.

Peppercorns. For the best flavor, keep whole black peppercorns in a pepper grinder so you can grind fresh pepper. It tastes worlds better than the preground stuff. The same goes for all dried spices. If you can, grind them yourself in a mortar and pestle or small spice grinder (coffee grinder). You will get more flavor from them.

Salt. We use fine or medium ground sea salt for most cooking. Sometimes, we use Maldon flake salt for finishing dishes, and our "table salt" is Himalayan pink salt, which is full of beneficial minerals. It's also nice to have some smoked salt on hand for flavor. When sautéing vegetables, I like to season them with a little sea salt right when they go in the pan. Then I taste the dish at the end of cooking, and season with a little more salt if it's needed. Get in the habit of cooking this way, and you'll notice that your food tastes seasoned all the way through instead of just on the surface. Salt tolerance is personal, so we use a minimal amount for seasoning the recipes in this book. You can always add more at the table. To reduce your sodium intake, get flavor from ingredients like olives, capers, pickles, miso, and sea greens. It helps to make liberal use of spices, too. Keep a few seasoning mixes in shakers on your table, including Gomasio (page 171) and Pumpkin Dulse (page 173).

Sea greens. Kelp, kombu, arame, wakame, hijiki, and other sea vegetables (sea weeds) are basically the winter greens of the Ayurvedic diet because that is when they are harvested. Although they come from the sea instead of the soil, sea greens are full of B vitamins and beneficial minerals such as iodine, potassium, calcium, and magnesium. They also have a very satisfying savory or umami flavor. They are dried, have an almost indefinite

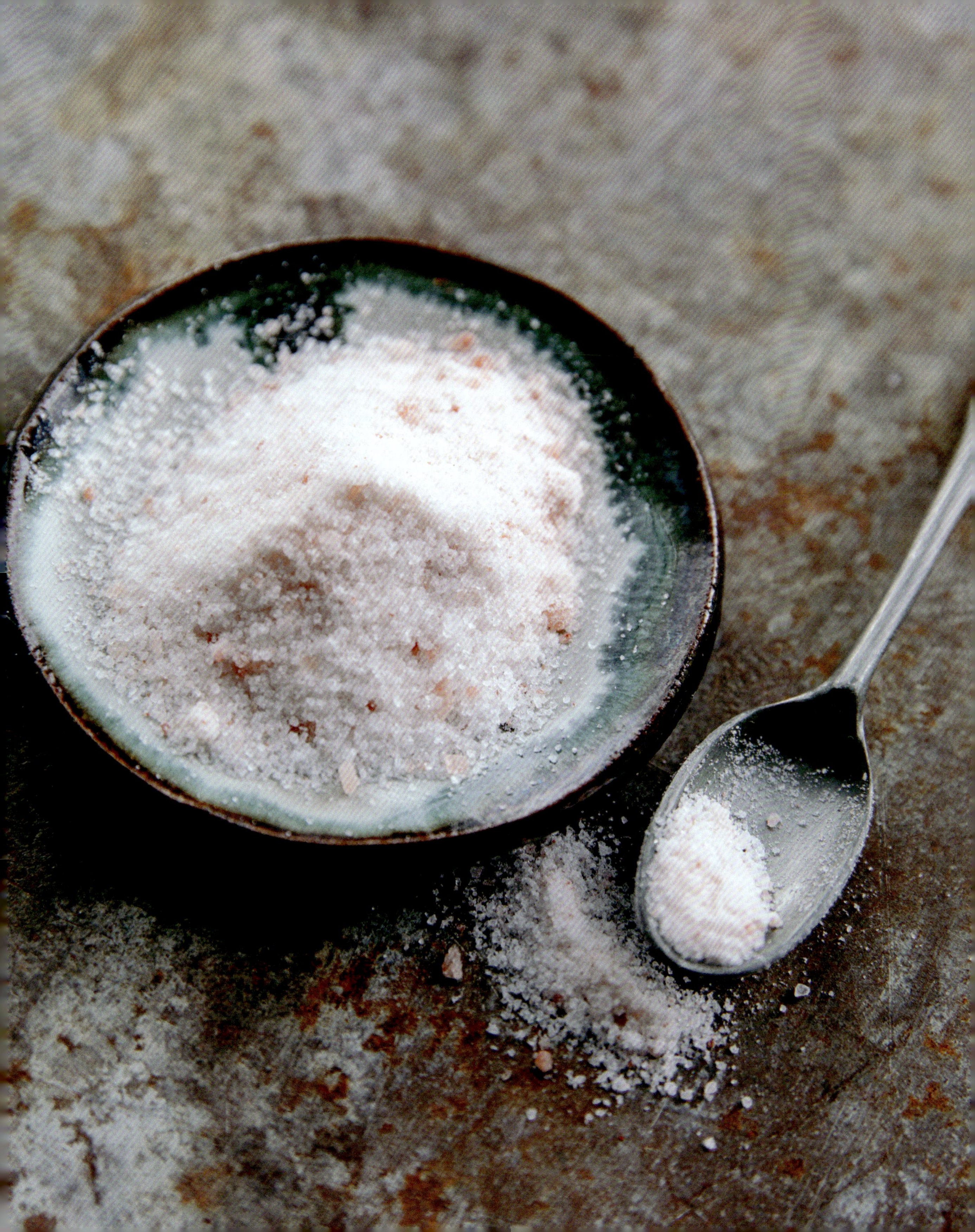

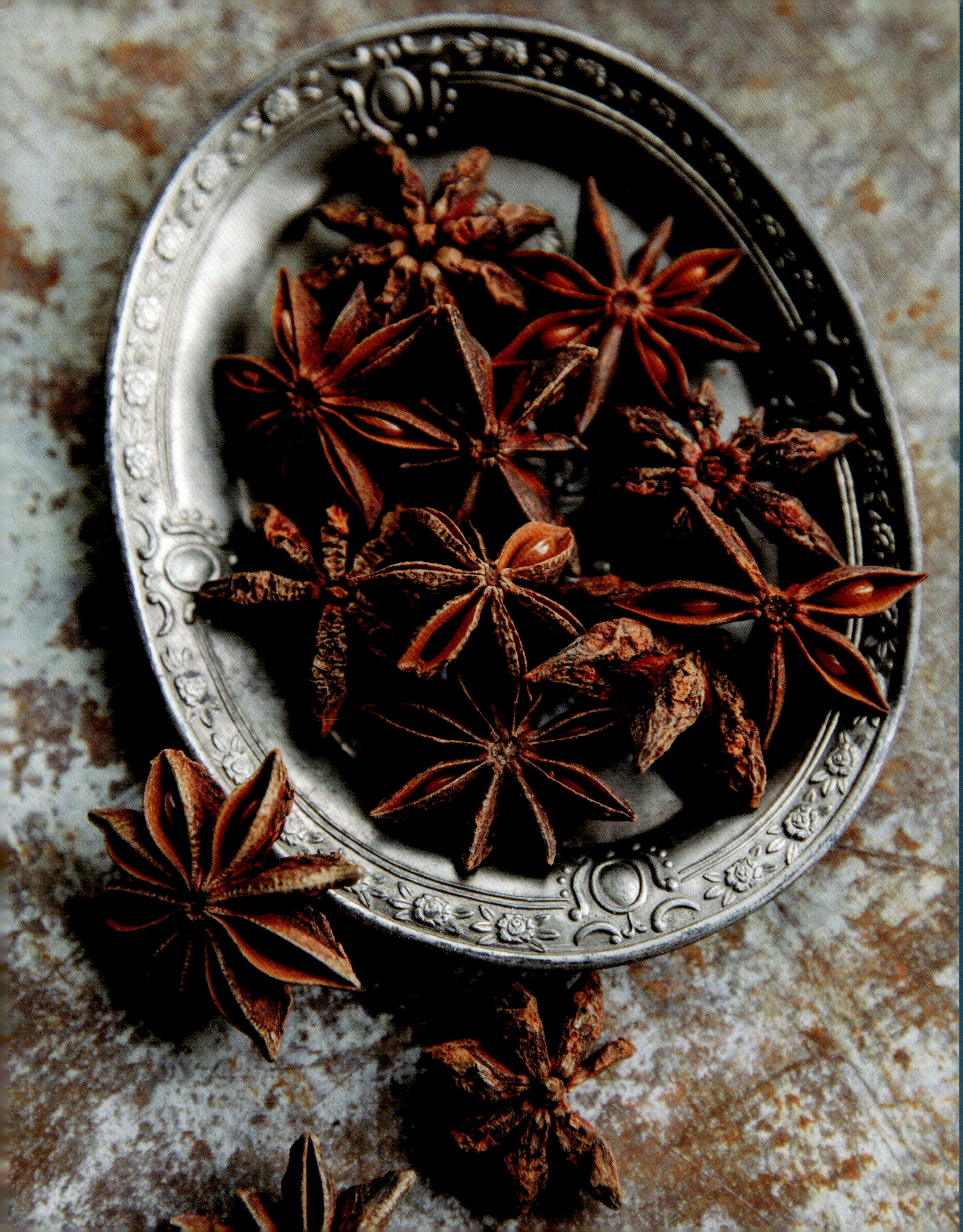

shelf life, and are good to keep on hand for dishes like Morning Broth (page 279), Arame and Tempeh (page 160), and Tofu in Tamari Ginger Broth (page 158).

Seeds. Like nuts, seeds are packed with protein, minerals, and vitamins . . . basically, everything needed to grow a healthy new plant—and a healthy new you! Keep a variety of seeds on hand for snacking and cooking, including sunflower seeds, pumpkin seeds, sesame seeds, chia seeds, and flax seeds.

Spices. Ayurvedic cooking uses various spices because most spices improve digestion and many of them are anti-inflammatory. Plus, they do wonders for the taste of plant-based foods. For flavor and nutrition, it's best to grind spices whole rather than buy them preground. We know that's not always practical for home cooks. The most important ground spices to keep on hand are turmeric, cumin, coriander, cinnamon, nutmeg, allspice, cardamom, and paprika. Among whole spices, keep some fennel seeds, cumin seeds, and mustard seeds in your pantry.

Sweeteners. Pure maple syrup is Kripalu's sweetener of choice. It's minimally processed and we get incredible-tasting local maple syrup up here in the Berkshires. We also use organic cane sugar (sparingly), Sucanat (evaporated sugar cane juice), agave nectar, and raw honey. We prefer raw honey over commercial pasteurized honey because pasteurization (or heating of any kind) makes the honey less healthy. Raw honey is a living food, packed with beneficial enzymes and probiotic bacteria such as acidophilus that help to make this food easier for us to digest. Pasteurizing or heat-treating honey deactivates these beneficial bacteria and enzymes. Look for raw honey and avoid heating it. We prefer to drizzle it on at the end of cooking, as in dishes like Sautéed Barramundi with Harissa, Toasted Almonds, and Honey (page 212).

Teas. Keep a variety of black and herbal teas on hand to make hot or iced tea, depending on the time of year. Black tea can be used to make Kripalu Chai (page 282) and Iced Lavender Black Tea (page 286), while herbal mint tea makes a fabulous summer beverage in Moroccan Mint Iced Tea (page 290).

Yogurt. Fermented foods like yogurt improve digestion by filling our bellies with probiotic lactic acid bacteria such as *L. acidophilus* and *L. bulgaricus*. As with our grass-fed milk, we use yogurt that comes from a local organic farm that raises cows on grass. Many health food stores stock this kind of yogurt, including Whole Foods Market.

Vinegar. Along with sweet, salty, bitter, and "umami," sour is a key flavor in cooking. Keep a variety of vinegars in your pantry to enliven the taste of your dishes, including balsamic vinegar, red and white wine vinegar, brown rice vinegar, and cider vinegar. On occasion, we also use umeboshi vinegar, a traditional Japanese ingredient squeezed from pickled plums (umeboshi). Umeboshi vinegar has a pale pink color and tastes not only sour but also fruity, salty, and savory. Try it in Umeboshi Pickled Radishes and Greens (page 166).

Xanthan gum. If you eat gluten-free, here's the secret to better texture in gluten-free baked goods. Xanthan gum is the slippery outer layer of an inactive bacterium called *Xanthomonas campestris*. Its ability to bind together small food particles makes it a great substitute for wheat gluten. You only need a tiny amount, about ¾ teaspoon per cup of gluten-free flour. Xanthan also emulsifies and thickens liquids like vinaigrettes. There, just ¼ teaspoon per cup of liquid will do the job. Xanthan gum is sold as a dry powder and most grocery stores carry it in the natural foods or baking aisle.

A FEW EQUIPMENT NOTES

Basic home kitchen equipment is all you need to make the recipes in this book. But we do have a few preferences, such as glass storage containers instead of plastic. Here's a quick roundup of essential cooking equipment and tips on what you will and won't need.

Bakeware. A basic 18 x 13-inch sheet pan (technically called a half-sheet pan) has many uses, including baking cookies, roasting vegetables, and toasting nuts. For other recipes in this book, you may want a 13 x 9-inch pan, an 8-inch square pan, a 12-cup muffin tin, a 9 x 5-inch loaf pan, and maybe some 8-inch round cake pans, all preferably stainless steel.

Blender. Immersion blenders and upright countertop blenders both work well. An immersion blender is a bit more versatile, often including attachments such as whisks and mini choppers. And it's easier to clean. We use blenders for pureed soups, sauces, and more.

Bowls. Keep small, medium, and large mixing bowls on hand for mixing and marinating. A colander and/or strainer is also useful for straining pasta and washing greens.

Cutting boards. We prefer wood. The larger the better, so you don't feel cramped when prepping vegetables. If you eat fish or meat, it's useful to have two boards: one for plant foods, and one for raw meat.

Food processor. If I had to choose between a countertop blender and a food processor, I'd get the food processor. It can handle more kitchen tasks, such as making pesto, chopping vegetables, and pureeing sauces. Plus, I'd get a handheld immersion blender!

Knives. Most home cooks don't need a full set of knives. Just get the three basics: a chef's knife, paring knife, and serrated knife. A Japanese santoku (vegetable cleaver) is a good all-around chef's knife for the food prep in this book. Put your money into that one good chef's knife. The most important thing is that the knife feels good and balanced in your hand. Like shoes, you have to actually try on a few to make sure the knife fits you comfortably. Go to a gourmet store and handle the chef's knives until you find one that feels right.

Knife sharpener. Most home cooks need to sharpen their knives only once or twice a year. But you should "hone" your knife every other cooking session. For that, you just need a honing steel. To actually sharpen the blade, it's easiest to enlist a professional. Go to your market and talk to the butcher. A lot of butchers operate knife sharpening services, or they can point you to a professional sharpener.

Mandoline. If your knife skills aren't up to snuff, a mandoline will make you look like a pro. This device shaves paper-thin slices of garlic, ginger, onions, fennel, beets—almost anything—quickly, easily, and evenly. Pick up an inexpensive Japanese style mandoline (less than $20), and you'll be shaving elegant vegetable salads in no time. Just watch your fingers!

Measuring devices. Basic measuring cups and spoons are all you need. For liquids, a 2-cup glass measure also comes in handy. If you do a lot of baking—especially yeast breads—I recommend buying an inexpensive digital scale. Powdery ingredients like flour compact easily, and weight measurements are much more accurate than volume measurements.

Grater/shredder. Stock a knuckle taker (box grater) for shredding carrots, cabbage, and cheese. A Microplane is also helpful for finely grating things like ginger and citrus zest. Keep a vegetable peeler on hand, too.

Pots and pans. I'm not a big fan of those giant sets you see in department stores. You need only a few sizes of two key pans: sauté pans and saucepans. Beyond that, a large stockpot or pasta pot is all you really need. We also don't recommend nonstick pans. They are not designed for high-heat searing and always scratch or wear out too soon. Stainless steel is the way to go. It's lightweight, durable, and versatile. Look for stainless pans with a core of either aluminum or copper, both of which improve the pan's responsiveness to heat. Buy pans with heatproof handles so you can easily transfer them to the oven after, say, searing a piece of fish, chicken, or tofu. If you don't have an outdoor grill, you might also want a cast-iron grill pan or a griddle that does double duty—a grill pan on one side and a flat griddle on the other. That's useful for things like pancakes, French toast, and home fries.

Storage containers. We prefer glass over plastic. Pint- and quart-size mason jars work great.

Thermometer. If you eat meat, a digital instant-read thermometer is a must. There is no other reliable way to judge the internal doneness of meat, especially chicken. Better safe than sorry.

Towels. Skip the oven mitts. Just handle your hot pans with a folded-up cotton towel. Cotton towels can also be used to clean up spills, wipe down countertops, and dry your wet hands.

Utensils. Keep a variety of wooden spoons, spatulas, ladles, and whisks on hand. Rubber spatulas are also useful for scraping batters, doughs, and pureed sauces out of bowls.

CREATE A KITCHEN WITH GOOD FLOW

Remember when you started driving? What was the first thing you learned? How to set yourself up in the driver's seat. Maybe you changed the seat position so you could reach the pedals. Tilted the steering wheel up or down, or adjusted the mirrors so you could see what was around you. Basically, you got everything in place to make it easier to drive. It's the same with cooking. Before you even turn on a burner, take a moment to set up your kitchen to make the process of cooking easier. Here's how.

Set up stations. Pro cooks call them stations, but these are just areas of your kitchen. You should have three main stations: prep, cooking, and cleaning. Ideally, the prep station will have the most counter space and your mixing bowls, cutting boards, knives, and other prep tools will be stored nearby. Your cooking area is near the stove, and that's where you want your pots, pans, wooden spoons, tongs, and other cooking equipment. The closer the cooking area is to the prep area, the better. That keeps you from running back and forth too much in the heat of the moment. Near the sink, the cleaning area should have some cupboards for your clean dishes and glassware, and drawers for utensils and such. If you have room, it also helps to set up a dedicated baking station to keep together all the flours, sweeteners, extracts, and your electric mixer. You could even set up a beverage station with glassware, pitchers, mugs, and teacups. Either way, setting up stations makes cooking more efficient because whatever you need at any given moment is within easy reach.

Arrange your pantry. Cooking takes forever when you can't find what you're looking for.

It's like hunting down your medical receipts when doing your taxes. Skip the headache. Organize your pantry so all the similar items are kept together. Designate one shelf for pasta and grains. Another for dried beans and nuts. One for sauces and condiments. Another for canned items like tomatoes and coconut milk. And one for oils and vinegars. You might even want to label your shelves so these items are returned to the right place. If you're feeling super organized, set up your refrigerator and freezer the same way. Just like an office where the files are arranged for easy access, your kitchen should be organized for efficiency. Believe me, it saves loads of time when you're trying to get a meal on the table quickly.

Buy only what you need. Most cooks don't need a complete set of spices or drawers full of every kitchen gadget imaginable. Just buy small jars of spices as you need them, and replace them when they get old—every six to twelve months. Yes, that means getting rid of the ones you bought on vacation ten years ago! Do you really need an avocado slicer? Probably not. But a Y-shaped peeler is a must—it peels potatoes lightning fast!

Maximize counter space. You will never have enough. Get as many things off the counter as you can. Keep small appliances that you rarely use, such as your waffle maker, stored away in cabinets. To make the most of the counter space you do have, think vertical. Store your knives on the wall on a magnetic rack. Maybe even install shelves to hold cookbooks and other items that would otherwise take up valuable counter space.

MINIMIZE FOOD WASTE

The United States leads the world in wasted food, throwing away approximately 60 million tons every year, according to the U.S. Department of Agriculture. Most of that food waste is produce that sits discarded in landfills. Here are some strategies to use up all the vegetables and fruits in your kitchen.

Use everything. If a soup recipe calls for ½ cup chopped onion and you happen to cut ¾ cup, just use it all. The soup will be fine. Also, many cooks take a half inch off the tip of carrots and other vegetables before chopping them. If the tip is usable, just wash it and use it.

Keep the peels. If you buy organic produce, you don't necessarily have to peel it. Many of the beneficial nutrients are in the peel, so try to keep the peels on. Hard vegetables like butternut squash obviously need to be peeled, but apples? Leave on the apple skins. Or bake the apple skins at 400°F to make a quick snack. You can also leave the peel on thin-skinned potatoes such as Yukon Golds. For thicker-skinned russet potatoes, toss the peels with a little oil and bake at 400°F. Then season them with a little salt or Pumpkin Dulse (page 173) for a quick snack of potato peel chips.

Keep a stock bag. After prepping vegetables, put the scraps in a freezer bag and stick it in the freezer. When you have enough veg scraps, use them to make Vegetable Stock (page 281). Or use the scraps to doctor up store-bought stock. Just simmer the veg scraps in the stock for an hour or so, then strain them out.

Save the stems. Herb stems and other vegetable stems can be tossed in your stock bag. Or add herb stems to a simple syrup when making drinks like Thai Basil Lemonade (page 289). You can pulse cauliflower stems in a food processor to make cauliflower "rice." You can shred broccoli stems to make broccoli slaw. Chard and kale stems can be chopped and sautéed before the greens to add some crunch. Or save up all the stems from leafy greens, keep them in the fridge, then add them to your juicer when making green juice such as Cucumber, Kale, Ginger, and Apple Juice (page 292).

Make fruit water. Trimmings from pineapples, mangos, melons, kiwis, and other fruit can be soaked in water for a few hours, then strained out to make fruit water. Sweeten the fruit water with a little maple syrup and cider vinegar for an easy beverage, or use it instead of plain water to make drinks like Moroccan Mint Iced Tea (page 290).

Make pesto. If your fresh herbs are on the way out, don't let them rot. Make pesto and freeze the pesto for later. Think beyond basil. That parsley or cilantro in your produce drawer, and even the kale, can be pureed to make pesto or a similar sauce, such as Kale Pesto (page 195), Arugula Chèvre Pesto (page 153), or Cilantro Mint Chutney (page 151).

Make herb oil. Here's another way to rescue wilted herbs: Place them in a saucepan with some olive oil. Steep the herbs and oil over low heat for an hour or so, then strain out the herbs, and you've got a nice, aromatic herb oil to drizzle over a dish of pasta, rice, or quinoa.

CENTER YOURSELF TO SAVE TIME

Each time you cook, it also helps to get yourself organized so the actual cooking goes quickly and you don't feel lost halfway through a recipe. What happens *before* you turn on the heat is incredibly important. The French call it *mise en place*, which translates to "things in place." You get yourself situated before diving in—just like you do in yoga! Gather all your ingredients, get out the pots and pans you'll need, chop all the vegetables, mix up the sauces, and have everything measured out and ready to go before turning on a single burner. This prevents you from frantically chopping garlic while the onions are burning away in the sauté pan. Don't be in a rush to start the actual cooking. Relax into the prep. That's where some of the real magic of cooking happens. Good prep makes cooking so much easier and more fun. Here's how to put the concept of *mise en place* into practice.

Know your game plan. Read recipes all the way through before cooking. That way you won't waste time in the middle of a recipe running to the store for an ingredient you didn't know you needed.

Time out the meal. If you're cooking a couple of recipes, get the long-cooking items going first. Preheat the oven. Light the grill. Boil the pasta water. Then, while those things are under way, you can chop the vegetables.

Group similar tasks together. Instead of constantly going back and forth from the fridge to the prep area, assemble all the necessary ingredients at once on a big sheet pan. Then gather all the equipment. Chop or prep all your ingredients. If you're making two different dishes for dinner and both call for chopped onions, chop all the onions at once. When you group similar tasks together, you streamline prep time.

Clean as you go. Believe it or not, this strategy actually saves time. A crusty pot can be soaking while you're finishing up the meal, which makes the pot cleanup much quicker later on. As you are cooking, move pots, pans, and utensils to the sink to soak. Put away pantry ingredients. Wipe down counters. Think of it not as "cooking" but as "cooking and cleaning." Of course, there will be a certain amount of cleanup afterward, but cleaning as you go greatly reduces it.

Do it together. Want to make cooking more fun? Do it with other people. Get your family and friends to help out. One person can rinse vegetables. One can peel potatoes. One can wash dishes. When you're all in the kitchen together, cooking becomes a fun, social experience. And it gets the job done faster. Plus, when everyone has a stake in the meal, you are all more likely to appreciate the food that is laid before you on the table.

GOOD KNIFE SKILLS MAKE A DIFFERENCE

The way you cut your food is important. It changes not only how the food looks but also how it cooks. Thicker foods take longer to cook. Thinner ones cook faster. That's why chefs add finely chopped garlic *after* sautéing vegetables like diced onions and peppers. If you add everything to the sauté pan at the same time, the smaller garlic will burn before the larger diced onions and peppers are cooked.

Knife cuts matter for presentation too, especially in salads. Evenly cut cubes or strips just look more appetizing than oddly cut and mismatched pieces. For the best results, cut your ingredients as described in the recipe. And hold the knife with authority. Choke up on the handle. Your thumb and forefinger should actually hold the back of the blade itself just above the heel. That gives you better control of the knife. With your other hand, hold the food, and arch your fingers like a claw, tucking your thumb behind your fingers. With a proper claw hold, you'll never cut yourself.

Here's a brief look at how to slice, dice, and julienne your way to culinary greatness. Be patient with your knife skills. Like perfect yoga positions, perfect knife cuts take practice. It can be frustrating at first, but every time you cook, your knife skills will improve. Take your time. Focus. Try to do it right. When you approach it this way, you may find that ingredient prep actually becomes relaxing, like meditation. You focus your hands on perfecting a singular task, and then your mind is free to wander.

DICE. This means to cut the food into cubes, just like the playing dice for which the cut is named. Technically, a medium dice is a ½-inch cube (the exact size of playing dice). A small dice is a ¼-inch cube, and a large dice is a ¾-inch cube. A superfine dice of ⅛ inch is known as "brunoise." When the ingredients will be visible in the dish, as in a salad or chunky soup, aim for perfect, even cubes. But don't waste your time making perfect cubes when the ingredients will be pureed, as in Vegan Butternut Squash Bisque (page 105). A rough chop is fine there.

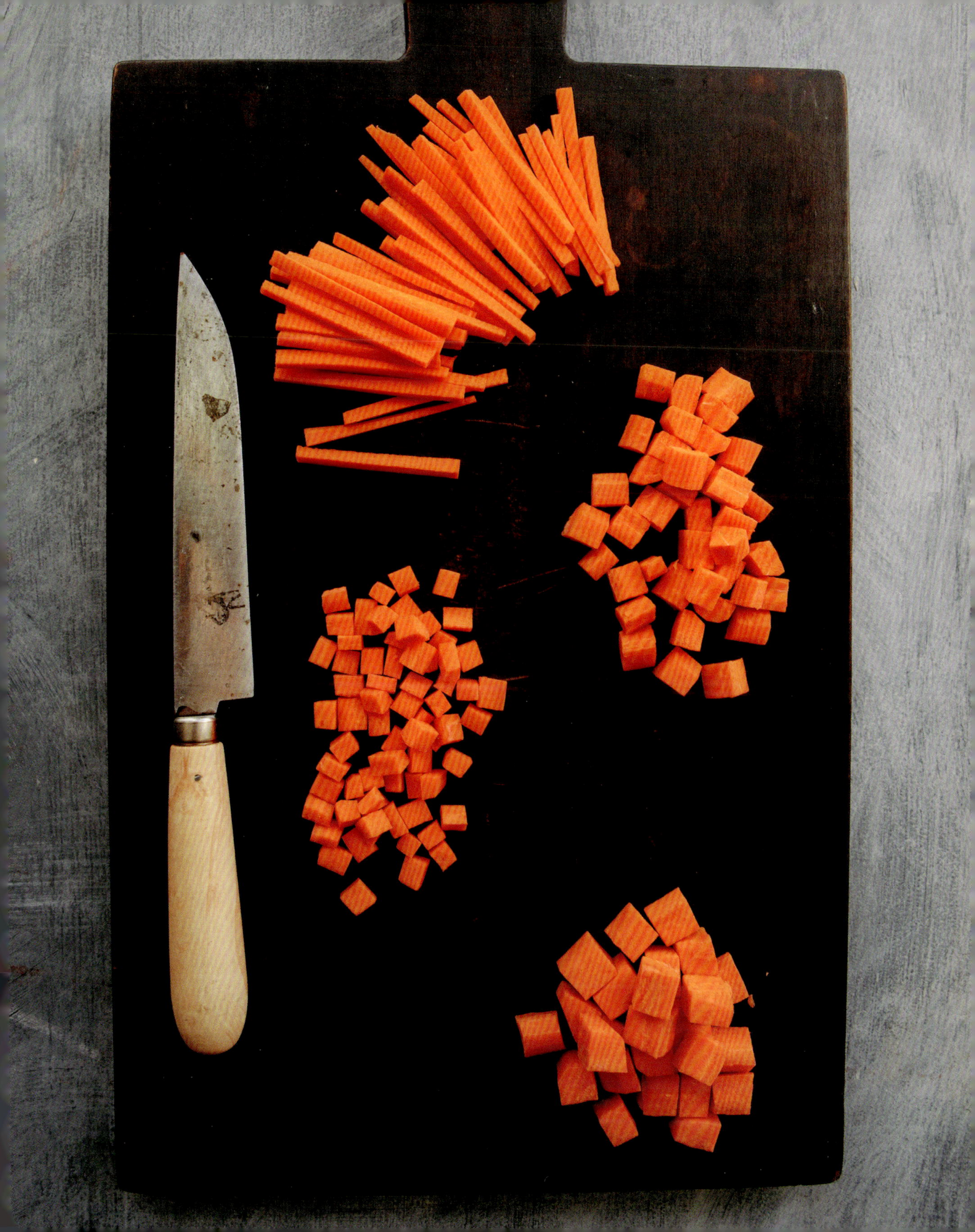

JULIENNE. Cut the food into long, thin rectangular strips resembling matchsticks (aka matchstick cut). This cut increases the food's surface area, which releases more flavor and exposes more of the food to heat, so it cooks faster. The matchstick cut is great for quick-cooking stir-fries and looks fantastic in salads. Technically, a julienne is ⅛ inch wide by 1½ inches long.

CHIFFONADE. This is the term used when leafy herbs like basil or greens such as kale are julienned. They are "shredded" into thin strips. For these leafy foods, a chiffonade cut looks much more appealing than a simple chop. To chiffonade, stack four or five leaves and roll the stack into a cigar. Then thinly slice the cigar crosswise. To separate the chiffonaded leaves, pick them up and shower them over your cutting board. For things like cabbage, you can make thin strips simply by cutting across the entire head. To make cutting a head of cabbage easier, halve the head first to create a flat surface on which to stabilize it.

SHAVE. Cut the food paper thin. For this cut, it's easiest and fastest to use a mandoline—even an inexpensive handheld one. Some julienne/spiralizer machines can also slice foods paper thin. Either way, shaving vegetables like fennel and radishes makes it very easy to put together a quick, fresh, crunchy salad.

ON THE BIAS. Cut the food on an angle. You've probably seen this cut used on scallions in Chinese stir-fries. It makes food look very attractive. Cutting on an angle also increases the surface area on vegetables like carrots, which is important for stir-fries, so the vegetables release more flavor during the short cooking time.

MAKE HEALTHY MEALS EASIER

Professional chefs sometimes start a dish on Thursday that they won't serve until Saturday. They may simply marinate a piece of chicken in the fridge. But come Saturday, that chicken will taste incredible. This is one of the biggest differences between pro chefs and home cooks. They don't think of each meal as an isolated event. Shifting your mind-set in this way can save time on meal prep. The pasta you make for dinner tonight doesn't have to be limited to tonight's dinner. If you make extra, it could also become tomorrow's pasta salad.

Think ahead. Every food in your kitchen can be viewed as a potential meal or component of a future meal. If you stockpile your fridge with prepped or cooked ingredients, a healthy meal will never be far away.

Prep ahead. Ever wonder how restaurants turn out hundreds of meals a day? They don't make everything from scratch right before it's served! Most vegetables are chopped hours ahead of time, sometimes a day ahead. If you cook mostly on weekends and you're chopping carrots on Saturday, chop some extra. You'll probably use them on Sunday. Spice mixes can be stirred up and pestos can be blended hours or days in advance. Get in the habit of prepping ahead.

Cook ahead. You can partially or fully cook food ahead of time, too. Steamed rice, cooked beans, and many cooked sauces can be made one, two, or three days ahead, refrigerated, and then reheated as necessary. Shock cooked beans or rice in cold water, then refrigerate until needed. Shocking cooked food in cold water quickly stops the cooking, preserves the food's integrity, and lengthens its useful life. Vegetables like steamed broccoli can also be shocked and cooled to streamline kitchen time later on. Without a doubt, vegetable prep and cooking take the most time when you are eating healthfully. Get a jump-start by prepping and cooking as much as you can ahead of time.

Batch cook. Why cook beans or grains for just one meal? Make a big batch so you have some ready for the next meal. Cooked cannellini beans can be today's side dish as well as tomorrow's Creamy Cannellini and Roasted Cauliflower Soup (page 115). If you're making pesto for Linguine with Pumpkin Sage "Alfredo" and Kale Pesto (page 192), make a double batch, and freeze the rest for a future meal.

It takes no more effort to make a double batch. If tonight's dessert is Gluten-Free Whole-Grain Vegan Brownies (page 261), double the recipe and freeze some for something sweet at a moment's notice.

Create components for different diets. Pesto sauce. Cooked rice. A seasoning mix. These are all "components" of a completed dish. Think of them as separate components, and you'll have greater flexibility in customizing meals for different diets. Let's say your teenage daughter has decided to eat vegan but you still eat meat because you are very athletic and crave protein. Plus, you want to use up those chicken breasts in the fridge. Make Adobo-Rubbed Chicken with Avocado Crème (page 217), but for your daughter, substitute tofu for half of the chicken component. Both the chicken and tofu get marinated in the same adobo seasoning, but they are cooked separately. The avocado crème component is already vegan, so the tofu version of the dish will be completely vegan. Splitting the recipe so it's half vegan makes mealtime much simpler. At Kripalu, this is how we avoid preparing different meals for the dietary preferences of every guest who walks through the door. We cook several different components and present guests with a multitude of options. Sauces are served on the side. Whipped creams are offered in both dairy cream and nondairy versions (using coconut milk). When you are planning meals at home for various dietary preferences, try to break each dish into its component parts, such as seasoning, sauce, protein, side, vegetable, and so on. That allows you to mix and match components in a single meal without having to create two or three entirely different meals to satisfy everyone at the table. Most of the recipes in this book are written so these kinds of options are easy to offer at home.

Keep it simple and attainable. If cooking is new for you, don't overdo it. Maybe you only "cook" one meal a day. Perhaps breakfast is just scrambled eggs and toast, and lunch is tuna salad on a big plate of greens. Then dinner can be something that you spend a little more time prepping and cooking. There is nothing wrong with eating simply. At home, you don't have to be Top Chef 24/7. Remember: The goal is to eat healthfully. If cooking sometimes gets in the way of that, keep it simple. Have a salad.

MASTER BASIC COOKING TECHNIQUES

We could write a whole book on this subject. But here are a few key techniques that crop up in the Kripalu kitchen. Knowing these terms and procedures will make it easier to cook the recipes in this book.

Blooming. I use this technique to boost the aroma of spices. You basically heat the spices in oil. After preheating a sauté pan, swirl in some oil along with ground spices and gently heat them over medium-low heat. The oil should only shimmer. If it bubbles, the ground spices will scorch and burn. The goal here isn't to toast the spices but to open them up or "bloom" their aromas. Many of the aromatic compounds in spices are fat-soluble, so blooming the spices in oil gives you more bang for your buck: you can use less spice and get more flavor.

Browning. This technique is the key to creating complex flavor in protein-based foods. When protein is seared, roasted, or otherwise cooked with high heat, the surface gradually turns a darker and darker brown. The protein actually breaks down into smaller compounds that react with each other, creating deeply savory, roasted, toasted, and satisfying flavors. To experience the incredible flavor of browning, try the recipe for Harissa Cauliflower Steaks with Castelvetrano Olive, Raisin, and Caper Tapenade (page 184). Remember: Browning = flavor.

Caramelizing. Similar to browning, this technique creates amazing flavor by heating the sugars in food until they turn caramel brown. Just think of the crunchy surface on crème brûlée. That is literally caramelized sugar. Most produce, including vegetables, also contains some sugar, and caramelizing the sugar in vegetables creates very complex, satisfying flavors. This technique is one of the secrets to making vegetables taste great. It's why grilled vegetables taste so much better than steamed vegetables. To see what I mean, check out the recipe for Caramelized Brussels Sprouts with Kimchi Sauce (page 235).

Cleaning leeks and greens. Grit and sand love to hide between the leaf layers of leeks and greens like kale. Even a little grit can ruin a meal, so make sure you clean them thoroughly. For leeks, remove the root end and the dark green tops (save them for stock!), and use only the light green and white parts of the leek. Cut the leeks or greens as directed for your recipe, then drop them into a bowl of cool water. Give them a quick swish, then let gravity do the work of pulling out the grit. Once the dirt falls to the bottom of the bowl, skim the leeks or greens off the top. If necessary, repeat the process until the water is clean.

Deglazing. This is simply a process of adding liquid to a hot pan after sautéing, searing, browning, or caramelizing other foods. The liquid dissolves the browned bits or glaze (aka the fond) from the pan, capturing all of the amazing flavors of browning. Consider this an essential step for maximizing flavor. Plus, it cleans the pan for you!

Fluffing rice. Does your rice come out clumpy? Fluffing can help. After cooking and resting rice, if you just stir it all together, the rice will clump up. Instead, start by using a fork to gently scrape the top of the rice, then continue scraping layer by layer until all the rice is loosened from itself. Only then, gently fold the rice with many small movements. Avoid the urge to stir, which causes the rice to clump.

Grilling. Some cooks fire up the grill until it's blazing hot, then wonder why their food comes out burnt. Medium to medium-high heat works best for most vegetables, fish, and seafood. High heat can also create some unhealthy compounds, so try to stick with medium heat. To prevent sticking, keep your grill grate clean and well lubricated. Scrape the hot grill grate right after you are done cooking on it. Then next time, after you preheat the grill, scrape the grate again while it's hot. To keep the cooking surface lubricated, rub an oily

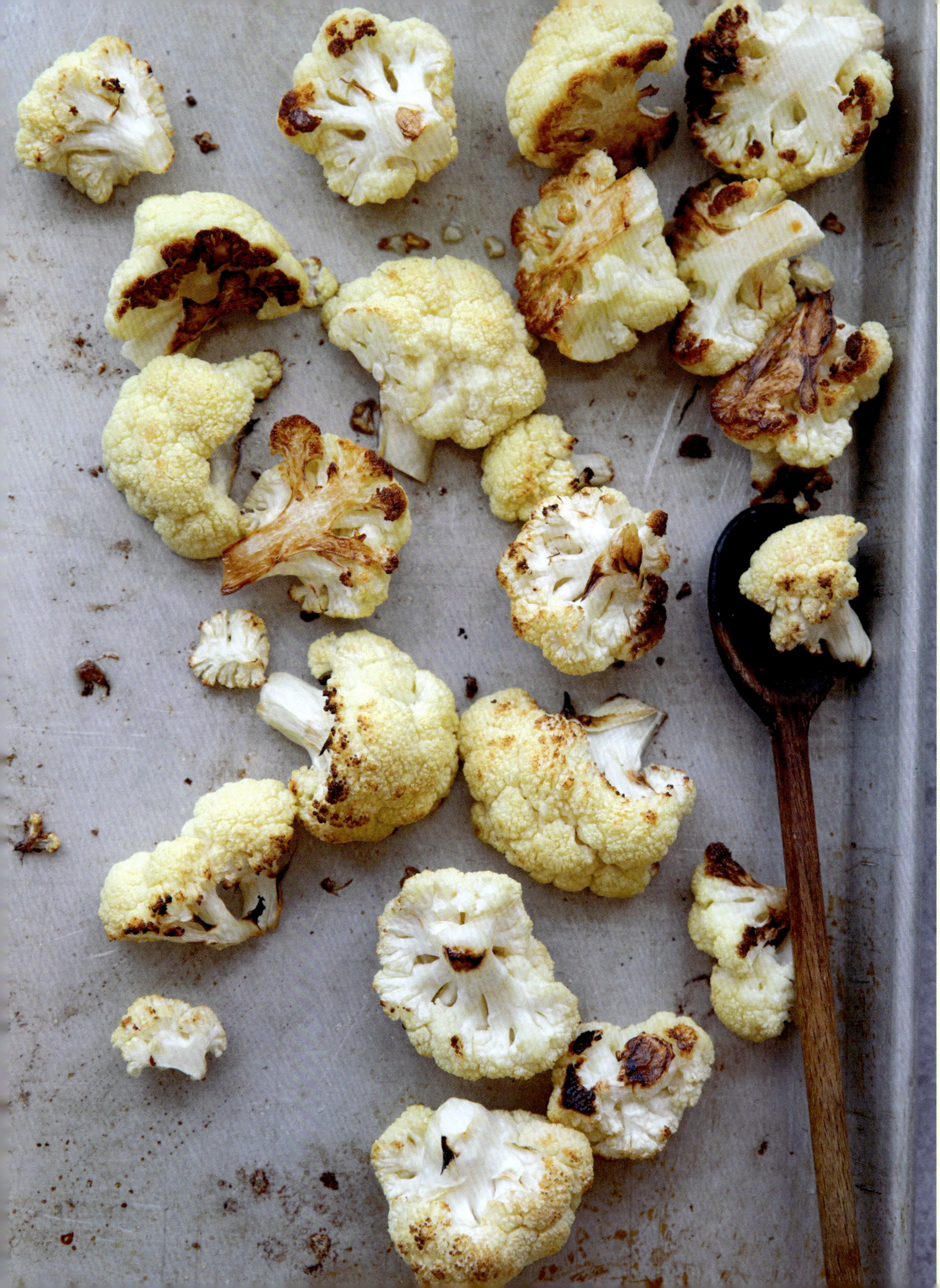

paper towel over the grates just before arranging the food. For delicate foods like fish, it may also help to lightly oil the food itself to prevent sticking.

Marinating. We avoid marinating in plastic bags or tubs. Instead, we recommend marinating in stoneware or glass and pressing parchment paper on top to get complete coverage of the marinated ingredient. It also helps to turn the ingredient a few times for deeper flavor penetration. Most foods should marinate in the refrigerator to avoid spoilage.

Preheating pans. Many cooks put oil in their sauté pans, put the oiled pan over the heat, then wait for everything to heat up before adding the food. But the oil usually overheats that way. (Hint: If you see smoke, the oil is breaking down, overheating, and creating some unhealthy compounds in the process.) It's best to preheat the pan naked for a few minutes before adding anything else. When the pan is good and hot, then add the oil and your vegetables or protein. That way, your healthy olive oil or sunflower oil stays healthy. Plus, if you forget about the hot pan for a minute, it's okay because there's nothing in it yet. Preheat your pan just a little hotter than the temp you want to cook at, because the cold food will briefly drop the pan temperature when it goes in. When the food is settled in the pan, adjust the heat as necessary.

Pressing tofu. Tofu is full of water. Pressing out the water firms up the texture and makes it more chewy. Pressing also allows the tofu to take on more flavor from marinades and spices because there's less water to dilute the flavor. To press a block of tofu, simply place it in a colander in the sink. Put a bowl over the tofu and put a heavy weight inside the bowl (a large can of tomatoes works well). Then let the weight press the excess liquid from the tofu for at least 30 minutes. An hour will press out even more liquid and make the tofu firmer.

Sweating. This technique is essentially sautéing with a lid over low heat. It is a gentler type of cooking that causes the ingredients to "sweat" before they start browning. After sweating vegetables, if you want to caramelize them, simply remove the lid and keep cooking.

Toasting nuts and seeds. Don't skip this step. Remember: Browning = flavor, and that goes for nuts and seeds, which consist primarily of protein and fat. When you toast nuts and seeds, they turn golden brown and delicious or, as chefs say, GBD. For the most even browning, toast nuts and seeds on a sheet pan in a 350°F oven (a toaster oven works fine). Shake the pan once or twice to make sure all sides are evenly browned. You can also toast nuts and seeds in a dry pan on the stovetop over medium heat, but you have to shake the pan more often to ensure even heat and browning.

HOW TO SEAR PROTEINS

Do you suffer from FOF (Fear of Fish)? Many cooks shy away from cooking delicate proteins like fish because they can easily overcook and stick to the pan. Here's how to make perfectly seared fish, tofu, and chicken that doesn't stick.

Cut evenly thick pieces. Even pieces will cook at the same rate. Also, four 4-ounce portions of fish will be much easier to handle than one large fillet. If necessary, pound chicken breasts so they are evenly thick.

Leave the skin on. For fish like snapper, trout, and barramundi, leave the skin on, but score it (especially for thin fillets) to keep the fish from curling up as it cooks. Leave the skin on chicken breast and thighs, too. It will get deliciously crisp in the pan. The healthiest fats reside just under the skin anyway.

Dry the protein surface. Start by letting your fish, chicken, or tofu sit at room temperature for 15 to 20 minutes to take off the chill. Then pat it dry with a paper towel. Both of these steps give you better browning and less "stiction."

Use a heavy pan. For stick-free searing, cast-iron pans work best, but well-seasoned stainless steel pans also do the job. Get the pan good and hot, then swirl in a little oil to coat the bottom.

Season the bottom side only. Season the food right before laying it in the hot pan, and season only the bottom side of the food that will touch the hot metal. Salt draws out moisture, which causes sticking, so wait to season the other side. For skin-on fish and chicken, season the skin side, then cook it skin down first.

Avoid overcrowding. When you add the protein, the pan temperature will drop. Adding too much food at once can drop the pan temp so low that your food steams and sticks instead of searing. Use two pans if necessary to prevent overcrowding.

No touchy. Once it's in the pan, just let the protein cook. For many cooks, this is a practice unto itself. Let it be! After a minute or two, the food will begin to shrink, tighten away from the pan, and unstick itself. If you try to move it too early, the food will be stuck to the pan. Once the food is golden brown on the bottom, it should unstick itself. If it isn't golden brown, let the food sear a bit longer.

Use two hands. To flip the food, hold both the pan and the spatula, so you can gently roll and flip the food. Avoid trying to pick up the food and slam dunk it back into the pan. A fish spatula makes it easier to flip fish fillets. Either way, think of pushing the spatula into the pan rather than into the food to help prevent any tearing.

Finish in the oven. Once the food is flipped, transfer the whole pan to a 350°F oven. The oven heat will surround the food and cook it more evenly. Fish and tofu are done when they reach an internal temperature of 135°F (residual heat will carry over the final temp to 140°F as the food rests); chicken should reach 160°F to carry over to 165°F.

Let it rest. After it's done, let your seared protein rest for a few minutes so the juices have a chance to settle. It's like a cool-down period after a run. Then serve.

KEEP PRACTICING

From shopping to prepping to cleaning, cooking is a practice. Keep at it, but be patient. The rewards of being able to cook healthy food are well worth the effort in the long run. In fact, the number one thing you can do to improve your health is to cook your own meals from whole foods rather than rely on packaged foods, takeout, and restaurant meals. Learn to cook well, and you will eat well.

It may help to reframe your perspective. Some people think of cooking as a luxury and a privilege. In reality, cooking is a necessity. Like knowing how to drive a car, cooking is something that every adult should know how to do reasonably well. At first, mistakes will be made, and you will learn quickly from them. Relax and keep cooking. When you get better at it, you'll find that cooking delicious, nourishing meals for yourself and your family or friends not only improves your health. It also increases your enjoyment of life itself.

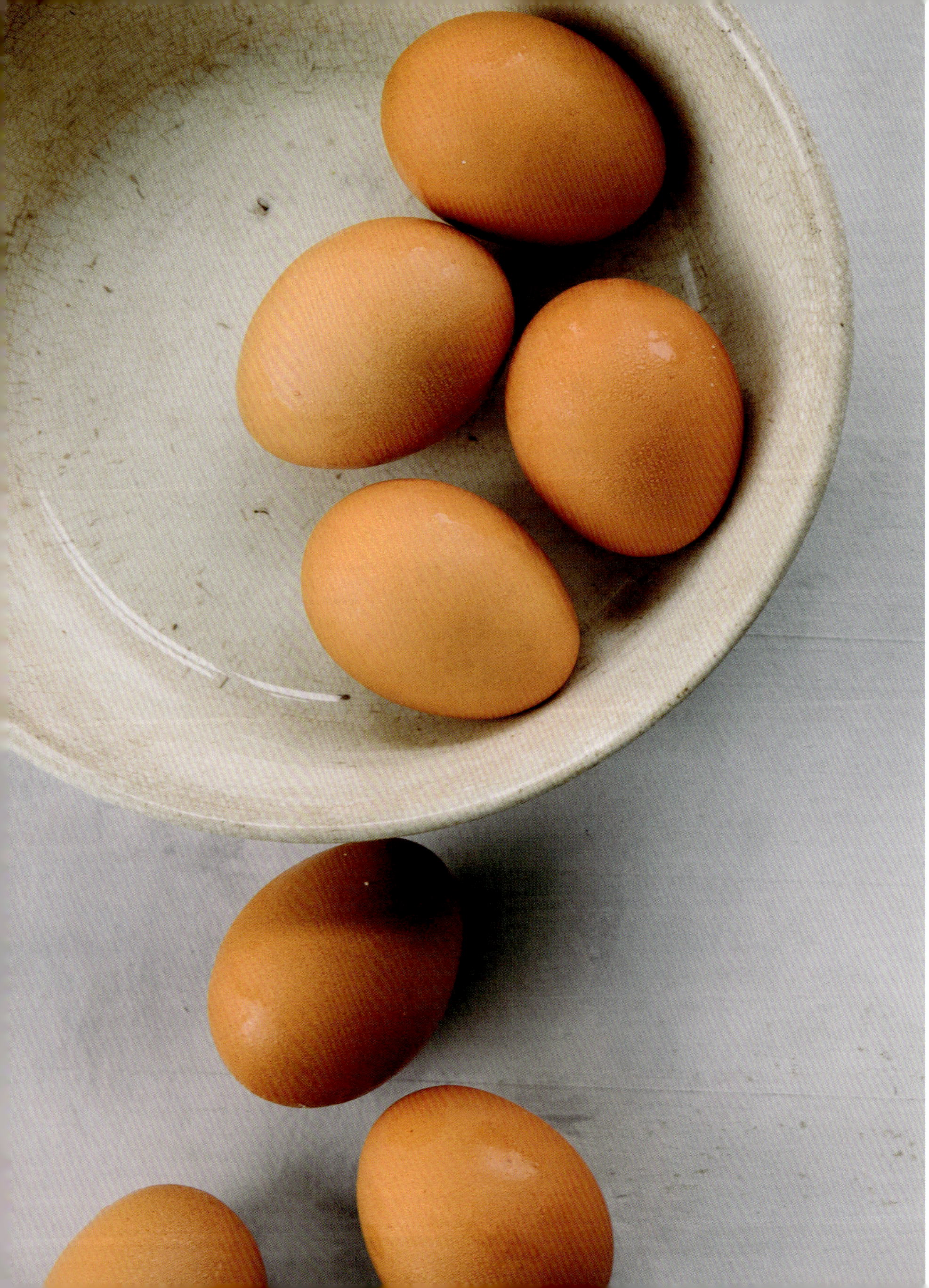

BREAKFAST

Despite what you may have heard, it turns out that breakfast may not be the most important meal of the day. Scientific studies have finally begun to verify what Ayurveda has advised for centuries: not everyone must eat a big meal in the morning. According to Ayurveda, what you eat in the morning, and how much, depends on whether you are hungry and how active you have been since rising.

Ayurveda measures overall digestive health by *agni*, which is Sanskrit for "digestive fire." Agni lives in the gastrointestinal track and is the metabolic fire or energy that absorbs nutrients in the body, eliminates what is unnecessary, generates warmth, and transforms physical matter into energy required for vitality. When your digestive fire is balanced, agni will naturally generate mild feelings of hunger. When it is low, you will have low appetite. When it is high, you will be ravenously hungry. The goal is to keep your digestive fire burning steadily and calmly throughout the day without great spikes of hunger followed by deep troughs of low energy.

How does this translate to breaking the fast? Both Ayurveda and recent clinical studies provide similar answers: if you are hungry, eat. If not, don't. Listen to your gut in the morning, and eat to your appetite. When you eat, take in just enough to stay full until lunch without a snack.

Breakfast is the ideal time to quietly reflect and check in with yourself, setting an intention for the day ahead. This is why at Kripalu, breakfast is a silent meal. Whether you do it silently or not, however, setting an intention while you feed your body is a great way to nourish your soul and prepare to embark on the day's journey.

Morning is also a time when most Kripalu guests are coming out of yoga or about to go into it, so we recommend simple foods that are easy to digest. Morning Broth (page 279) or miso soup and steamed vegetables compose a basic yogic morning meal.

For those in need of heartier food in the early part of the day, we offer egg dishes such as Leek, Tarragon, and Chèvre Scramble (page 60) and Gold Potato and Kale Pesto Frittata (page 59). Guests often request familiar yet healthy food for weekend mornings, and we provide dishes like Gluten-Free Sweet Potato Pancakes (page 53), Vegan Sourdough Buckwheat Pancakes (page 61), and Coconut French Toast with Thai Ginger Maple Syrup (page 62). We also set out cooked whole grains and cereals such as the traditional south Indian porridge Upma (page 70), hot oatmeal, and Spiced Quinoa Cream Cereal with Dates (page 67) and Raisin Sauce (page 69).

Gluten-Free Sweet Potato Pancakes

WE ALWAYS ASK OURSELVES: How can we get more healthy vegetables into unexpected places? Sometimes we make beet pancakes, but dropping sweet potato chunks roasted in coconut oil and cinnamon into pancake batter works exceptionally well. Plus, there is some evidence that cinnamon may help lower blood sugar levels.

Ayurvedic Insight: Moderation is key for all flour-based foods. Here, sweet potato adds a vata-balancing aspect to the dry quality of all flours, while warming spices heat up the inherent coolness of the rice flours.

Makes 10 to 12 pancakes
(5 to 6 inches in diameter)

↓V ↓P ↑K

SWEET POTATOES

3 tablespoons coconut oil

2 cups peeled, 1/4-inch diced sweet potatoes

1 teaspoon ground cinnamon

1/4 teaspoon fine sea salt

PANCAKE MIX

1/2 cup plus 2 teaspoons brown rice flour

1/2 cup plus 2 teaspoons white rice flour

1/3 cup almond flour (almond meal)

3 tablespoons potato starch

2 tablespoons plus 1 teaspoon tapioca flour

1 tablespoon sweet rice flour

1 tablespoon organic cane sugar

1 teaspoon fine sea salt

1 teaspoon baking powder

1/2 teaspoon baking soda

1/4 teaspoon xanthan gum

WET INGREDIENTS

2 large eggs

2 tablespoons sunflower or coconut oil

5 cups buttermilk

2 tablespoons coconut oil or ghee, for the pan

1. For the sweet potatoes, preheat the oven to 375°F.

2. Heat a medium cast-iron skillet or oven-proof sauté pan over medium heat for 2 to 3 minutes. Melt the coconut oil in the pan and add the sweet potatoes, shaking the pan to coat the potatoes. Cook until the sweet potatoes begin to soften, 2 to 3 minutes. Stir in the cinnamon and salt and transfer the pan to the oven. Roast until the sweet potatoes are tender all the way through but not too mushy, 8 to 10 minutes. Transfer the potatoes to a plate and reserve.

3. For the pancake mix, whisk everything together in a large bowl. For the wet ingredients, whisk the eggs, sunflower oil, and buttermilk in a medium bowl. Pour the wet ingredients into the dry and whisk gently until no lumps remain. Let the batter sit for 5 to 10 minutes to thicken.

4. Heat a large cast-iron griddle or skillet over medium heat for 2 to 3 minutes. Put 1 table-

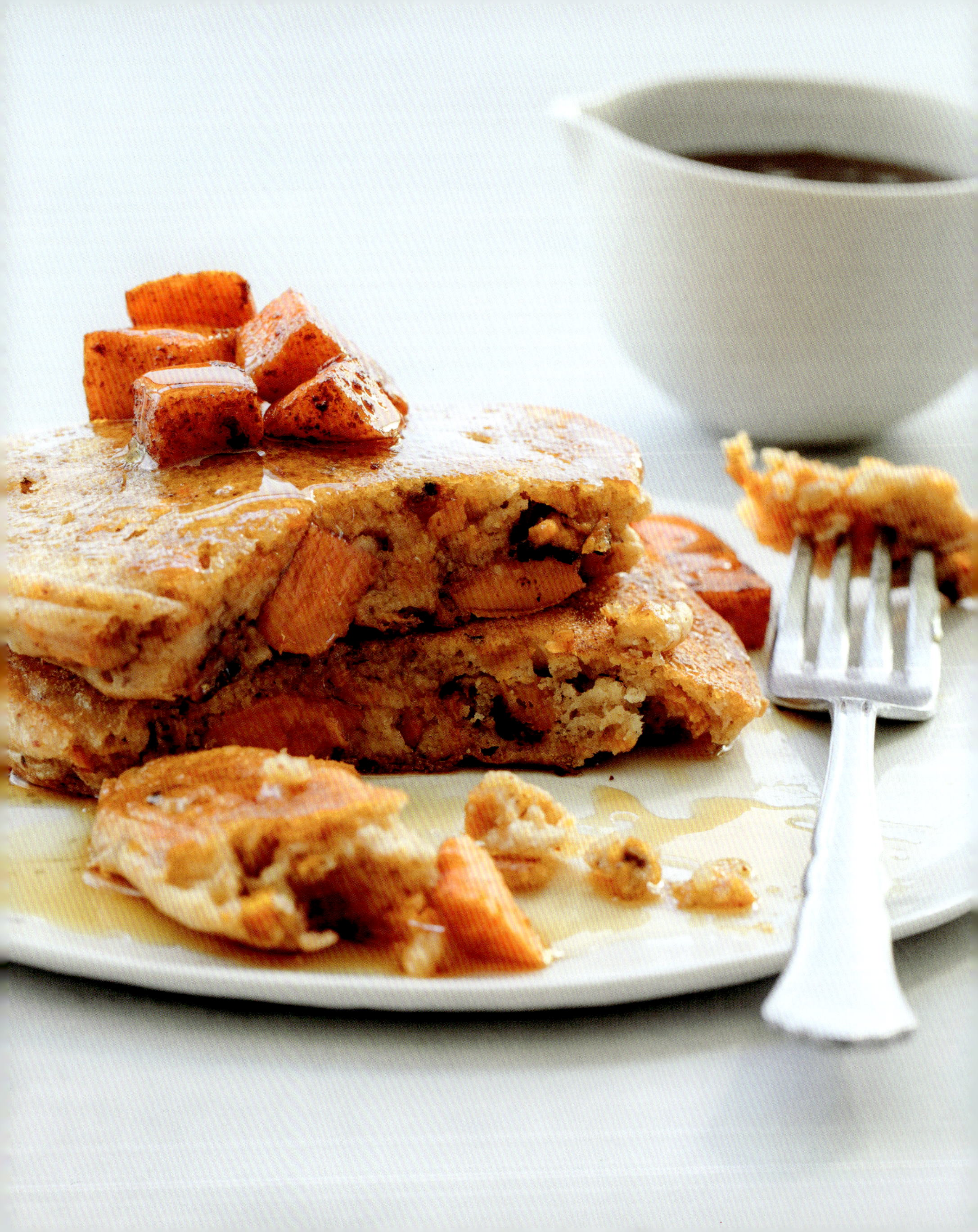

spoon of the coconut oil in the pan, swirling or spreading to coat the bottom. Pour in ½ cup batter for each pancake, and immediately top each pancake with 1 to 2 tablespoons of the sweet potatoes. Let cook until bubbles appear on the surface of each pancake, 1 to 2 minutes. Flip and cook until the batter is set, 1 to 2 minutes more. Repeat with the remaining coconut oil and batter.

OPTIONS

- You can prepare the dry pancake mix ahead of time and store it in an airtight container in the refrigerator for up to a week.
- For a dairy-free version, replace the buttermilk with 4¾ cups nondairy milk (such as soy milk or almond milk) mixed with ¼ cup fresh lemon juice. Let sit for 10 minutes to thicken.
- If you can't find tapioca flour but have pearl tapioca on hand, grind the pearl tapioca to a fine powder in a spice grinder or clean coffee mill.

Thai Scrambled Tofu

↓V
↑P
↓K

ONE OF THE ORIGINAL Kripalu scrambles using tofu instead of eggs, this dish works equally well as breakfast, brunch, lunch, and breakfast-for-dinner. Coconut milk adds moisture so the tofu doesn't dry out and a bit of sweetness to balance the spices.

Ayurvedic Insight: Tofu is best served warm for vata and kapha. The warming spices—turmeric, curry paste, and ginger—also make this dish perfect any time of day in winter or on cool mornings the rest of the year.

Serves 4

8 ounces firm tofu
1/2 cup 1/4-inch diced red bell peppers
1/2 cup freshly cut or frozen corn kernels
1/4 cup 1/4-inch diced onions
1 tablespoon toasted sesame oil
1 teaspoon ground turmeric
1 teaspoon ground cumin
1 teaspoon prepared green curry paste, such as Taste of Thai
1/2 cup grated carrots
1 teaspoon minced fresh ginger
1 tablespoon tamari
1/2 cup canned full-fat 100% coconut milk
1/2 teaspoon fine sea salt
2 tablespoons chopped fresh cilantro

1. Drain the tofu and place it in a colander in the sink. Place a small bowl on the tofu and then put a large can of tomatoes or beans in the bowl. Let the tofu press for 20 minutes to drain excess water. Crumble the pressed tofu until it resembles scrambled eggs and set aside.

2. Heat a large sauté pan over medium-high heat for 2 minutes. Put in the peppers, corn, onions, and sesame oil, shaking the pan to coat the vegetables. Cook until the vegetables are just beginning to get tender, about 2 minutes. Stir in the turmeric, cumin, and curry paste, stirring to distribute the curry paste. Cook until the spices smell fragrant, about 2 minutes.

3. Stir in the crumbled tofu, carrots, and ginger and cook, stirring occasionally, until the carrots soften up a bit, 2 to 3 minutes. Stir in the tamari, coconut milk, and salt, and simmer until the liquid thickens up some, 2 to 3 minutes. Remove from the heat, stir in the cilantro, and serve.

OPTION

- You could replace the tofu here with 6 eggs. Just sauté everything but the tofu in the sauté pan, including the tamari, coconut milk, and salt, then remove them from the pan and scramble the eggs in the pan. Add back the sautéed veg and you have a nice Thai egg scramble.

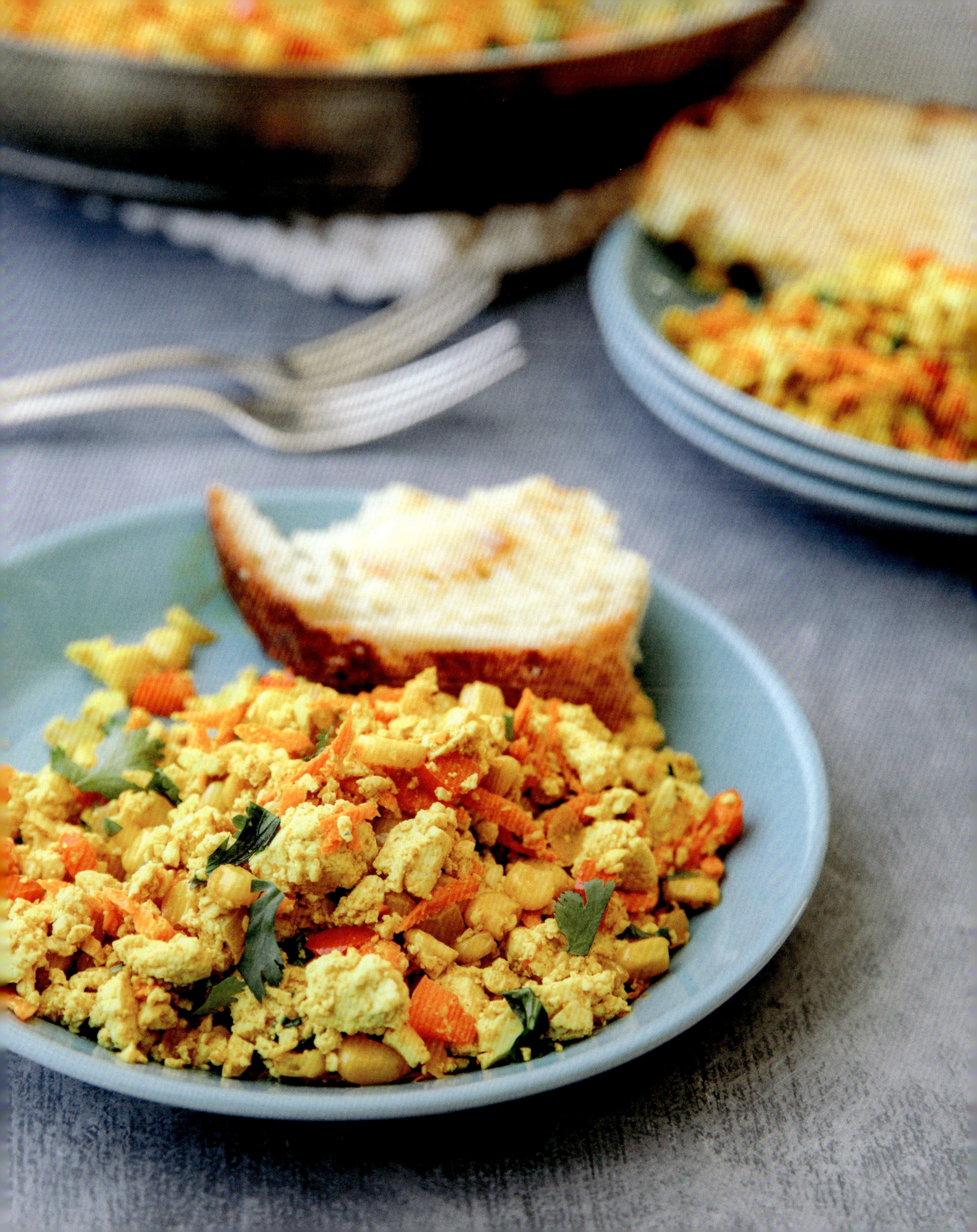

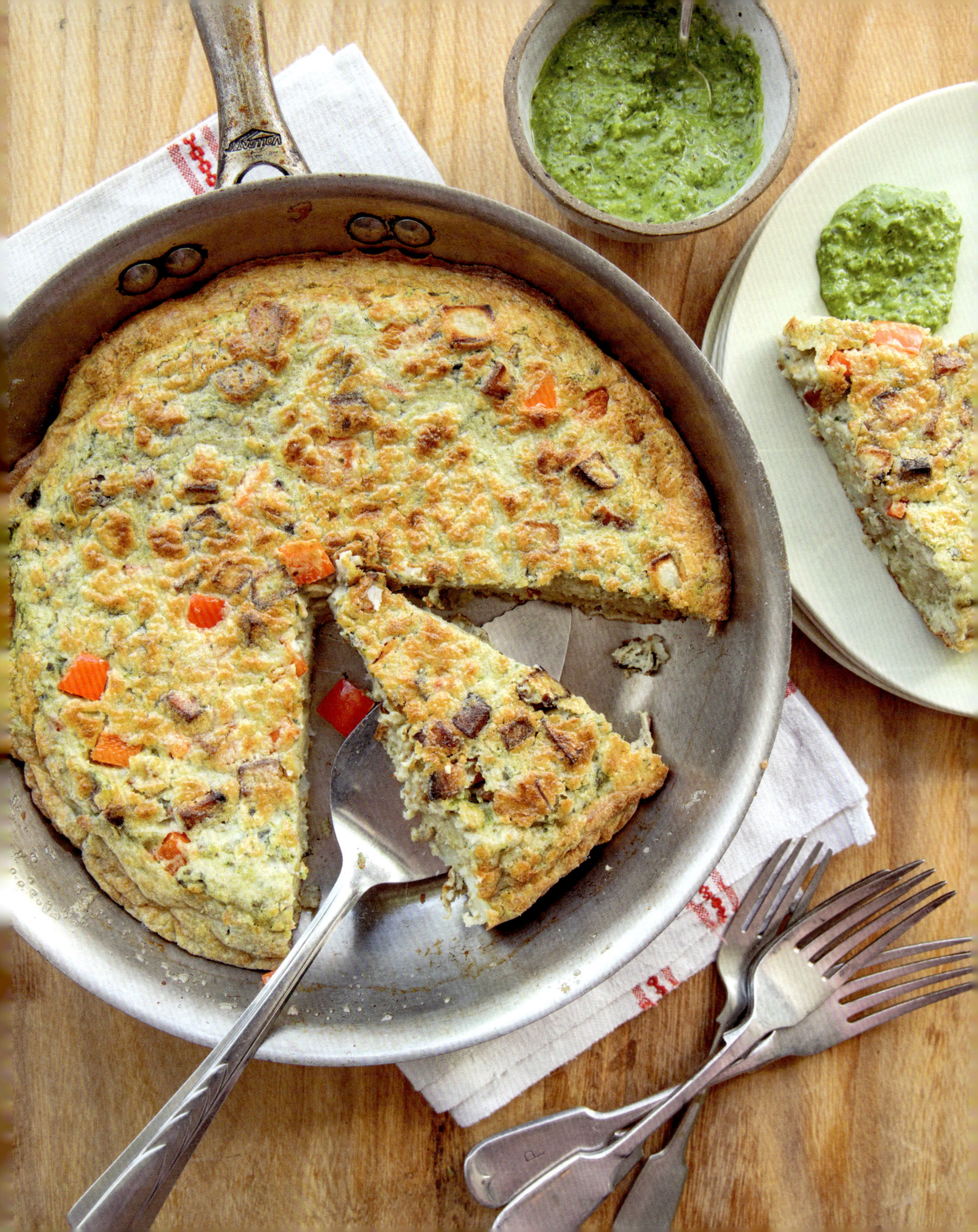

Gold Potato and Kale Pesto Frittata

=V

=P

=K

FRITTATAS WORK WELL any time of year and for any meal. Roast or sauté whatever vegetables you have on hand, add blended eggs to the pan, and bake. We use heavy cream here because we serve this version in winter when richer ingredients are welcome. At other times of year, you could use milk instead, or even water or stock.

Ayurvedic Insight: Kale pesto adds a light quality to balance the heavier potato, cheese, and eggs here. Kapha types should use water, stock, or milk in place of cream.

Serves 6

1/2 cup Kale Pesto (page 195), made without lemon

2 tablespoons extra-virgin olive oil

2 cups 1/4-inch diced Yukon Gold potatoes with skin

1/4 cup 1/4-inch diced red bell peppers

9 large eggs

1/2 cup heavy cream

1/2 cup grated Parmesan cheese

1/2 teaspoon fine sea salt

1/4 teaspoon freshly ground black pepper

1. Preheat the oven to 325°F. Make the pesto so it's ready to go.

2. For the frittata, heat a medium cast-iron skillet or ovenproof and reasonably nonstick pan over medium heat for 3 minutes. Swirl in the oil and add the potatoes, shaking the pan to coat the potatoes. Cook until the potatoes are lightly browned all over and tender, 6 to 8 minutes. Stir in the peppers and cook for 2 minutes.

3. Meanwhile, whisk together the eggs, cream, Parmesan, salt, pepper, and 2 tablespoons of the pesto. Pour the egg mixture into the pan, gently stirring everything together and scraping the pan bottom for about 1 minute. The eggs will begin to cook but still be very wet and liquid. Transfer the pan to the oven and cook until the middle of the frittata is firm to the touch, 8 to 10 minutes.

4. Remove from the oven and let stand for 3 to 4 minutes. Loosen the frittata by running a rubber spatula around the perimeter of the pan and under the frittata. Cut into 6 wedges and drizzle some of the remaining pesto over each wedge.

OPTIONS

- Try sweet potatoes instead of Yukon Gold potatoes.
- For a nice presentation, completely loosen the frittata from the pan, then place a large plate on top of the pan and invert the frittata onto the plate.
- For a dairy-free or paleo version, replace the cream with Vegetable Stock (page 281) and omit the Parmesan.

Leek, Tarragon, and Chèvre Scramble

↓V
=P
↑K

WHEN I FIRST put this dish on the Kripalu menu, I named it Eggs Bagnulo after John Bagnulo, the nutritionist who introduced it to me and shared the ingredient combination on social media. He thought I was joking when I said I would name it after him! It's been hugely popular with our guests ever since. Fresh goat cheese is easy for many to digest, and the tropical aroma of coconut oil marries well with the flavors of tarragon and leeks.

Ayurvedic Insight: Herbs tend to lighten the heaviness of eggs. This dish is especially good in cool weather to help soothe the cold and dry qualities of the weather.

Serves 4

1 1/2 cups thinly sliced cleaned leeks

2 tablespoons coconut oil

8 large eggs

1/2 teaspoon fine sea salt

1/4 teaspoon freshly ground black pepper

3 tablespoons chèvre (soft goat cheese)

1 teaspoon chopped fresh tarragon

1. Heat a large cast-iron or other reasonably nonstick skillet over medium-low heat for 5 minutes. Put in the leeks and 1 tablespoon of the coconut oil, shaking the pan to coat the leeks. Cover and sweat until the leeks are soft and translucent, 3 to 4 minutes. Transfer the leeks to a plate and reserve. Place the pan back over medium heat.

2. Using a fork, whip the eggs, salt, and pepper. Place the remaining 1 tablespoon of coconut oil in the pan, then pour in the eggs. Slowly cook the eggs, stirring periodically with a rubber spatula or wooden spoon so they cook evenly. When the eggs are barely set and still glistening and moist, fold in the leeks.

3. Remove the pan from the heat and fold in the chèvre and tarragon. Serve hot.

OPTIONS

- If you find fresh spring ramps at your farmer's market, use them in place of the leeks. You can use the green tops of the ramps, too.
- For a dairy-free or paleo version, omit the chèvre.

Vegan Sourdough Buckwheat Pancakes

↓V

=P

=K

OUR BAKERS LOVE sourdough and use it to leaven as many baked goods as possible. When they added some sourdough starter to these vegan pancakes, it worked beautifully with the earthy flavor of buckwheat. Enjoy this hearty breakfast in the colder months.

Ayurvedic Insight: Buckwheat and sourdough are both sour, which can increase heat in a pitta type. This dish is best for vata types, who tend to love sour flavors.

Makes 10 to 12 pancakes (5 to 6 inches in diameter)

- 1/3 cup (3 ounces) active Sourdough Starter (page 82)
- 1 2/3 cups whole-wheat flour
- 1 1/2 cups buckwheat flour
- 1 teaspoon rye flour
- 3 1/2 teaspoons flax meal
- 2 1/2 tablespoons unsweetened applesauce
- 1 tablespoon plus 1 teaspoon pure maple syrup
- 1 tablespoon plus 1 teaspoon sunflower oil
- 1/3 cup unsweetened soy milk
- 1/4 teaspoon baking soda
- 1/4 teaspoon fine sea salt
- Scant 1/4 teaspoon ground allspice
- 2 tablespoons coconut oil

1. In a large bowl, stir the starter and 3¾ cups cold tap water, mixing well.

2. Whisk the whole-wheat flour, buckwheat flour, and rye flour in a small bowl. Gradually stir the flour mixture into the starter, mixing until the starter is fairly smooth. Loosely cover and let the batter sit at room temperature until it begins to get bubbly, at least 1 hour. To let the batter ferment overnight for more flavor, put it in the refrigerator.

3. In a medium bowl or a 2-cup measure, whisk together the flax meal, applesauce, maple syrup, and sunflower oil, and then whisk in the soy milk. Scatter the baking soda, salt, and allspice over the top and whisk until smooth. Stir the soy milk mixture into the starter just until combined.

4. Heat a large cast-iron griddle or skillet over medium heat for 2 to 3 minutes. Put 2 teaspoons of the coconut oil in the pan, swirling or spreading to coat the bottom. Pour in ½ cup batter for each pancake, and let cook until bubbles appear on the surface of each pancake, 1 to 2 minutes. Flip and cook until the batter is set, 1 to 2 minutes more. Repeat with the remaining coconut oil and batter.

Coconut French Toast with Thai Ginger Maple Syrup

↓V
=P
↑K

WE LOVE COCONUT MILK in the Kripalu Kitchen. It's creamy, fragrant, dairy-free, and rich in calcium, potassium, and magnesium. It makes the perfect substitute for cow's milk in French toast. For a Thai twist, we flavor our local maple syrup with lime, orange, ginger, and a touch of mild red curry paste called Lan Chi. Look for Lan Chi in Asian food markets or online.

Ayurvedic Insight: Spicy maple syrup heats up the heavy, dense French toast here. This dish will sit best in winter or with vata types who are digesting really well. To make it more kapha friendly, use gluten-free bread. Kapha and wheat have the same sticky qualities, and too much wheat can create excess kapha, leaving one lethargic with excess mucus.

Serves 4

SYRUP

1/4 cup pure maple syrup
1 teaspoon fresh lime juice
1 teaspoon minced fresh ginger
1 teaspoon grated orange zest
2 teaspoons orange juice
1/8 teaspoon Lan Chi chili paste or other red chili paste

FRENCH TOAST

2 large eggs
3/4 cup canned full-fat 100% coconut milk
1/2 teaspoon ground cinnamon
1/4 teaspoon ground allspice
1 teaspoon vanilla extract
Pinch of fine sea salt
2 teaspoons coconut oil or plant-based butter
6 thick slices (about 10 ounces) Sourdough Semolina Bread (page 87) or other country bread
Citrus Mango Compote (recipe follows; optional)

1. For the syrup, combine the maple syrup, lime juice, ginger, orange zest, orange juice, and chili paste in a small saucepan. Gently warm over low heat.

2. For the French toast, whisk together the eggs, coconut milk, cinnamon, allspice, vanilla, and salt in a wide, shallow bowl.

3. Heat a large skillet or griddle over medium heat. When hot, pour in the oil and distribute it evenly in the pan. Dip the bread slices in the coconut milk mixture long enough for the bread to absorb the liquid but not get soggy, about 2 minutes. Shake off any excess liquid and place the bread in the pan. Cook until golden brown, 2 to 3 minutes per side.

4. Cut each piece of bread in half diagonally and divide the pieces evenly among 4 plates. Serve with the syrup and compote, if using.

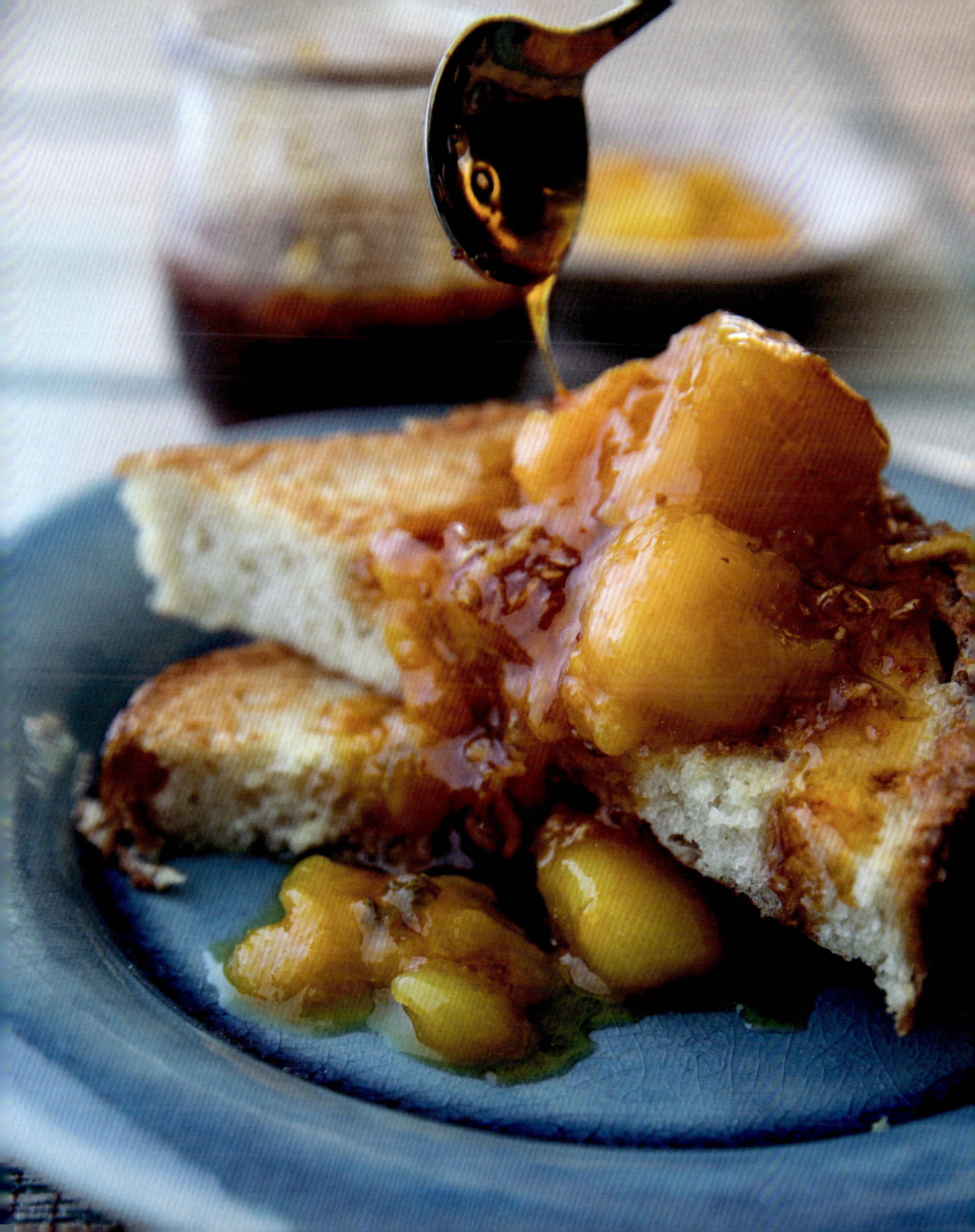

CITRUS MANGO COMPOTE

WE OFFER THIS as a topping for our Coconut French Toast. It works well on pancakes, too, and if you have extra, it keeps refrigerated for several days. Just warm it up a little before using.

Makes about 4 cups

1 orange

2 tablespoons fresh lime juice

4 cups fresh or frozen cubed mango

1 tablespoon chopped fresh cilantro (optional)

Grate the orange zest into a small saucepan. Squeeze in ¼ cup of the orange juice, then add the lime juice and mango. Bring to a simmer over medium heat, then simmer gently until the mango just starts to break down and the compote thickens, about 5 minutes. Remove from the heat and stir in the cilantro, if using.

Tempeh Potato Sausage

YES, THIS IS HIPPIE vegan breakfast food. But don't knock it until you try it! The key step is simmering the tempeh to remove any bitterness. With sage, rosemary, and other herbs, these patties have an aroma similar to other breakfast sausages and the texture gets nice and crisp in the oven.

Ayurvedic Insight: These sausages make a filling breakfast for pitta types. They are best when you are quite hungry, as the rich tempeh and heavy potatoes will sustain you until your next meal. Use sweet potatoes to make these more vata balancing.

Makes 8 to 10 patties
(3 inches in diameter)

Oil spray
4 ounces tempeh
2 1/4 cups 1/2-inch diced Yukon Gold potatoes with skin
1/4 cup tamari
1 tablespoon extra-virgin olive oil
1 1/2 teaspoons minced fresh garlic
1 teaspoon chopped fresh sage
1/2 teaspoon chopped fresh rosemary
1/2 teaspoon chopped fresh thyme
1/2 teaspoon chopped fresh oregano
1/4 teaspoon freshly ground black pepper

↑V
↓P
↑K

1. Preheat the oven to 400°F. Lightly coat a baking sheet with oil spray.

2. Place the tempeh in a small sauté pan with water to cover. Bring to a boil over high heat, then reduce the heat and gently simmer the tempeh for 10 minutes to remove any bitterness. Drain the tempeh and place it in a medium bowl to cool. When cool enough to handle, use your hands to crumble the tempeh into small beads.

3. Meanwhile, place the potatoes in a small saucepan with water to cover. Bring to a boil over high heat, then reduce the heat and gently simmer the potatoes until they are just fork-tender, 3 to 5 minutes. Avoid overcooking the potatoes or the sausage mixture will become too wet.

4. Drain the potatoes and add to the tempeh along with the tamari, oil, garlic, sage, rosemary, thyme, oregano, and pepper. Mash with a potato masher or fork until the mixture is fairly smooth, with only small chunks remaining. The potatoes should bind everything together. Taste the mixture and add more tamari, pepper, or other seasonings if you think it needs them.

5. Using a ¼-cup measure, form the mixture into 3-inch round patties (about ½ inch thick). Place the patties on the oiled baking sheet and spritz them all over with oil spray. Bake until

they are browned and slightly crisp on the outside yet still tender in the center, 12 to 15 minutes.

OPTIONS

- You can freeze the bulk sausage mixture. You can also form the patties and refrigerate them for up to 1 day.
- Use a baked potato from the night before. Or use sweet potatoes.

Spiced Quinoa Cream Cereal with Dates

↓V ↓P ↓K

THE KRIPALU DINING room buffet is an exercise in liberty, and this hot breakfast cereal illustrates that freedom. Here, we provide a basic cooked grain with dried fruit, nuts, and spices. But we encourage you to customize these elements to your heart's content.

Ayurvedic Insight: This is a tridoshic breakfast that anyone can enjoy. To fine-tune it for your own doshic balancing, see the optional mix-ins. Pitta and kapha should favor seeds, while vata should favor nuts. Raisins are also more kapha balancing than dates.

Serves 4

1 cup quinoa
1/4 cup chopped dates
2 teaspoons pure maple syrup or Raisin Sauce (recipe follows)
1 to 1 1/2 teaspoons ground cinnamon
1/2 teaspoon ground cardamom
1/4 teaspoon fine sea salt
1/2 cup milk, any kind
6 tablespoons slivered almonds, toasted (or whole roasted and chopped)

1. In a medium saucepan, combine 4 cups water with all the ingredients except the milk and almonds. Bring the mixture to a boil over high heat. Cover, reduce the heat to low, and simmer until the grains are almost tender, about 10 minutes, stirring now and then as the cereal thickens.

2. Uncover and let simmer gently until most of the remaining liquid is absorbed, about 5 minutes. Remove from the heat and stir in the milk and almonds. Serve hot.

OPTIONS

- Amaranth Cream Cereal: Use 1 cup amaranth and 4 cups water.
- Millet Cream Cereal: Use 1 cup millet and 3 cups water.
- Creamy: Use milk, almond milk, soy milk, hemp milk, and/or coconut milk.
- Spicy: Use cinnamon, cardamom, ground or fresh ginger, turmeric, nutmeg, and/or allspice.
- Sweet: Use dried fruit (dates, figs, cherries, apricots, etc.), maple syrup, coconut sugar, or Raisin Sauce (recipe follows).
- Nuts and seeds: Use flax, chia, sunflower and/or pumpkin seeds; or walnuts, pecans, almonds, cashews, pistachios, and/or hazelnuts.

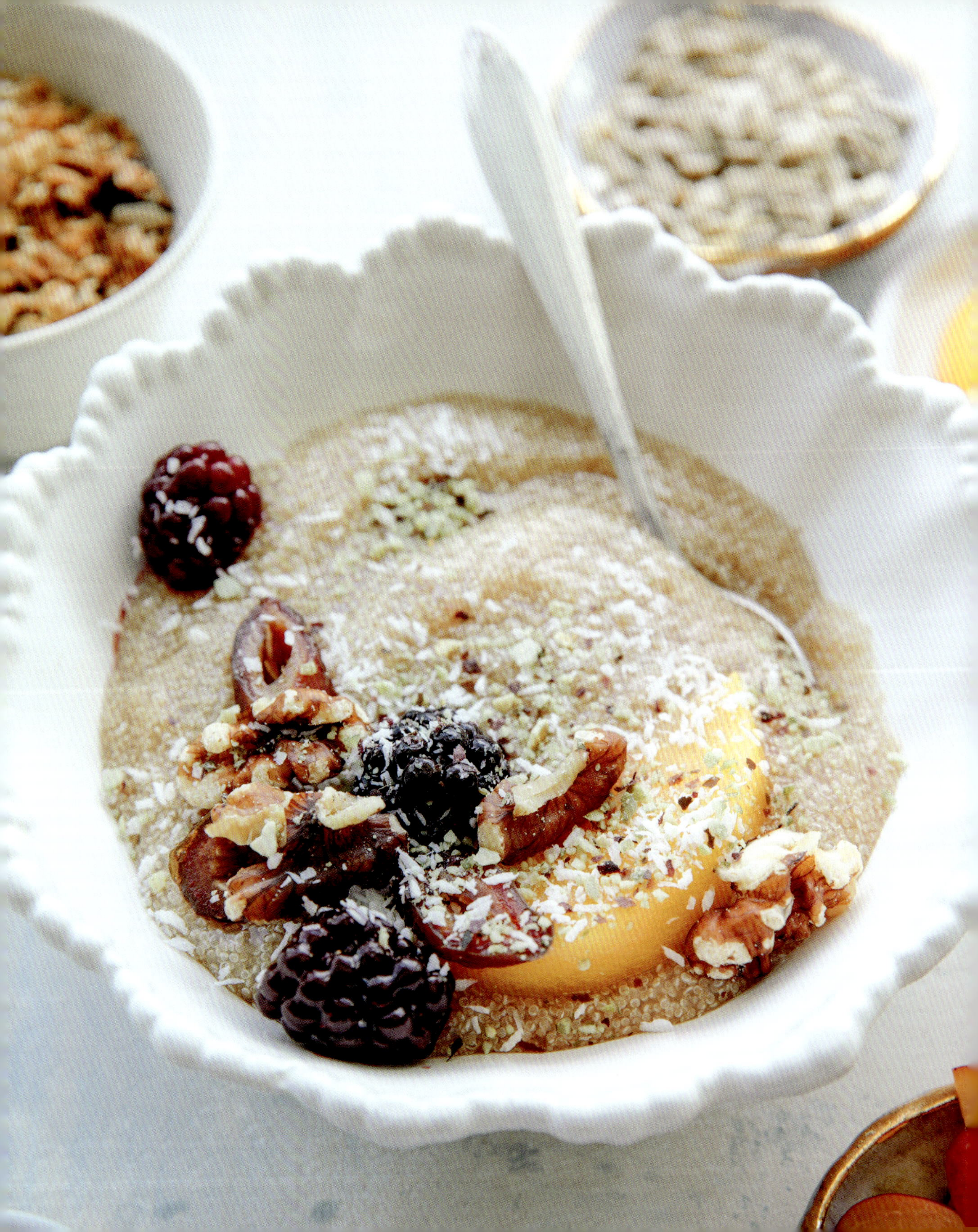

RAISIN SAUCE

HERE IS THE most magical asked-for recipe at Kripalu. It is our basic cereal topping, and we go through a ton of it. We actually make it in 5-gallon buckets. Assuming you don't need that much, simply cover 1¼ cups raisins with 1½ cups tap water and let sit overnight. The next day, puree everything with an immersion blender or food processor. That's it. Simple. Use it immediately or refrigerate it for up to 5 days.

Upma

↓V
↓P
↓K

ON THE KRIPALU MENU for at least two decades, upma is a classic south Indian porridge made from cream of wheat. The mix of broth, sugar, salt, vegetables, dried fruit, and spices gives you a perfect balance of sweet, creamy, spicy, and savory flavors. Why quinoa here? We ran out of cream of wheat one morning at 5 A.M., and one of our chefs made the upma with quinoa instead. Now, it's even better.

Ayurvedic Insight: Using quinoa makes this dish lighter and balancing for all three doshas. The warmth of the spices balances out the dryness of the potatoes, making this a balanced dish for all.

Serves 4

3/4 cup quinoa

3 cups Vegetable Stock (page 281) or store-bought stock

1/3 cup peeled, 1/4-inch diced Yukon Gold potatoes

1 tablespoon coconut sugar

1/2 teaspoon fine sea salt

2 1/2 tablespoons 1/4-inch diced carrot

2 1/2 tablespoons 1/4-inch diced green bell pepper

2 tablespoons ghee

1 1/4 teaspoons ground turmeric

3/4 teaspoon cumin seeds

3/4 teaspoon brown mustard seeds

Pinch of cayenne pepper

Pinch of asafetida (hing)

1/4 cup dark raisins

1 tablespoon fresh lemon juice

1/4 cup cashews, toasted and coarsely chopped

1 tablespoon chopped fresh cilantro

1. Pour the quinoa into a spice grinder or clean coffee mill (or a high-speed blender) and grind it to fine bits, similar to the texture of cream of wheat.

2. In a small saucepan, combine the stock, potatoes, coconut sugar, and salt. Bring to a gentle simmer over medium heat and simmer until the potatoes are just fork-tender, 3 to 5 minutes.

3. Meanwhile, heat a medium saucepan over medium heat for 1 minute. Put in the carrots, peppers, and ghee, shaking the pan to coat the vegetables. Sauté until the carrots begin to get tender, 3 to 5 minutes. Stir in the turmeric, cumin seeds, mustard seeds, cayenne, and asafetida and cook until the spices are fragrant, 1 to 2 minutes.

4. Stir in the ground quinoa, raisins, and lemon juice. Raise the heat to high and pour in the stock and potato mixture, stirring constantly. Continue cooking and stirring rapidly until the upma is just thick enough to stick to the spoon, like porridge, 3 to 4 minutes. The potatoes and

ground quinoa will bind everything together, but avoid letting the upma become too dry.

5. Remove from the heat and stir in the cashews. Divide among 4 bowls and garnish with the cilantro.

OPTION

- For a sugar-free version, omit the sugar.

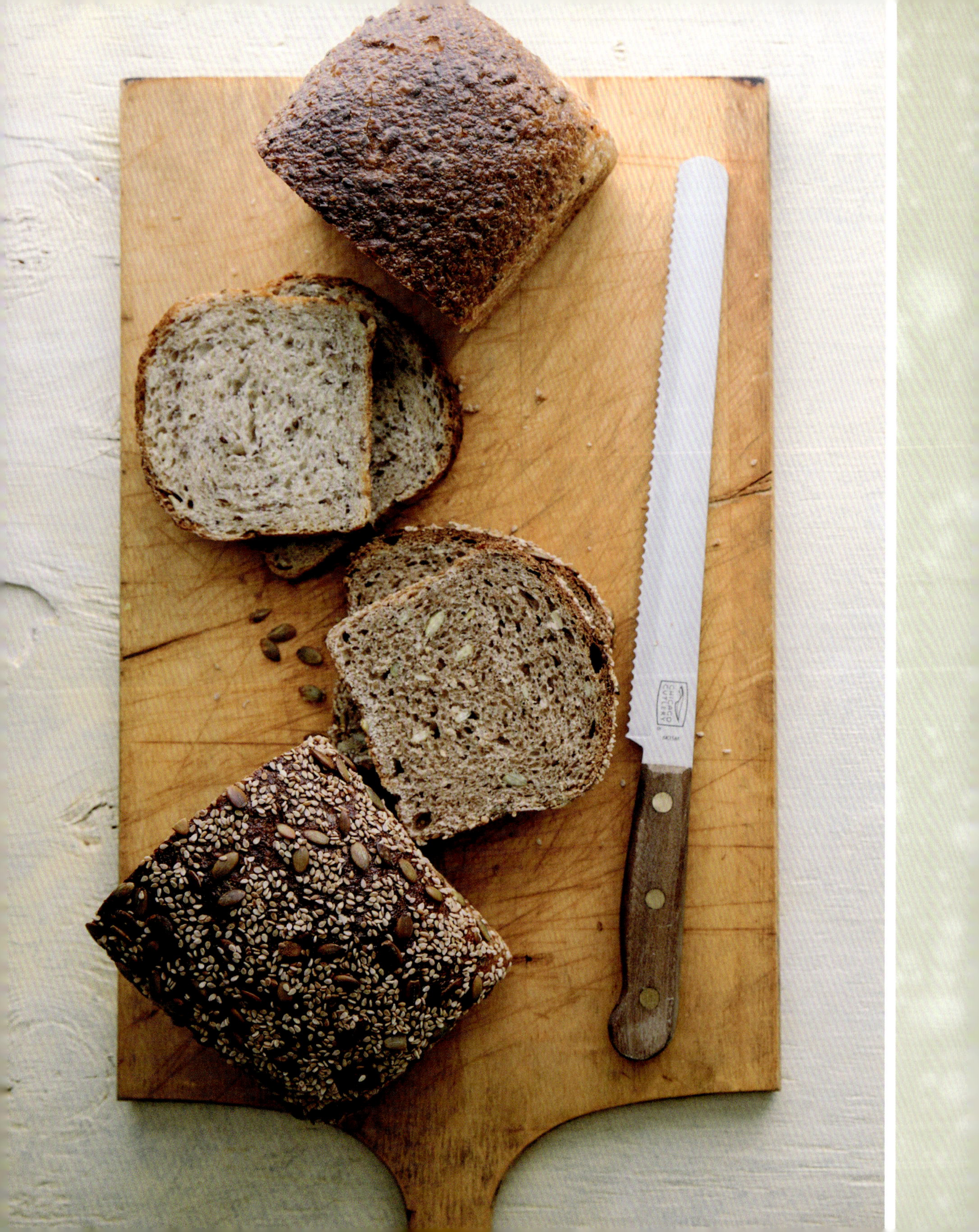

MUFFINS, SCONES, *and BREADS*

Bread has gotten a bad reputation, but undeservedly so. Most of bread's potential ill effects are due to cheap loaves that are made with refined wheat flour, refined fats, and commercial dry yeast, pumped up with dough conditioners, and given very little time to ferment properly. Whole-grain bread, on the other hand, is a cornerstone common to thriving civilizations around the world. The first grinding stones were constructed in Egypt around 8,000 B.C.E. to grind whole grains such as einkorn and emmer into flour for simple breads. Made from unleavened wheat dough, modern Indian chapattis still resemble the nourishing breads made at that time. Over the course of several thousand years, leavened sourdough breads began to spread from Egypt to the Middle East and the Mediterranean. These whole-grain sourdough breads helped to feed and advance many diverse societies all over the globe.

In the Kripalu bakery, we use whole grains and natural sourdough yeasts whenever possible. Leavening breads the old-fashioned way with wild yeast and natural lactic acid bacteria brings more flavor to the bread and fully ferments the flour, making the bread easier to digest. Recall that, according to Ayurveda, the sour taste quickens our digestive fire, promoting healthy digestion. For those avoiding gluten and wheat, we use several alternative grains in our gluten-free baked goods, including oat flour, coconut flour, quinoa flour, and rice flour. Whether baked goods are made with wheat or other grains, using whole-grain flours is the key to providing your body with much-needed fiber, minerals, and other nutrients that can help to regulate digestion, prevent constipation, and ward off cancer risk.

It's not a stretch to say that our Vegan Ginger Scones (page 80) are probably the most beloved food item at Kripalu. As a healthier version of a familiar food, guests find them supremely comforting and nourishing all at once. If you are someone who eats gluten-free but longs for a tasty breakfast treat, try our Gluten-Free Blackberry Chocolate Chip Muffins (page 77). Coconut flour makes them easy to digest, moist, and mouthwatering. This chapter also includes recipes for Sourdough Sunflower Flax Bread (page 83) and Sourdough Semolina Bread (page 87), two naturally leavened breads that our guests love to use for making sandwiches and toast. Our Gluten-Free Pizza Dough and Sourdough Whole-Grain Pizza Dough recipes (pages 91 and 90) are included as well so you can enjoy pizza no matter what your dietary preferences or restrictions may be.

Whether you enjoy gluten-free or wheat-based baked goods, keep in mind that the grains in these foods may challenge your digestive system. It is best to enjoy breads in the colder months of fall, winter, and early spring when digestion is dialed up. Find a cozy chair and savor these nourishing baked goods with a hot beverage to help warm your body and soothe your digestion.

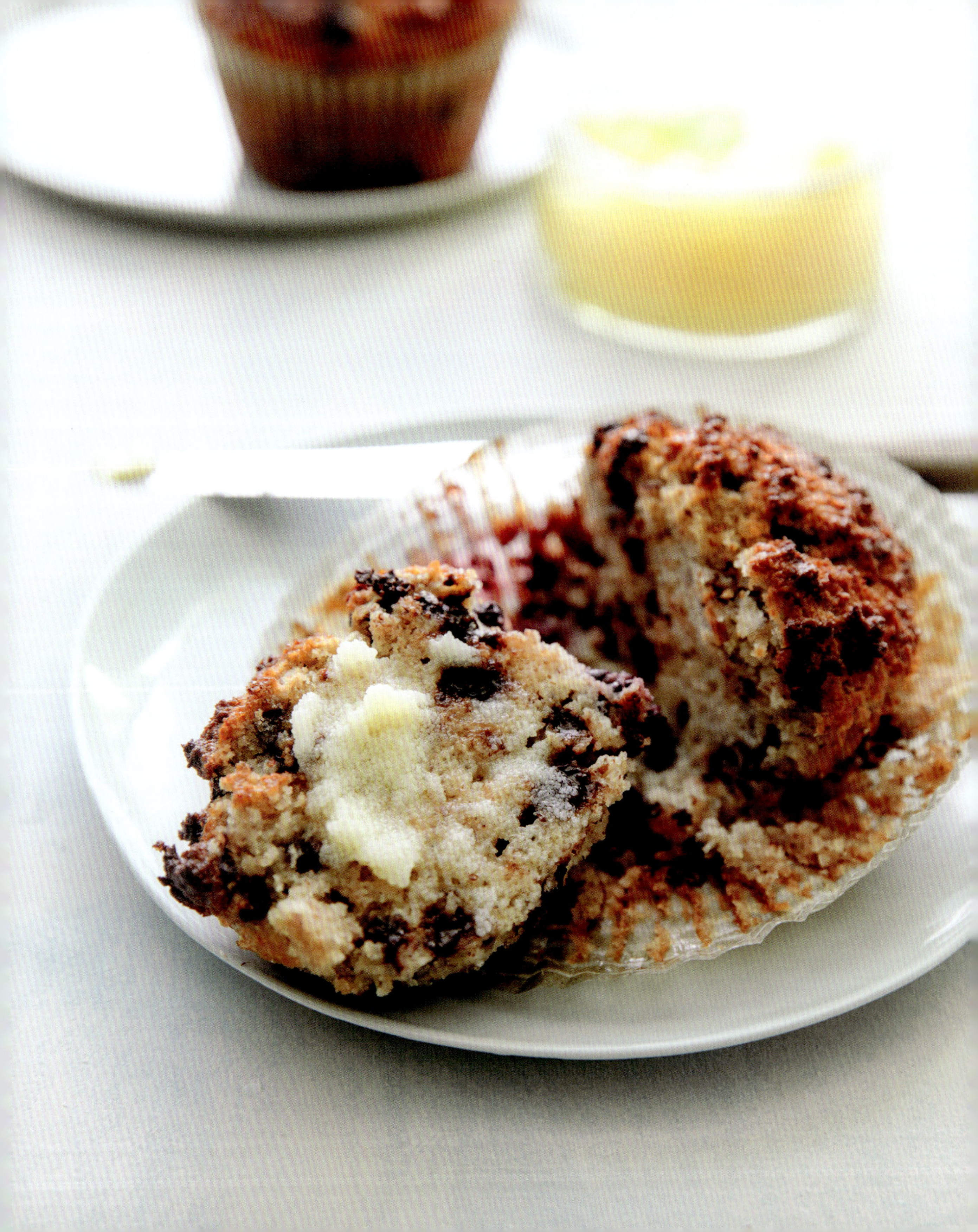

Gluten-Free Blackberry Chocolate Chip Muffins

↓V ↓P =K

VERY MOIST AND SATISFYING, but not overly sweet, these handy treats are perfect for a light breakfast, a midday hike, or late afternoon pick-me-up.

Ayurvedic Insight: The coconut flour and coconut oil here are wonderfully satisfying for pitta types without being overheating. Coconut oil also helps support digestive health and proper brain functioning.

Makes 12 muffins

Oil spray
1/2 cup unsweetened applesauce
1/4 cup flaxseed meal
2/3 cup coconut oil
6 large eggs
2/3 cup pure maple syrup
1 tablespoon vanilla extract
2/3 cup coconut flour
1 teaspoon baking powder
1 teaspoon fine sea salt
1/2 cup chocolate chips
1 cup blackberries (about 3 ounces)

1. Preheat the oven to 350°F. Line a 12-cup muffin tin with paper liners and coat the papers with oil spray.

2. In a large bowl, stir together the applesauce and flaxseed meal. Let soak for at least 20 minutes and up to 1 hour.

3. If your coconut oil is solid, liquefy it on a sunny windowsill or by briefly heating then cooling it. Stir the cooled liquid oil, eggs, maple syrup, and vanilla into the applesauce mixture.

4. In a small bowl, combine the coconut flour, baking powder, and salt. Mix the dry ingredients into the wet, stirring well until everything is evenly incorporated. Let sit until the mixture thickens up some, 3 to 5 minutes. Fold in the chocolate chips and blackberries. The batter will be a bit thinner than muffin batter made with wheat flour. That's okay.

5. Spoon the batter into the prepared muffin tin and bake until a toothpick inserted into the center of a muffin comes out clean, about 30 minutes. Let cool at least 15 minutes before serving.

OPTIONS

- Use whatever berries you like.
- For a paleo version, use dairy-free and soy-free chocolate chips such as the Enjoy Life brand.

Vegan Maple Walnut Scones

=V

=P

=K

FOR VEGAN BAKING, we use palm shortening instead of butter. Look for palm shortening from companies committed to sustainability, such as Spectrum. It's also important to use 100% palm shortening because some brands use a mix of palm oil, coconut oil, and other fats that may alter the texture of these scones.

Ayurvedic Insight: Maple syrup is our preferred natural sweetener in baked goods, not only because it is made locally but also because honey loses its nutritive qualities when heated.

Makes 12 scones

- 3/4 cup cold 100% palm shortening, such as Spectrum
- 1 cup old-fashioned rolled oats
- 2/3 cup whole-wheat pastry flour
- 2/3 cup all-purpose flour, plus more for dusting
- 1/4 cup organic cane sugar
- 1 3/4 teaspoons baking powder
- 1/2 teaspoon fine sea salt
- 1/3 cup soy, almond, or other milk
- 1/3 cup pure maple syrup
- 2/3 cup chopped walnuts

1. Preheat the oven to 350°F. Line a sheet pan with parchment paper.

2. Partially freeze your shortening until it is stiff enough to shred, about 20 minutes. Use a box grater to grate the cold shortening into shreds onto a plate, then keep the shreds cold in the refrigerator.

3. In a large bowl, mix the rolled oats, whole-wheat pastry flour, all-purpose flour, sugar, baking powder, and salt.

4. Using your fingertips, a pastry cutter, a food processor, or an electric mixer with a paddle attachment, cut the shredded shortening into the dry ingredients until the mixture looks mealy. Gently stir in the milk and maple syrup until the dry ingredients are barely moistened. Then stir in the walnuts, mixing just enough to form a wet, heavy dough. Mix gently and briefly at all times to ensure tender scones.

5. Lightly flour a work surface and turn the dough out onto it. The dough will be somewhat wet. With floured hands, pat the dough into a circle about 1 inch thick. Cut the dough into wedges like a pie (or cut into 2-inch rounds and gently re-pat, then cut any remaining dough). Place the scones on the prepared sheet pan and bake until golden brown, 35 to 40 minutes. Serve warm or within 8 hours. Scones are best enjoyed the day they are made.

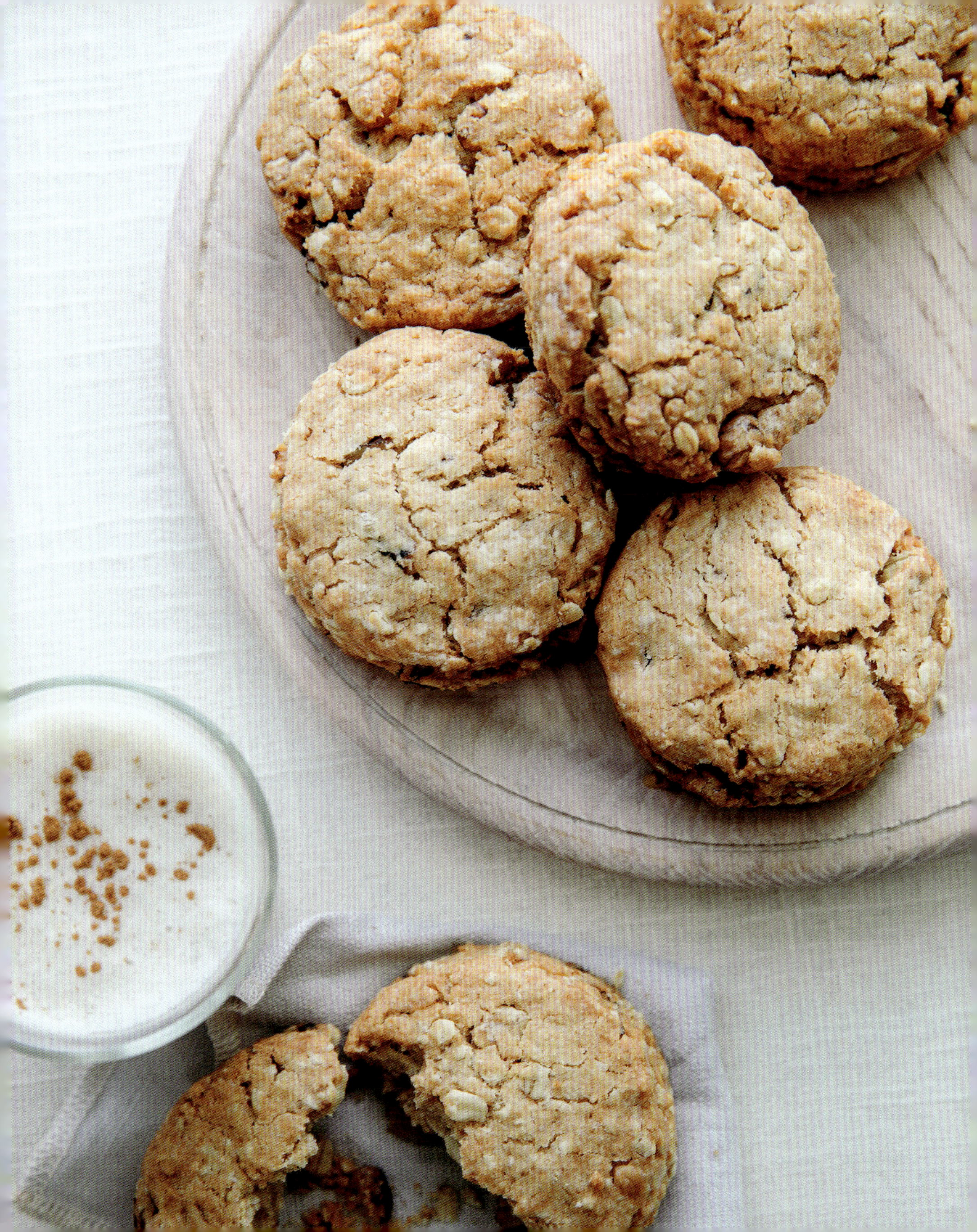

Vegan Ginger Scones

=V

=P

=K

AMONG OUR BREAKFAST BREADS, ginger scones are far and away the most popular. They are moist and rich, pair well with hot tea, and travel well so you can pack one in your work bag for a snack later in the day. I have found these scones stashed by guests in cubbies outside our program rooms!

Ayurvedic Insight: The ginger in these scones balances the sugar and flour with just the right amount of heating spice. Whole-wheat flour also provides fiber to aid digestion.

Makes 12 scones

- 3/4 cup cold 100% palm shortening, such as Spectrum
- 1 cup old-fashioned rolled oats
- 2/3 cup whole-wheat pastry flour
- 2/3 cup all-purpose flour, plus more for dusting
- 1/4 cup organic cane sugar
- 1 3/4 teaspoons baking powder
- 1/2 teaspoon fine sea salt
- 2/3 cup soy, almond, or other milk
- 2/3 cup chopped candied ginger

1. Preheat the oven to 375°F. Line a sheet pan with parchment paper.

2. Partially freeze your shortening until it is stiff enough to shred, about 20 minutes. Use a box grater to grate the cold shortening into shreds onto a plate, then keep the shreds cold in the refrigerator.

3. In a large bowl, mix the rolled oats, whole-wheat pastry flour, all-purpose flour, sugar, baking powder, and salt.

4. Using your fingertips, a pastry cutter, a food processor, or an electric mixer with a paddle attachment, cut the shredded shortening into the dry ingredients until the mixture looks mealy. Gently stir in the milk until the dry ingredients are barely moistened, then stir in the candied ginger, mixing just enough to form a wet, heavy dough. Mix gently and briefly at all times to ensure tender scones.

5. Lightly flour a work surface and turn the dough out onto it. With floured hands, pat the dough into a circle about 1 inch thick. Cut the dough into wedges like a pie (or cut into 2-inch rounds and gently re-pat, then cut any remaining dough). Place the scones on the prepared sheet pan and bake until golden brown, 30 to 35 minutes. Serve warm or within 8 hours. Scones are best enjoyed the day they are made.

OPTION

- Make a double batch and freeze half on a sheet pan. When frozen, put the scones in a freezer bag.

Sour Cream Coffee Cake

PART OF THE CHARM of this comforting coffee cake is that some of the streusel topping falls into the batter, creating a surprise layer of sweetness, cinnamon, and crunch right in the middle.

Ayurvedic Insight: Due to the refined white flour and refined sugar here, it's best to enjoy this cake only occasionally and with a cup of black tea or coffee. The bitterness of the tea or coffee balances the sweetness of the cake.

Makes one 8 x 4½-inch loaf, about 10 slices

STREUSEL TOPPING

1/4 cup packed light brown sugar

3/4 teaspoon ground cinnamon

3 tablespoons cold unsalted butter

CAKE

1/2 cup (1 stick) unsalted butter, softened, plus more for greasing the pan

1 1/4 cups all-purpose flour, plus more for dusting the pan

1/4 teaspoon baking powder

1/2 teaspoon baking soda

1/2 teaspoon fine sea salt

1/2 cup organic cane sugar

1/2 cup sour cream, at room temperature

3 large eggs, at room temperature

1 teaspoon vanilla extract

=V
=P
=K

1. Preheat the oven to 350°F. Butter an 8 x 4½-inch loaf pan. Cut a piece of parchment paper to fit the bottom and just up the sides of the pan. Grease the paper, then dust the entire pan with flour. Gently tap out the excess flour.

2. For the streusel, mix the brown sugar and cinnamon in a medium bowl. Using your fingertips or a pastry cutter, cut in the cold butter to make a crumbly mixture. Pop the bowl in the fridge to keep the butter cold while you make the cake.

3. For the cake, mix the flour, baking powder, baking soda, and salt in a small bowl.

4. Put the butter and sugar in the bowl of an electric mixer fitted with the paddle attachment. Beat on medium speed until well mixed but not yet light and fluffy, about 1 minute. Turn the mixer to low speed and gradually add the dry ingredients, beating just until smooth. Scrape down the sides of the bowl and return the mixer to medium speed. Add the sour cream and beat until smooth. Then add the eggs, one at a time, scraping down the sides of the bowl at least once. Add the vanilla and mix until smooth.

5. Scrape the batter into the prepared pan and sprinkle the streusel evenly over the top. Bake until golden brown and a toothpick inserted into the center comes out clean, 55 to 60 minutes. This cake keeps for a day or two at room temperature. You can also freeze it for a month or two.

Sourdough Starter

↓V
↑P
=K

WE LOVE TO BAKE SOURDOUGH breads at Kripalu. You can get a sourdough starter going from scratch in your own kitchen (simple instructions can be found online), but there is nothing like getting a well-established starter that has a proven track record. Renowned baker Richard Bourdon of Berkshire Mountain Bakery provided the one we use. You can also buy established starters online from retailers such as King Arthur. Once you get a starter, here's how to activate it and keep it going. This recipe makes 1 pound, which gives you plenty of starter to bake with and to keep going for future baking.

Ayurvedic Insight: Sourdough breads are generally easier to digest than breads made with commercial dry yeast. For that reason, this sourdough starter allows many of our guests to enjoy bread again.

Makes 1 pound

2 ounces established starter

8 ounces bread flour or all-purpose flour

1. In a large bowl, mix the starter, flour, and 6 fluid ounces (¾ cup) cold water. If you want active starter to use for baking, cover loosely and let it ferment at warm room temperature (about 72°F) for 6 to 8 hours, depending on the temperature and humidity. The starter should roughly double in size over that time as the wild yeast feeds on the flour and water.

2. If you want to save the starter for later use, instead of letting it get very active, cover it loosely and let it ferment at room temperature for only 2 to 3 hours, then refrigerate it to slow down its activity.

3. Either way, to keep the starter going, it needs to be fed fresh water and flour. Most bakers take out the amount of starter they need for baking, and feed the rest, discarding any excess. Once you have taken out what you need, feed 2 ounces of starter with 8 ounces flour and 6 ounces water as described above. We like to feed ours every 3 days. You can also let it go for up to 5 days in the fridge. The longer you let the starter ferment, the stronger its sour flour will become. You can use the starter when you like, depending on your flavor preferences and your schedule. Simply remove it from the refrigerator, feed it, and let it become very active again as described above.

Sourdough Sunflower Flax Bread

=V

↓P

=K

WHY DO WE PREFER sourdough breads at Kripalu? The longer fermentation period in this breadmaking process creates more complex flavor in the bread. It also introduces beneficial bacteria and yeast, which make the gluten and other components in the bread easier to digest while increasing the availability of various nutrients. Guests love to make sandwiches with this whole-grain bread.

Ayurvedic Insight: The oily warmth of flax seeds and sunflower seeds balances the sticky qualities of the refined flour here. A fair amount of whole-wheat flour also adds fiber and minerals to aid digestion.

Makes two 2-pound 9 x 5-inch loaves

1/2 cup sunflower seeds

1/2 cup flax seeds

2/3 cup (6 ounces) active Sourdough Starter (page 82)

4 1/2 cups bread flour

1 1/4 cups whole-wheat flour

2 tablespoons rye flour

2 cups water (preferably nonchlorinated), about 70°F

1 tablespoon fine sea salt

Vegetable oil, for oiling the bowl and dough

Oil spray

1. Day 1: Soak the sunflower seeds and flax seeds in ¾ cup water in the refrigerator overnight.

2. Day 2: If your starter is cold, let it warm up at room temperature for 1 to 3 hours.

3. Drain the seeds of any residual water and place them in a large mixing bowl. You can mix the dough in a stand mixer or by hand. Either mix on low speed with a dough hook or gently stir in the bread flour, whole-wheat flour, and rye flour. Then gradually mix in all but ¼ cup of the water. Mix until a dry dough forms, 1 to 2 minutes. Let the dough rest at room temperature for 20 to 30 minutes. This important step, known as autolyse, doesn't change the look of the dough much but it allows the flour to absorb water and the enzymes in the flour to activate, both of which reduce the total kneading time required.

4. After the autolyse, add the active starter, gently kneading it into the dough on low speed until it is well incorporated. Mix the salt into the reserved ¼ cup water, then mix the salty water into the dough until it is incorporated. At this point, you may want to add more water, depending on the wetness of your dough. A wetter dough makes a moister bread, but if it is too wet, it won't have the structure to rise well. The wetness of your dough will change according to variables like the ambient humidity in the room and the moisture content of your flour and starter. Start with the amount of water given

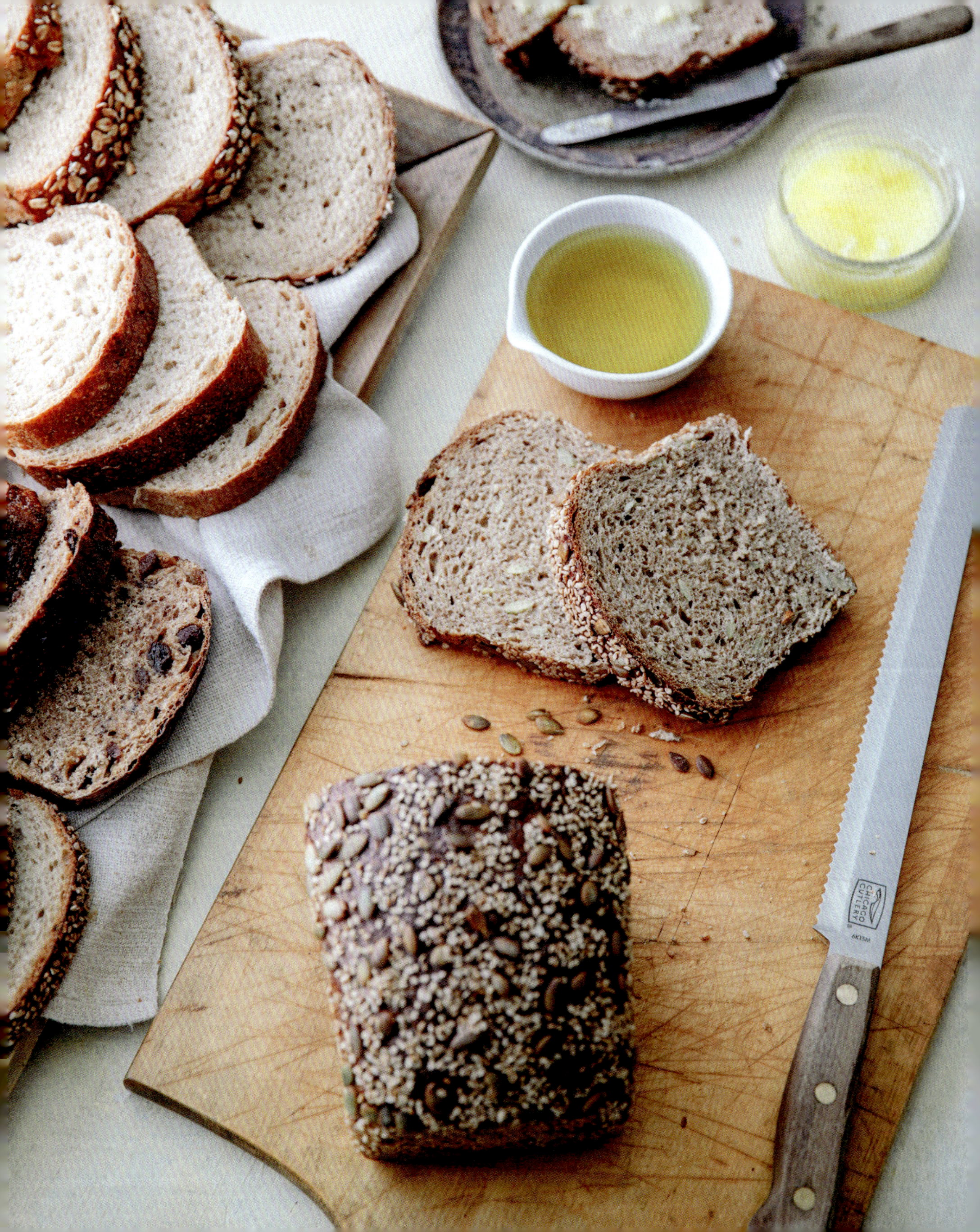
CHICAGO CUTLERY

here (these are the exact proportions we use at Kripalu) and adjust as necessary.

5. Knead the dough in the mixer or on a work surface until it is shiny, smooth, and elastic, 8 to 10 minutes. The smoothness and elasticity are signs of strong gluten development and structure in the dough. The next period of rising will also smooth out the gluten, so it is better to slightly underknead than overknead the dough.

6. Place the dough in an oiled bowl and brush it with a little more oil to prevent the dough from drying out. Cover the bowl and let the dough rise at warm room temperature for 1½ to 3 hours, until you can feel bubbles of gas in the dough when you gently pull a bit off with your fingers. When you pull it, the dough should feel light, warm, and lively, rather than like a heavy piece of putty. The total rising time will vary according to the temperature and humidity of your environment.

7. Coat two 9 x 5-inch loaf pans with oil spray.

8. When the dough has risen, turn it out onto a work surface and cut it into 2 equal pieces. Loosely cover and let rest for 5 to 10 minutes. Form each piece into an oblong loaf shape and place the loaves in the prepared pans. Cover the pans loosely with plastic (at Kripalu, we use recycled plastic vegetable bags from the produce section of the grocery store). At this point, you can refrigerate the dough or let it rise at room temperature a bit longer. If your dough rose quickly and you can see small bubbles right under the surface of the dough, refrigerate it immediately. If the dough rose slowly and didn't develop as many bubbles of gas, let it rise at room temperature for about 1 hour, then refrigerate it. Refrigerate the dough for 8 to 16 hours, during which time it will slowly rise and develop flavor.

9. Day 3: Pull the loaves from the refrigerator and let them rest at warm room temperature (80°F to 90°F) until they rise up and look puffy, and you can see bubbles under the surface, 1 to 3 hours. To check, press the dough gently with a fingertip. If the dough yields, the gluten is no longer supporting further expansion, and the loaves are ready to bake. If the dough bounces back, the gluten is too strong and more rising time is needed. Again, it all depends upon time, temperature, and humidity. You can also adjust these factors. We prefer a warm and humid final rise, though sometimes the dough has already fully risen in the refrigerator and the loaves are ready to bake straight from the fridge. In general, slow to moderate and gentle rising yields the best results.

10. Preheat the oven to 425°F. Place a pan of water on the lower oven rack.

11. Place the pans in the oven, and quickly mist the dough and the oven with a few sprays of water from a spray bottle. A steamy environment helps prevent the dough from forming a crust too quickly, which helps the bread rise fully in the oven.

12. During the first 10 to 15 minutes of baking, mist the dough again a couple of times. Bake for a total of about 45 minutes, misting the dough once more about 15 minutes before the bread is done. This misting helps to create a beautifully browned crust. When finished, the bread should be fully risen and deeply browned, and the internal temperature should register about 200°F on an instant-read thermometer. Turn out onto a rack immediately to cool. Once cooled, this bread will last 5 to 7 days at room temperature.

OPTIONS

- For a richer bread, mix in up to 3 tablespoons oil along with the salty water.
- If you find yourself making sourdough bread on a regular basis, you might want to consider investing in a wooden breadbox. Your bread will keep for over a week and be perfectly moist and delicious.

Sourdough Semolina Bread

HERE'S KRIPALU'S TAKE on healthier "white" bread that comes with my kids' stamp of approval. It's light, airy, and perfect for toasting. Make grilled cheese with it or simply slather it with nut butter and jam.

Ayurvedic Insight: Semolina flour looks like fine cornmeal, but it is actually the ground endosperm of durum wheat, which gives it a yellow color. This yellow flour is full of antioxidant carotenoids that can help improve your eye health.

↑V ↓P ↑K

Makes two 2-pound 9 x 5-inch loaves

3⅓ cups bread flour

2¾ cups fine golden semolina flour

¾ cup (7 ounces) active Sourdough Starter (page 82)

1 tablespoon fine sea salt

Vegetable oil, for oiling the bowl and dough

Oil spray

1. Day 1: You can mix the dough in a stand mixer with a dough hook or by hand. Either mix the bread flour and semolina flour on low speed or gently stir them together. Then gradually mix in 2½ cups water. Mix until a tacky dough forms, 1 to 2 minutes. Let the dough rest at room temperature for 20 to 30 minutes. This important step, known as autolyse, doesn't change the look of the dough much, but it allows the flour to absorb water and the enzymes in the flour to activate, both of which reduce the total kneading time required.

2. After the autolyse, add the active starter, gently kneading it into the dough on low speed until it is well incorporated. Dissolve the salt in ¼ cup water, then mix the salty water into the dough until it is incorporated. At this point, you may want to add more water, depending on the wetness of your dough. A wetter dough makes a moister bread, but if it is too wet, it won't have the structure to rise well. The wetness of your dough will change according to variables like the ambient humidity in the room and the moisture content of your flour and starter. Start with the amount of water given here (these are the exact proportions we use at Kripalu) and adjust as necessary.

3. Knead the dough in the mixer or on a work surface until it is shiny, smooth, and elastic, 8 to 10 minutes. The smoothness and elasticity are signs of strong gluten development and structure in the dough. The next period of rising will also smooth out the gluten, so it is better to slightly underknead than overknead the dough.

4. Place the dough in an oiled bowl and brush it with a little more oil to prevent the dough from drying out. Cover the bowl and let the dough rise at warm room temperature for 1½ to 3 hours, until you can feel bubbles of gas in the dough when you gently pull off a bit of dough with your fingers. When you pull it, the dough should feel light, warm, and lively, rather than like a heavy piece of putty. The total rising time

will vary according to the temperature and humidity of your environment.

5. Coat two 9 x 5-inch loaf pans with oil spray.

6. When the dough has risen, turn it out onto a work surface and cut it into 2 equal pieces. Loosely cover and let rest for 5 to 10 minutes. Form each piece into an oblong loaf shape and place the loaves in the prepared pans. Cover the pans loosely with plastic (at Kripalu, we use recycled plastic vegetable bags from the produce section of the grocery store). At this point, you can refrigerate the dough or let it rise at room temperature a bit longer. If your dough rose quickly and you can see small bubbles right under the surface of the dough, refrigerate it immediately. If the dough rose slowly and didn't develop as many bubbles of gas, let it rise at room temperature for about 1 hour, then refrigerate it. Refrigerate the dough for 8 to 16 hours, during which time it will slowly rise and develop flavor.

7. Day 2: Pull the loaves from the refrigerator and let them rest at warm room temperature (80°F to 90°F) until they rise up and look puffy, and you can see bubbles under the surface, 1 to 3 hours. To check, press the dough gently with a fingertip. If the dough yields, the gluten is no longer supporting further expansion, and the loaves are ready to bake. If the dough bounces back, the gluten is too strong and more rising time is needed. Again, it all depends on time, temperature, and humidity. You can also adjust these factors. We prefer a warm and humid final rise, though sometimes the dough has already fully risen in the refrigerator and the loaves are ready to bake straight from the fridge. In general, slow to moderate and gentle rising yields the best results.

8. Preheat the oven to 425°F. Place a pan of water on the lower oven rack.

9. Place the pans in the oven. Quickly mist the dough and the oven with a few sprays of water from a spray bottle. A steamy environment helps prevent the dough from forming a crust too quickly, which helps the bread rise fully in the oven.

10. During the first 10 to 15 minutes of baking, mist the dough again a couple of times. Bake for a total of 40 to 45 minutes, misting the dough once more about 15 minutes before the bread is done. This misting helps to create a beautifully browned crust. When finished, the bread should be fully risen and deeply browned, and the internal temperature should register about 200°F on an instant-read thermometer. Turn out on a rack immediately to cool.

OPTIONS

- For a richer bread, mix in up to 3 tablespoons oil along with the salty water.
- *Sourdough Ciabatta Rolls:* Add 3 tablespoons oil along with the salty water. Divide the dough into 12 pieces and roll each piece into

a ball about 3½ inches in diameter. Gently stretch the balls into slightly flattened disks, transfer to oiled sheet pans, and let the disks rise on the pans as directed. If the dough flattens dramatically, reshape it into slightly flattened balls before baking. Bake as directed until the rolls are lightly browned, about 20 minutes.

- If you find yourself making sourdough bread on a regular basis, you might want to consider investing in a wooden bread box. Your bread will keep for more than a week and be perfectly moist and delicious.

Sourdough Whole-Grain Pizza Dough

↑V
↓P
↑K

THIS PIZZA DOUGH is essentially bread dough with a little oil in it so the dough is easier to stretch thin. Don't be alarmed that it takes three days to make. You don't have to do much during that time besides mix and shape it. Three days gives the yeast and bacteria plenty of time to develop flavor in the dough and make the wheat gluten easier to digest.

Ayurvedic Insight: Moderation is a central concept in Ayurveda. With that in mind, pizza should be enjoyed on occasion. A single hot slice may be just the thing to keep your mind, body, and spirit in balance.

Makes 2 pounds,
enough for 1 sheet pan pizza or
two 12-inch round pizzas

- 2⅔ cups all-purpose flour
- ⅔ cup whole-wheat flour
- ⅔ cup (6 ounces) active Sourdough Starter (page 82)
- 1 tablespoon barley malt syrup, brown rice syrup, or honey
- 1½ teaspoons fine sea salt
- 1 tablespoon extra-virgin olive oil

1. Day 1: In a large bowl, mix the all-purpose flour, whole-wheat flour, and 1⅓ cups water to form a rough dough. Cover loosely and let rest at room temperature for 20 minutes. Mix in the active starter and knead it with your hands by pressing and folding the dough over itself continually until the dough starts to get smooth and shiny. Knead in the barley malt syrup and salt. When everything is well incorporated, gradually knead in the olive oil and continue kneading until the dough is very smooth and shiny. Cover and let rest at room temperature for about 1 hour. Form into a ball, place in an oiled bowl, cover, and refrigerate the dough overnight.

2. Day 2: The next day, in the morning, re-form the dough into a ball, or if making 2 pizzas, form the dough into 2 balls. Cover and refrigerate again. That evening, re-form the dough into a ball or balls again.

3. Day 3: Before using, again re-form the dough into a ball or balls and let rest for at least 45 minutes at room temperature before rolling out.

Gluten-Free Pizza Dough

THIS DOUGH MAKES a flatbread-like pizza crust that's quite tasty, and many guests prefer it to our sourdough pizza crust. The dough is wet and spreadable when raw; the key is to bake it without any toppings to firm it up. Then add your toppings and bake to crisp up the pizza. Go for drier sauces and toppings such as pesto and shredded mozzarella rather than wet sauces and toppings like tomato sauce and fresh mozzarella. Drier sauces and toppings help to keep the dough firm and crisp.

Ayurvedic Insight: If troubles with gluten have made pizza seem like a distant memory, try this crust. It gets crisp around the edges and is spiced just right to spark your digestive fire.

Makes about 2 pounds,
enough for 1 sheet pan pizza
or two 12-inch round pizzas

1/4 cup extra-virgin olive oil, plus more for oiling the pan
2 tablespoons flax meal
1 cup quinoa flour
1 cup gluten-free oat flour
1/2 cup brown rice flour
1 tablespoon instant dried yeast
2 teaspoons xanthan gum
1 1/2 teaspoons fine sea salt
2 teaspoons dried oregano
1 teaspoon dried basil
1/8 teaspoon freshly ground black pepper
1/2 cup soy milk
2 tablespoons agave nectar
1/2 teaspoon fresh lemon juice

=V
↓P
↓K

1. Preheat the oven to 400°F. Grease an 18 x 13-inch sheet pan or two 12-inch round pizza pans with olive oil.

2. You can mix the dough in an electric mixer or in a bowl with a spoon. Either way, mix the flax meal and ¼ cup water in a large bowl. Let soak for 20 minutes.

3. In a medium bowl, mix the quinoa flour, oat flour, brown rice flour, instant yeast, xanthan gum, salt, oregano, basil, and pepper.

4. Give the flax meal a quick stir, then gently mix in 1¼ cups water, the soy milk, agave, and lemon juice on low speed using a flat beater or stir in. Gradually add the dry ingredients, mixing on low speed or stirring for 2 to 3 minutes. Mix in the olive oil. The dough will be very loose and wet like a batter. You can use it immediately or cover it with plastic wrap and let it sit at room temperature for up to 30 minutes.

5. Dip an offset spatula in water, then use it to spread and press the dough onto the prepared pans in a thin, even layer all the way to the pan edges. Bake until the crust is set and the edges are lightly browned, 25 to 30 minutes. Check once or twice during baking: if

the dough puffs up, poke it all over with a fork to keep it flat.

6. Add your desired toppings and bake until they are heated through and the crust is crisp, another 15 to 20 minutes.

OPTION

- To make crackers, skip the toppings and bake the crust at 375°F until it is crisp, 20 to 30 minutes total. Break into pieces and serve with Mushroom Nut Pâté (page 129), Chickpea of the Sea (page 126), Herbal Tofu Spread (page 128), Trapenese Sauce (page 152), Arugula Chèvre Pesto (page 153), or Kale Pesto (page 195).

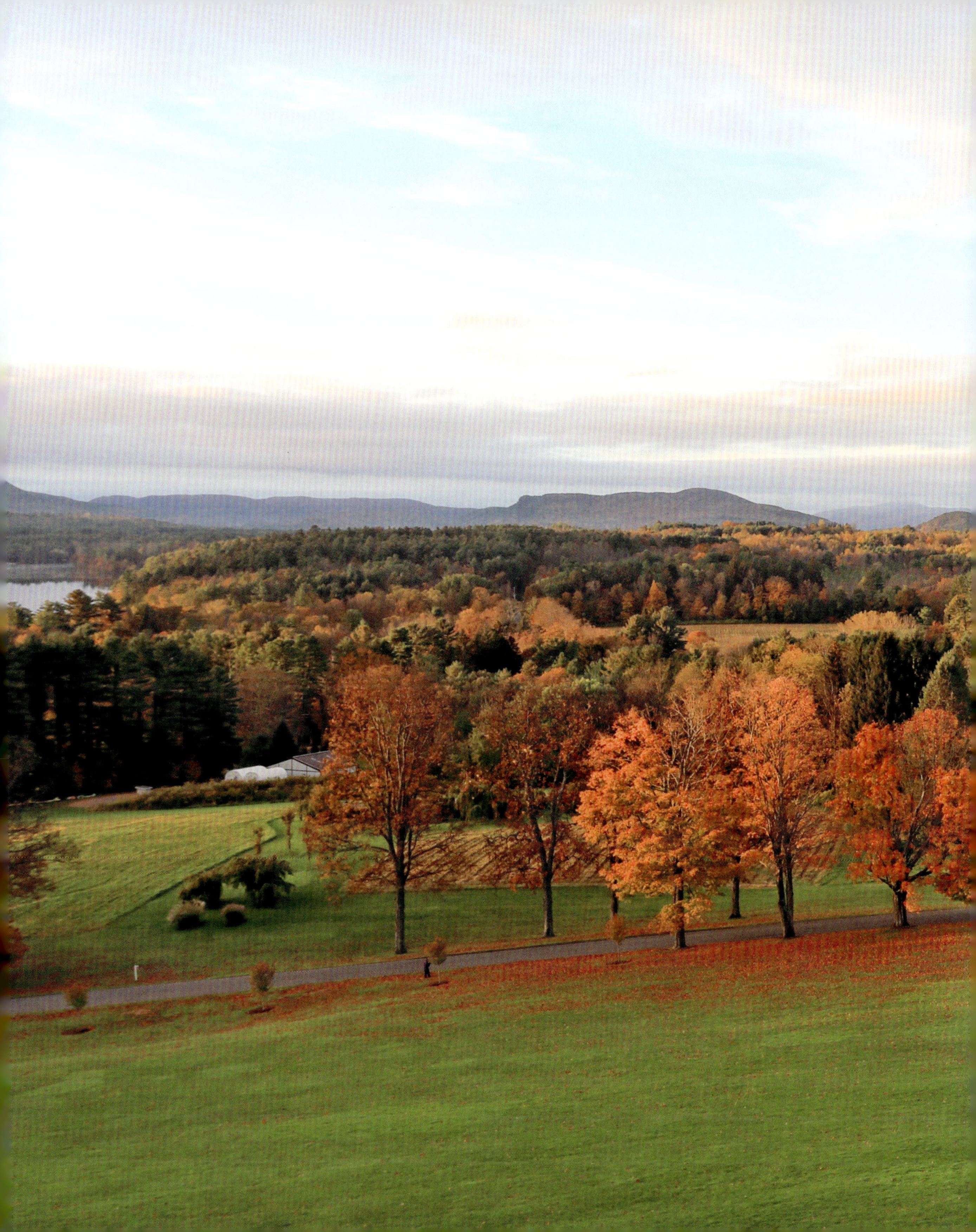

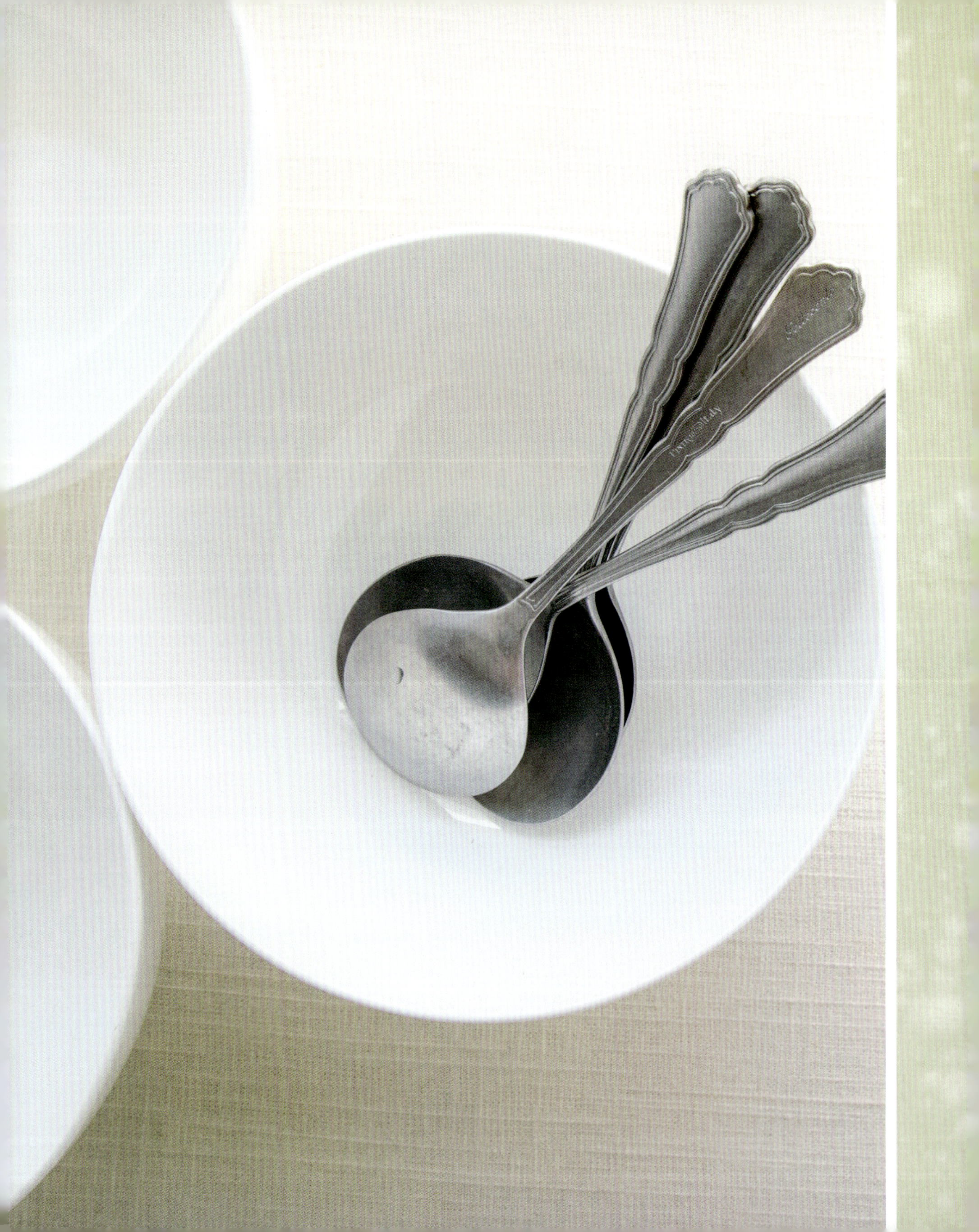

SOUPS

Both grandmothers and scientists know that soup is healing food, and that is why we serve it at every meal. The liquids help flush your system clean while supplying it with much-needed nutrients. For many people, soups are an afterthought or considered only in cold weather, but we encourage you to enjoy soup year-round, from Chilled Mango Soup (page 100) in the summer to warm Vegan Butternut Squash Bisque (page 105) in the fall to hearty Vegan Black-Eyed Pea Soup (page 119) in the winter.

At Kripalu, we call the giant soup kettles Pa, Ma, and Baby, names that were given to them way back when Kripalu was an ashram. To this day, Pa is cranked up every morning with forty gallons of Vegetable Stock (page 281) for the dozens of soups, sauces, and other dishes we serve every week. Ma and Baby handle big-batch soups, and smaller batches now go into three smaller kettles that are affectionately dubbed "the triplets."

In the summer, when the days are hottest, guests are often outside, and the midday meal occurs as the sun reaches its blinding peak in the sky. Chilled soup can offer incredible refreshment. Its cooling effect is similar to that of a cold smoothie. On the other hand, during the fall and winter months here in the chilly Berkshires, a warm bowl of Creamy Cannellini and Roasted Cauliflower Soup (page 115) or Middle Eastern Pumpkin Lentil Soup (page 117) can provide the restorative comfort you need. Temperature is one of the most beautiful aspects of soup. It can help balance the cold or hot nature of the environment around you.

All of our soup stock is vegan, and we tend to stick with vegetarian soups. For creaminess, we puree simmered vegetables like butternut squash or cooked beans like cannellini. Sometimes we drizzle in a little coconut milk for richness. On our buffet line, seasonal soup is the first thing you see, and guests often make it the centerpiece of their meals from noon to night.

One of Ayurveda's central dietary tenets is to make lunch your largest meal of the day. Depending on the weather, that idea could translate to enjoying a hearty soup for lunch or to having a light soup for dinner. At night, when you are less active, soup can provide a nourishing and filling meal without leaving you feeling stuffed. Either way, in the evening, try to eat your last meal of the day at least two hours before bedtime. That time allows for complete digestion, so your evening meal will not interrupt your sleep.

Raw Avocado and Romaine Soup

HERE WE HAVE DRINKABLE guacamole in a bowl. People love it, and it's the simplest soup to make. The avocado lends a rich and creamy texture, yet the soup still tastes healthy and light. For more color and vitamin C, I garnish the soup with chopped fresh tomatoes.

Ayurvedic Insight: This soup is a bit too cooling for kapha. But the oiliness of the avocado makes it okay for vata in moderation. Pitta will love the coolness of the watery vegetables.

Serves 4

2 cups sliced avocados (about 2 medium)
1 1/2 cups shredded romaine lettuce
1 1/2 cups chopped cucumber with skin
1/4 cup plus 2 tablespoons fresh lemon juice
2 tablespoons chopped fresh mint
1 1/2 teaspoons minced fresh garlic
3/4 teaspoon fine sea salt
3 cups cold Vegetable Stock (page 281) or water
1/2 cup 1/2-inch diced fresh tomatoes
1 tablespoon thinly sliced scallion greens
1 tablespoon extra-virgin olive oil

1. Chill 4 shallow soup bowls.

2. Combine the avocados, lettuce, cucumber, lemon juice, mint, garlic, salt, and stock in a blender or food processor. Puree until smooth. Use immediately or chill the soup for up to 3 hours.

3. In a small bowl, combine the tomatoes, scallions, and oil.

4. When ready to serve, divide the soup among the chilled bowls and garnish with the tomato mixture.

=V
↓P
↑K

OPTIONS

- Spice it up by adding ½ teaspoon ground cumin and/or coriander. For heat, add a small jalapeño, seeded and chopped. You could also use cilantro instead of mint.
- For a fun presentation, halve the avocados and scoop out the flesh, leaving the skins intact. Then serve the soup in the hollowed-out halves.

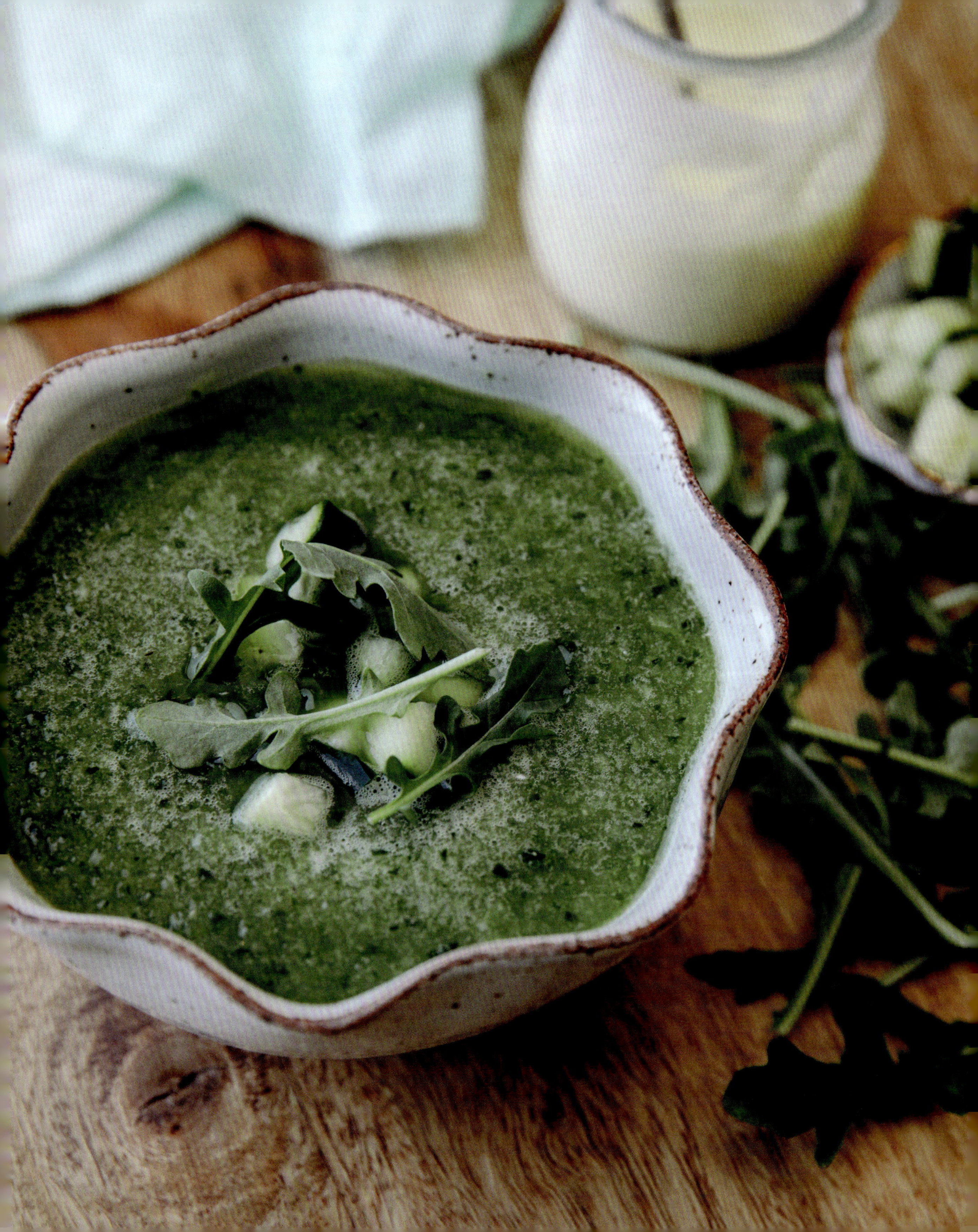

Chilled Cucumber and Arugula Soup

IN THE SUMMER, guests often ask for smoothies to cool off. I make smooth chilled soups instead. With cucumbers and lemon juice, this soup is exceptionally refreshing. Look for small thin-skinned cucumbers so you can leave on the skin, which provides beneficial nutrients for your own skin.

Ayurvedic Insight: In warm weather, cucumbers make the perfect cooling and rehydrating food, particularly for pitta types. If you are cold vata, add hot water to enjoy this soup.

Serves 4 to 6 (6 to 8 cups)

- 4 cups chopped seedless cucumbers with skin plus 1 cup 1/4-inch diced cukes (about 2 1/4 pounds total)
- 1/2 cup thin strips (chiffonade) of arugula, plus 1/4 cup for garnish
- 1/4 cup thinly sliced shallots
- 3 1/2 tablespoons fresh lemon juice
- 2 tablespoons thin strips (chiffonade) of fresh mint
- 1 tablespoon minced fresh garlic
- 1 1/2 teaspoons fine sea salt
- 1/2 teaspoon freshly ground black pepper
- 2 to 3 tablespoons plain yogurt, stirred until smooth (optional)

1. Chill 4 shallow soup bowls.

2. Combine the 4 cups cucumbers, 3½ cups cold water, the ½ cup arugula, shallots, lemon juice, mint, garlic, salt, and pepper in a blender or food processor. Pulse until almost pureed but still slightly chunky. You should still see small bits of cucumber in the soup.

3. Stir in the 1 cup diced cucumbers. Use immediately or chill the soup for up to 3 hours. If necessary, whisk the soup again just before serving. Divide the soup among the chilled bowls and garnish each with about ½ tablespoon yogurt, if desired, and 1 tablespoon arugula strips.

↓V
↓P
↑K

Chilled Mango Soup

↓V
↓P
=K

I LIKE TO SERVE this soup in the summer along with Indian meals. In many ways, it is a mango lassi, the popular Indian cold beverage. People get all crazy for this soup. Creamy, cold, and sweet with a hint of spice . . . what's not to love?

Ayurvedic Insight: Juicy, sweet mango is dreamy for vata and pitta, and the warmth of ginger and jalapeño balance the dairy products. To avoid the dairy altogether, pitta types may want to use coconut milk and coconut yogurt.

Serves 4

4 cups chopped fresh or frozen and thawed mango
1/2 cup plain yogurt
1/2 cup whole milk
2 1/2 tablespoons fresh lime juice
2 tablespoons chopped fresh mint, plus more for garnish
2 tablespoons chopped fresh cilantro, plus more for garnish
1 tablespoon agave nectar or honey
1 1/2 teaspoons minced fresh ginger
1/2 teaspoon minced jalapeño pepper
Pinch of ground allspice
1/4 teaspoon fine sea salt

1. Chill 4 shallow soup bowls.

2. Combine the mango, yogurt, milk, lime juice, mint, cilantro, agave, ginger, jalapeño, allspice, and salt in a food processor or blender. Pulse until the soup is somewhat smooth but still a bit chunky. You should see little bits of mango and herbs in the soup. Use immediately or chill the soup for up to 3 hours.

3. Divide the soup among 4 bowls and garnish with chopped mint and cilantro.

OPTIONS

- For a vegan or paleo version, replace the yogurt and milk with any type of nondairy yogurt and milk. Coconut milk works well.
- To make refreshing ice pops, blend in a little more agave and freeze the mixture in ice pop molds.

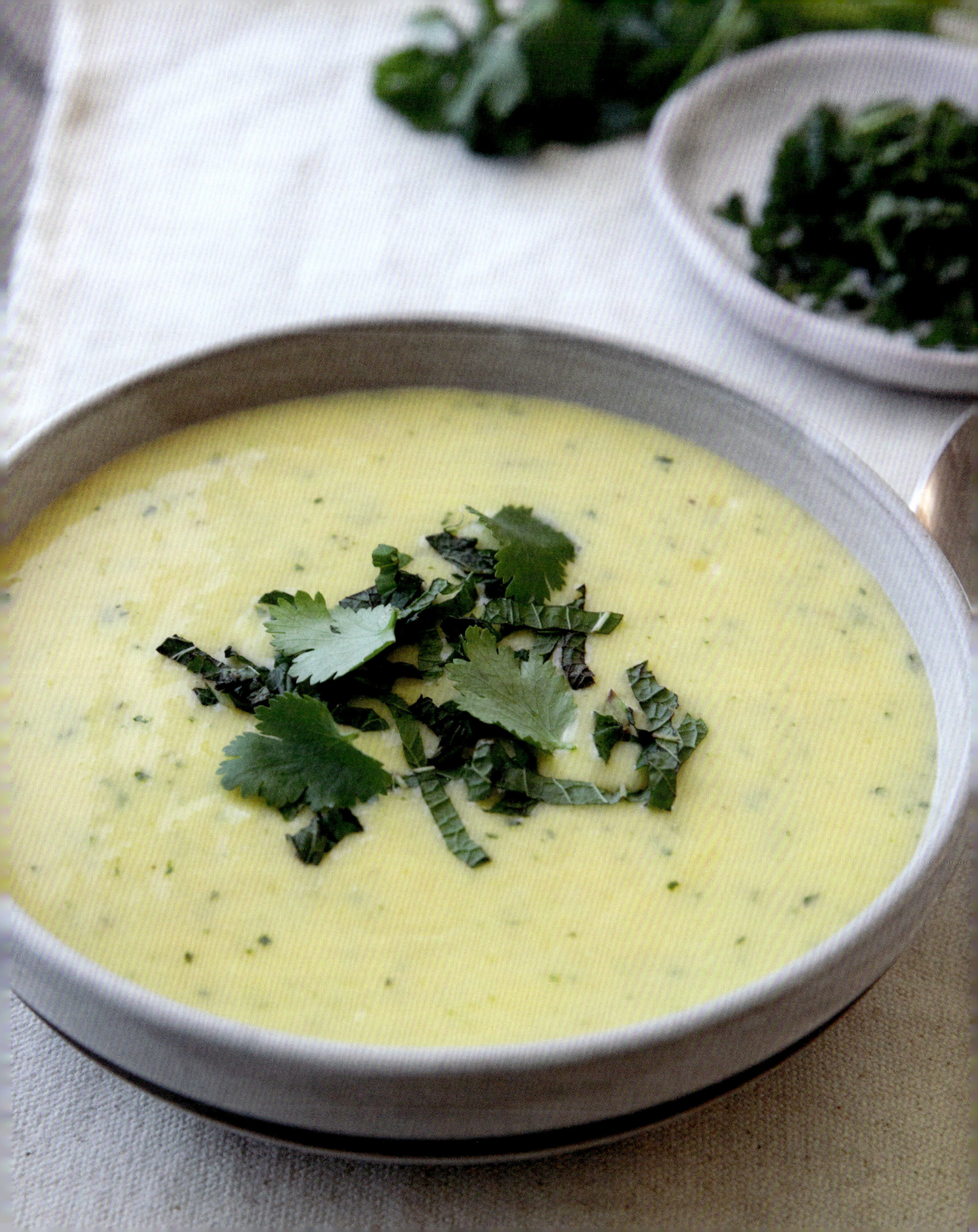

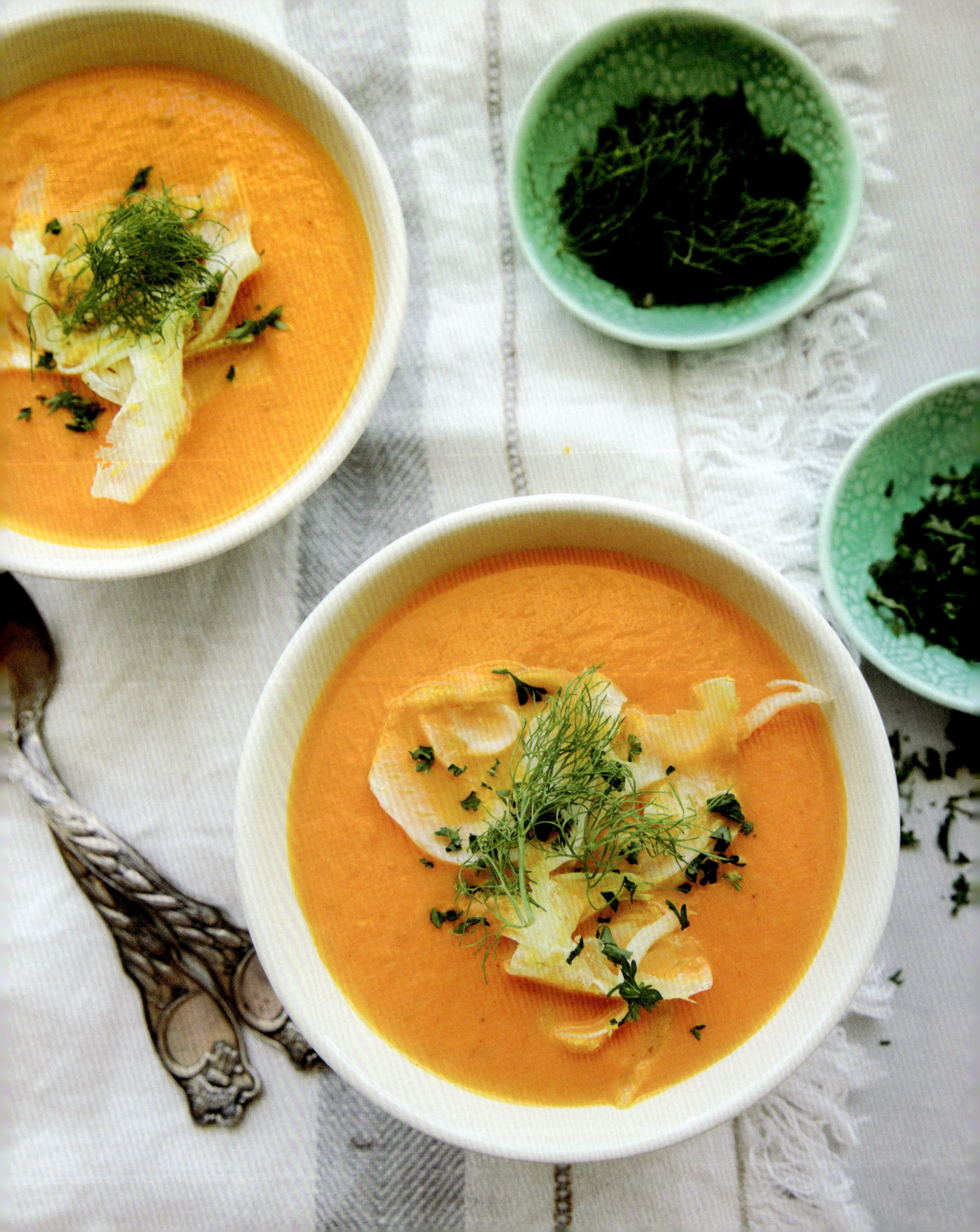

Lemony Carrot Soup

↓V
↓P
↓K

MAKE THIS SOUP when spring weather rolls around and you still have some carrots in the fridge. The fresh dill, lemon, and fennel make it bright and lively, while pureeing the carrots gives it a creamy, satisfying texture. I like to serve this one with a fresh fennel relish on top. You could even garnish it with a few lacy fronds from the fennel tops.

Ayurvedic Insight: This refreshing soup gives you the feel of a cream soup without the heaviness of cream. All doshas will sleep well with this one.

Serves 4

3 cups finely chopped carrots
1/2 cup minced onions
2 tablespoons finely chopped fresh fennel
1 1/2 tablespoons extra-virgin olive oil
1/4 teaspoon ground fennel seed
4 cups Vegetable Stock (page 281)
3 tablespoons fresh lemon juice
2 teaspoons chopped fresh dill
1/2 teaspoon fine sea salt
1/4 teaspoon freshly ground black pepper
Fennel Relish (recipe follows; optional)

1. Heat a medium soup pot over low heat. Put in the carrots, onions, fennel, and oil, shaking the pot to coat the vegetables. Cover and sweat gently until the carrots are almost tender, 8 to 10 minutes.

2. Uncover and stir in the ground fennel seed. Raise the heat to medium and cook until the spice is fragrant, 2 to 3 minutes. Add the stock and bring to a boil over high heat, then reduce the heat to medium-low and simmer gently until the flavors blend and the carrots are very tender, 8 to 10 minutes.

3. Puree the soup until smooth with an immersion blender or in an upright blender. If using an upright blender, avoid a blowout by slightly cooling the soup and partially removing the center lid of the blender.

4. Pour the soup back into the pot and stir in the lemon juice, dill, salt, and pepper. Serve hot with the relish if desired.

OPTION

- You can grind whole fennel seed in a mortar and pestle or crush it under a heavy pan such as a cast-iron skillet.

FENNEL RELISH

↓V
↓P
↓K

THIS RELISH MAKES a terrific garnish for our Lemony Carrot Soup. You could also serve it as part of an appetizer platter at room temperature.

Ayurvedic Insight: With just the right amount of sour from the lemon, fennel is cooling and soothing for all doshas.

About 1 cup

1 cup shaved fennel (from about 1 very small bulb)
2 teaspoons fresh lemon juice
1/2 teaspoon grated lemon zest
1 tablespoon extra-virgin olive oil
1/4 teaspoon fine sea salt
Pinch of freshly ground black pepper

Combine everything in a small bowl. Let macerate at room temperature for about 20 minutes to blend the flavors.

Vegan Butternut Squash Bisque

↓V ↓P ↓K

MOST BISQUE IS MADE with cream, but this one gets its silky texture from pureed butternut squash and a touch of coconut milk. You could even use coconut cream for a richer consistency. Apple cider and cinnamon make it the ideal autumn soup.

Ayurvedic Insight: With warming spices and earthy yams, this family-friendly soup balances all three doshas. Enjoy it as a light supper in the cooler months.

Serves 4

2 tablespoons extra-virgin olive oil

5 cups peeled, seeded, and cubed butternut squash (about 1 pound)

1/2 cup minced shallots

1 teaspoon finely chopped garlic

1 teaspoon ground cinnamon

1/2 cup apple cider

2 cups Vegetable Stock (page 281)

1/4 cup canned full-fat 100% coconut milk

1/2 teaspoon cider vinegar

1/2 teaspoon fine sea salt

1/8 teaspoon freshly ground black pepper

1/2 cup 1/2-inch diced red apples with skin

1 teaspoon chopped fresh flat-leaf parsley

1. Heat a medium soup pot over low heat. Swirl in the olive oil and add the squash, shaking the pot to coat the squash. Cover and cook until the squash is tender, 3 to 5 minutes. Uncover, raise the heat to medium, and cook, stirring occasionally, until the squash is lightly browned and caramelized, 2 to 3 minutes. Once the squash is caramelized, stir in the shallots, garlic, and cinnamon and cook for 2 minutes.

2. Add the cider and bring to a simmer, scraping the pot bottom to loosen any browned bits. Add the stock and bring to a boil over high heat, then reduce the heat to medium-low and simmer until the flavors blend, about 10 minutes.

3. Add the coconut milk and vinegar, and puree the soup until it is supersmooth with an immersion blender or in an upright blender. If using an upright blender, avoid a blowout by slightly cooling the soup and partially removing the center lid of the blender.

4. Pour the soup back into the pot (if you used an upright blender), bring to a gentle simmer, and season with the salt and pepper. Pour into 4 bowls and garnish with the apples and parsley.

=V
↓P
↓K

Spring Pea and Mint Soup

WITH FRESH MINT and spring peas, this vibrant green, silky-smooth soup is an homage to the season of rebirth. There are no spices here, so caramelizing the vegetables is a key step in developing the flavor.

Ayurvedic Insight: Peas are astringent and excellent for reducing kapha. Due to the pungent onions, leeks, scallions, garlic, and black pepper, vata types may prefer this soup at lunchtime, when digestion is strongest.

Serves 4

- 1 1/2 cups chopped cleaned leeks
- 1/2 cup chopped fennel
- 1/2 cup chopped scallions (green and white parts)
- 3 tablespoons extra-virgin olive oil
- 1 teaspoon finely chopped garlic
- 5 cups fresh or frozen peas
- 3 cups Vegetable Stock (page 281) or water
- 1/2 cup thinly sliced spinach (chiffonade)
- 1/4 cup chopped fresh mint
- 3/4 teaspoon fine sea salt
- 1/4 teaspoon freshly ground black pepper
- 1 1/2 teaspoons fresh lemon juice

1. Heat a medium soup pot over medium-low heat for 2 minutes. Put in the leeks, fennel, scallions, and oil and shake the pot to coat the vegetables. Cover and cook gently until the vegetables are translucent, 3 to 5 minutes.

2. Uncover, raise the heat to medium, and cook until the vegetables are lightly browned, 3 to 5 minutes more. Stir in the garlic and cook for 1 minute.

3. Add 4 cups of the peas and the stock, scraping the pot bottom to loosen any browned bits. Bring to a boil over high heat; then reduce the heat to low and simmer just until the peas are heated through but still bright green, about 3 minutes.

4. Puree the soup with an immersion blender or in an upright blender. If using an upright blender, avoid a blowout by cooling the soup slightly and partially removing the center lid of the blender. Puree the soup until it is supersmooth.

5. Pour the soup back into the pot (if you used an upright blender) and stir in the remaining 1 cup peas, the spinach, mint, salt, pepper, and lemon juice. Heat through and serve.

OPTION

- The soup can also be cooled, chilled for up to 1 day, and served cold.

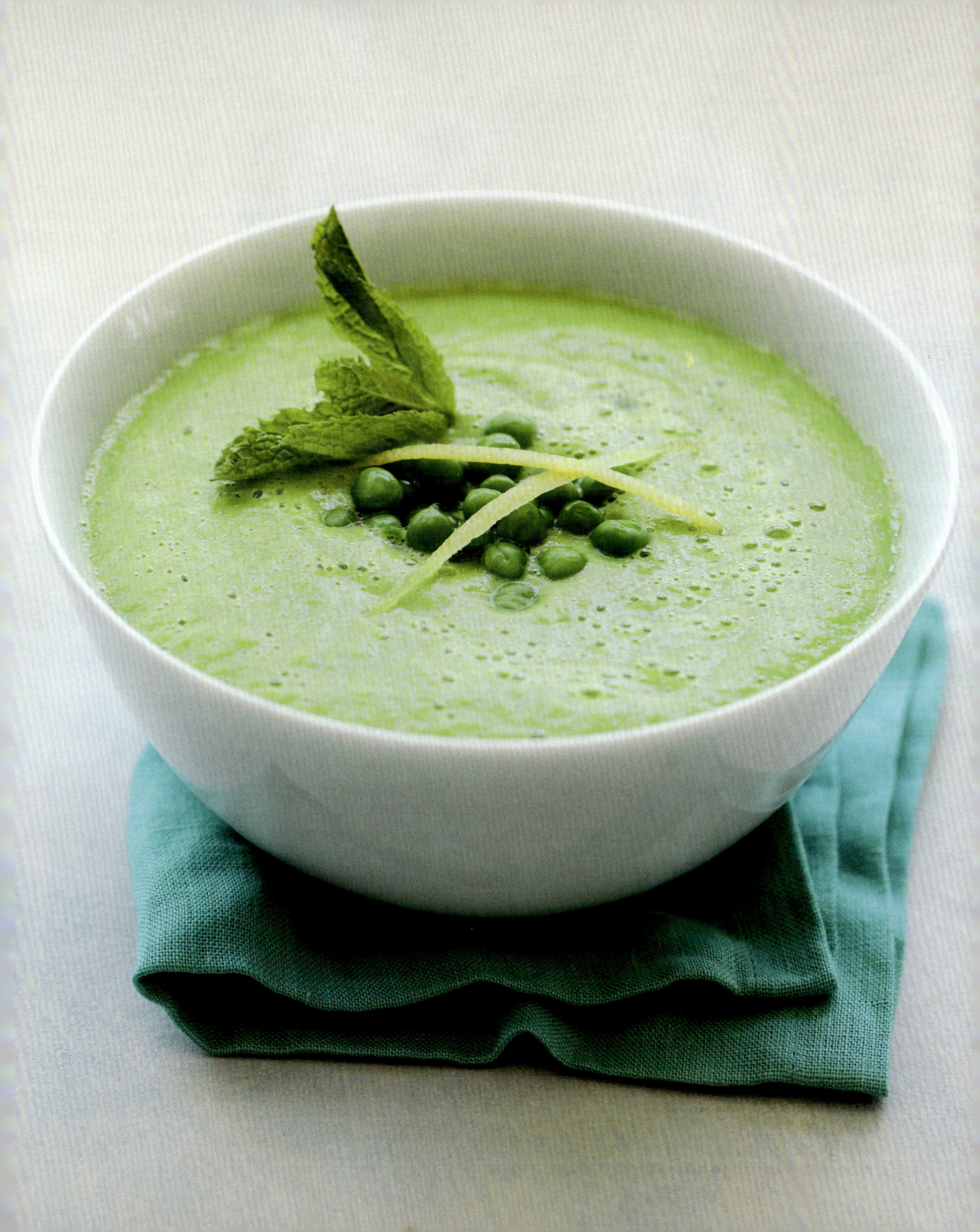

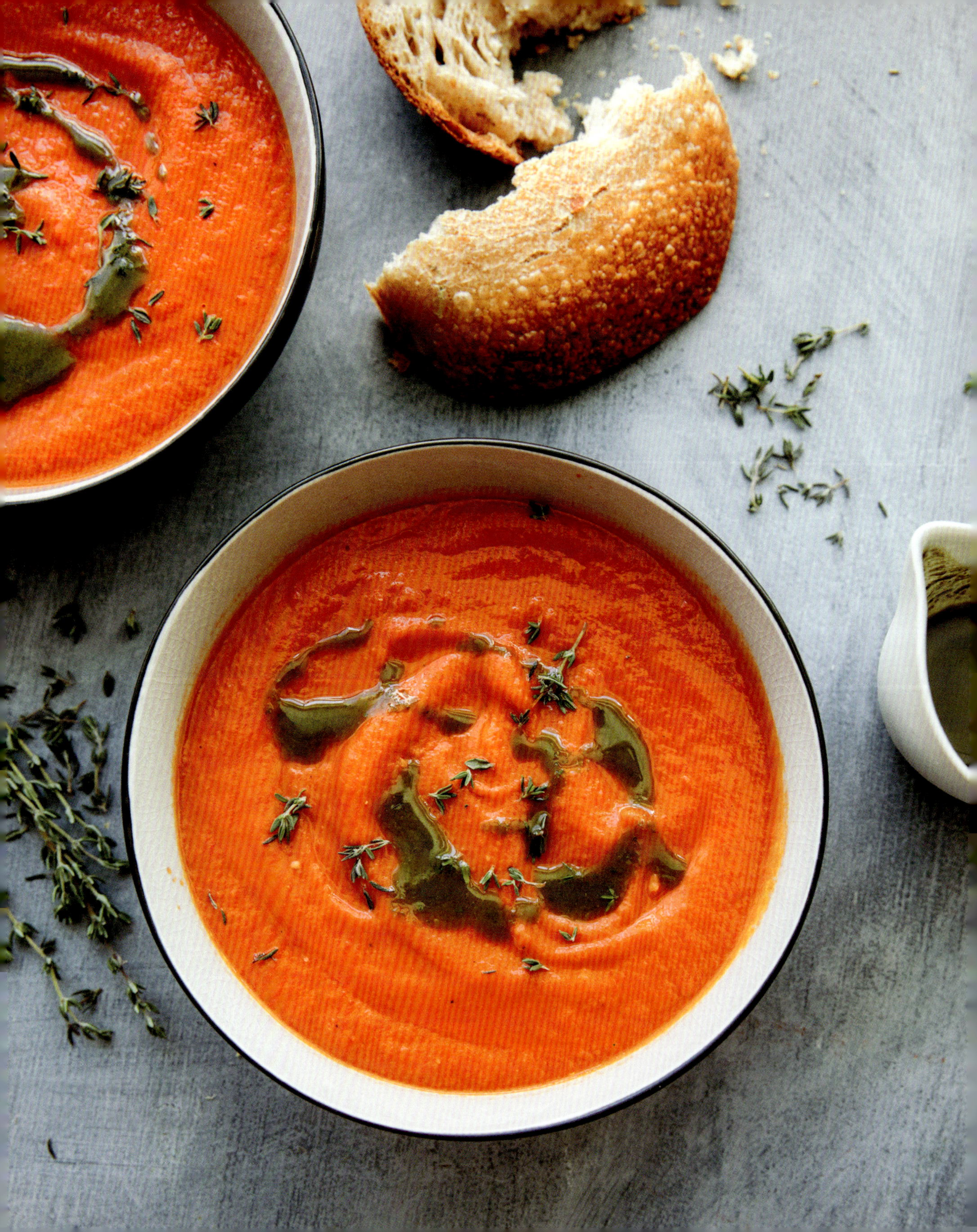

Smoky Tomato Soup

TOMATOES AND BASIL would make this a classic Italian soup, but we added cumin and smoky chipotle chiles to lend it the flavors of the American Southwest. Fresh, ripe tomatoes are best, but in wintertime, you can use canned plum tomatoes.

Ayurvedic Insight: Warm and pungent spices, onions, and smoky chiles make this soup excellent for warming cold vata and kapha.

↓V ↑P ↓K

Serves 4

1/2 cup minced fresh onions
1/4 cup finely chopped carrots
1 1/2 tablespoons extra-virgin olive oil
1/4 teaspoon ground cumin
1 tablespoon finely chopped garlic
1 teaspoon chopped chipotles in adobo sauce
1 tablespoon tomato paste
1 cup tomato puree
2 cups finely chopped fresh tomatoes
2 cups Vegetable Stock (page 281)
1/4 cup thin strips (chiffonade) of fresh basil, plus more for garnish
1/2 teaspoon chopped fresh thyme
1/2 teaspoon fine sea salt
Pinch of freshly ground black pepper

1. Heat a medium soup pot over low heat. Put in the onions, carrots, and oil, tossing to coat the vegetables. Cover and cook until the onions are translucent, about 5 minutes. Uncover, stir in the cumin and garlic, and raise the heat to medium. Let the spices bloom for 2 to 3 minutes.

2. Stir in the chipotles, tomato paste, and tomato puree. Reduce the heat to low, cover, and cook for 3 to 4 minutes, stirring now and then. Stir in the tomatoes and stock and bring to a boil over high heat. Reduce the heat to medium-low and simmer gently until the flavors blend, 15 to 20 minutes.

3. Puree the soup with an immersion blender or in an upright blender. If using an upright blender, avoid a blowout by slightly cooling the soup and partially removing the center lid of the blender. Puree the soup until it is supersmooth.

4. Pour the soup back into the pot (if you used an upright blender) and stir in the basil, thyme, salt, and pepper. Divide among 4 bowls and garnish with more basil.

OPTION

- To make the soup more substantial, fold in 1 cup cooked brown basmati rice.

Coconut Yam Soup

↓V
↓P
↑K

THIS BROTHY SOUP mirrors the brilliant display of fall foliage we get here in the Berkshires. Cubes of orange sweet potatoes and yellow yams float in a savory broth enriched with coconut milk. I like to add diced red bell peppers right at the end, so they stay nice and crunchy.

Ayurvedic Insight: The cooling coconut and earthy yam are perfect for vata and pitta types but a little too chilling and grounding for kapha.

Serves 4

1½ tablespoons coconut oil

¼ cup minced fresh onion

3½ cups peeled and diced yams and/or sweet potatoes

1 teaspoon minced fresh ginger

1½ teaspoons finely chopped garlic

3 cups Vegetable Stock (page 281)

1 cup canned full-fat 100% coconut milk

1 teaspoon mirin or brown rice vinegar

Grated zest and juice of 1 lime

½ cup ¼-inch diced red bell peppers

3 tablespoons thinly sliced scallions (green and white parts), preferably cut on an angle

1 tablespoon chopped fresh cilantro

½ teaspoon fine sea salt

⅛ teaspoon freshly ground black pepper

1. Heat a medium soup pot over low heat. Swirl in the oil and add the onion, shaking the pot to coat the onion. Cover and gently sweat the onion until translucent, 3 to 5 minutes. Add the yams and raise the heat to medium. Cook, uncovered, until the yams are lightly caramelized and just begin to soften, 6 to 8 minutes, stirring now and then.

2. Stir in the ginger and garlic, and cook until fragrant, about a minute. Add the stock and bring to a boil over high heat, then reduce the heat to medium-low and simmer until the yams are fork-tender, 5 to 7 minutes.

3. Stir in the coconut milk, mirin, lime zest, and lime juice. Bring to a simmer and simmer gently over medium-low heat for 5 minutes. Stir in the peppers, scallions, cilantro, salt, and pepper. Serve hot.

OPTION

- For more protein, sear 8 ounces peeled and deveined medium shrimp in the oil in the soup pot before cooking the vegetables. Remove the seared shrimp from the pan, then cut them in half and fold them into the soup along with the peppers and scallions at the end.

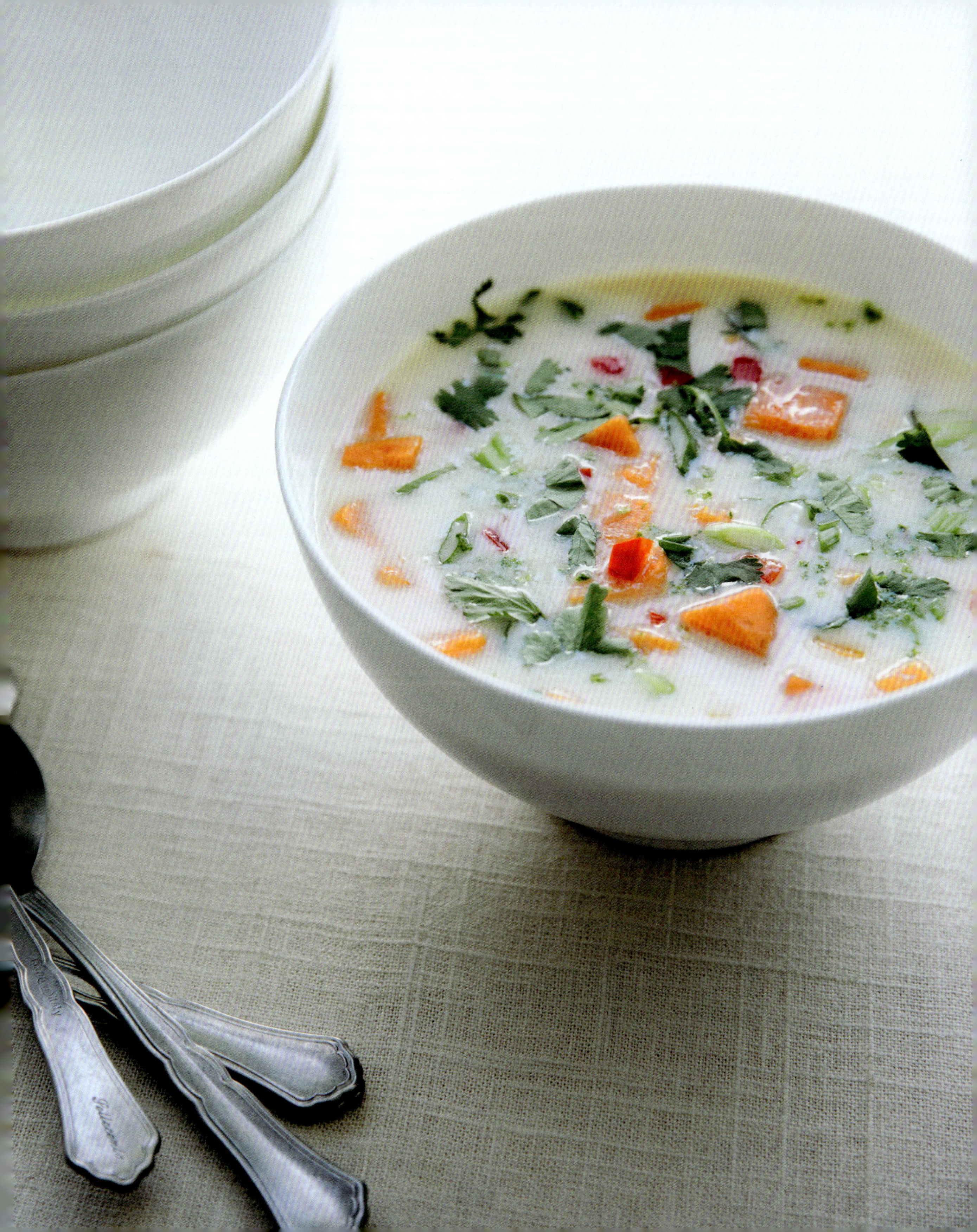

Sweet-and-Sour Cabbage Soup

↓V
↑P
↓K

THIS SOUP IS SIMILAR to traditional hearty German cabbage soup, minus the meat. Our local maple syrup and white wine vinegar tame the bitterness of the cabbage, while ground fennel seed provides a key flavor reminiscent of licorice.

Ayurvedic Insight: The three tastes that balance vata are sweet, sour, and salty. This soup provides them all and can be enjoyed by vata types all winter long. Pittas, on the other hand, may find the warming qualities of this soup to be overheating.

Serves 4

1/2 cup minced fresh onions
1/4 cup 1/4-inch diced celery
1/4 cup 1/4-inch diced carrots
1 1/2 tablespoons extra-virgin olive oil
2 cups shredded green cabbage
1/2 teaspoon ground fennel seed
1/2 teaspoon ground coriander
1 1/2 teaspoons finely chopped garlic
1/2 cup 1/2-inch diced fresh tomatoes
3 cups Vegetable Stock (page 281)
1 tablespoon plus 2 teaspoons white wine vinegar
1 tablespoon pure maple syrup
1/2 teaspoon fine sea salt
1/4 teaspoon freshly ground black pepper

1. Heat a medium soup pot over medium-low heat. Put in the onions, celery, carrots, and oil, shaking the pot to coat the vegetables. Cover and sweat gently until the carrots are tender, 3 to 5 minutes. Stir in the cabbage, cover, and sweat gently again until the cabbage is almost tender, about 5 minutes.

2. Uncover and stir in the fennel, coriander, and garlic. Allow the spices to bloom until fragrant, 2 to 3 minutes, stirring now and then.

3. Stir in the tomatoes, stock, vinegar, and maple syrup. Bring to a simmer over high heat, then reduce the heat to medium-low and simmer gently until the flavors blend, about 15 minutes. Season with salt and pepper. Taste the soup and adjust the sweet and sour flavors to your liking by adding more vinegar or maple syrup. Serve hot.

Roasted Parsnip and Apple Soup

PARSNIPS ARE AN UNDERRATED root vegetable. They're less sweet and more complex than carrots. This recipe gives them even more depth with warm hints of cinnamon and nutmeg. At Kripalu, the story goes that when this soup was first developed, a basket of fresh green apples was hanging out in the kitchen just begging to be used. The apples were quickly diced and roasted for a garnish. Their bright acidity and caramelized sweetness perfectly complemented the earthy parsnips.

Ayurvedic Insight: Ideal autumn foods, root vegetables and apples give this soup a balanced profile for all doshas to enjoy.

Serves 4 to 6

3 cups peeled and diced parsnips
2 tablespoons extra-virgin olive oil
1/4 cup 1/4-inch diced onions
1/4 cup 1/4-inch diced celery
1/2 cup 1/2-inch diced Yukon Gold potatoes
1/2 teaspoon ground fennel seed
1/2 teaspoon celery seeds
Pinch of ground nutmeg
1 teaspoon finely chopped garlic
2 tablespoons cider vinegar
1/2 cup apple cider
4 cups Vegetable Stock (page 281) or water
1 cup 1/2-inch diced green apples with skin
2 tablespoons chopped fresh flat-leaf parsley
1/2 teaspoon sea salt
1/4 teaspoon freshly ground black pepper

↓V ↓P ↓K

1. Preheat the oven to 375°F.

2. Toss the parsnips and 1 teaspoon of the oil on a rimmed baking sheet. Roast until soft, 15 to 20 minutes.

3. Meanwhile, heat a medium soup pot over medium-low heat. Put in the onions, celery, potatoes, and 1 tablespoon of the oil, shaking the pot to coat the vegetables. Cook, stirring occasionally, until the potatoes begin to get soft, about 8 minutes. Don't worry if the potatoes stick to the pot. Any crispy bits will get unstuck later. Stir in the roasted parsnips and cook for another 5 minutes.

4. Raise the heat to medium and add the ground fennel, celery seeds, and nutmeg. Add 1 teaspoon more oil and let the spices bloom in the oil until fragrant, 2 to 3 minutes. At this point, the vegetables will begin to caramelize, leaving a brown film of flavor on the bottom of the pot.

5. Stir in the garlic and cook for 1 minute. Add the vinegar and apple cider and cook for 2 to 3 minutes, stirring to deglaze the pot and capture all the flavors. Stir in the broth and simmer over low heat for 20 minutes.

6. While the soup simmers, toss the apples with the remaining 1 teaspoon olive oil on a

rimmed baking sheet and roast until browned on the edges, about 6 minutes. Remove from the oven and set aside.

7. Puree the soup until it is supersmooth with an immersion blender or in an upright blender. If using an upright blender, avoid a blowout by slightly cooling the soup and partially removing the center lid of the blender.

8. Pour the soup back into the pot (if you used an upright blender) and stir in the parsley, salt, and pepper. Serve garnished with the roasted apples.

OPTION

- For more flavor, toast the fennel seeds in the dry soup pot before sautéing the onions, celery, and potatoes. Then pour the toasted seeds into a mortar and pestle or clean coffee grinder, cool slightly, and grind to a powder.

Creamy Cannellini and Roasted Cauliflower Soup

WHEN COOKED AND PUREED, cauliflower gets amazingly creamy. The same goes for beans (that creaminess is one reason why people love hummus so much). Together, cannellinis and cauliflower make this pureed soup feel decadently rich and creamy. Yet it is entirely vegan and relatively low in calories.

Ayurvedic Insight: This soup is for the pitta and kapha who can handle hearty beans like cannellinis. The warming herbs, rosemary, sage, and thyme, help to ease the digestion.

↑V ↓P ↓K

Serves 4

HERB OIL

3 tablespoons extra-virgin olive oil

2 teaspoons chopped fresh thyme

2 teaspoons chopped fresh sage

2 teaspoons chopped fresh rosemary

SOUP

2 cups small cauliflower florets plus 1/2 cup chopped cauliflower

2 tablespoons extra-virgin olive oil

1/2 teaspoon fine sea salt plus a pinch

1/2 cup minced onions

1/2 cup finely chopped carrots

1/4 cup finely chopped celery

1 1/2 teaspoons finely chopped garlic

Pinch of crushed red pepper flakes

3 cups cooked or rinsed and drained canned cannellini beans

3 cups Vegetable Stock (page 281)

1 bay leaf

1 teaspoon finely grated lemon zest

1 tablespoon plus 1 teaspoon fresh lemon juice

1/4 teaspoon freshly ground black pepper

1. Preheat the oven to 350°F.

2. For the herb oil, combine the oil, thyme, sage, and rosemary in a small sauté pan. Heat over low heat just until the herbs become warm and fragrant, 30 to 60 seconds. Remove from the heat and let stand while you make the soup.

3. For the soup, rub the 2 cups cauliflower florets with 1 tablespoon of the oil on a rimmed baking sheet until thoroughly coated. Season the florets with a pinch of salt. Roast until lightly browned and soft with just a bit of crunch left, 8 to 10 minutes. Set aside.

4. Heat a medium soup pot over low heat. Put in the onions, carrots, celery, chopped cauliflower, and remaining 1 tablespoon oil, shaking the pot to coat the vegetables. Cover and gently sweat the vegetables until tender, 5 to 6 minutes. Uncover and stir in the garlic and red pepper flakes. Cook until the spices are fragrant, about a minute.

5. Stir in the beans, stock, and bay leaf and bring to a gentle simmer over medium heat. Reduce the heat to medium-low and simmer gently until the flavors blend, 10 to 15 minutes.

6. Remove the bay leaf and puree the soup until it is supersmooth with an immersion blender or in an upright blender. If using an upright blender, avoid a blowout by slightly cooling the soup and partially removing the center lid of the blender. Pour the soup back into the pot (if you used an upright blender) and stir in the reserved cauliflower, lemon zest, lemon juice, black pepper, and remaining ½ teaspoon salt.

7. Divide the soup among 4 bowls and drizzle each serving with some of the herb oil.

Middle Eastern Pumpkin Lentil Soup

MOST PEOPLE DON'T cook with pumpkin enough. It's a fantastic source of beta-carotene, which can help boost your immune system and reduce the risk of heart disease as well as various cancers. Plus, pumpkin is full of blood-building iron, and it's deliciously sweet. Along with tender French lentils and spices like cumin, cinnamon, and cardamom, pumpkin makes a very satisfying soup.

Ayurvedic Insight: All doshas can freely enjoy small legumes such as lentils, but vata types may want to soak the lentils overnight to reduce their gassiness.

↓V ↓P ↓K

Serves 4

- 1/2 cup minced onions
- 2 tablespoons extra-virgin olive oil
- 1/2 teaspoon ground cinnamon
- 1/2 teaspoon ground cumin
- 1/4 teaspoon paprika
- 1/4 teaspoon ground turmeric
- 1/4 teaspoon ground cardamom
- 1 tablespoon tomato paste
- 1 cup dry French green lentils
- 5 cups Vegetable Stock (page 281)
- 1 1/4 cups peeled 1/4-inch diced pumpkin or butternut squash
- 2 teaspoons fresh lemon juice
- 1/2 teaspoon fine sea salt
- 1/8 teaspoon freshly ground black pepper
- 1/2 cup thin strips (chiffonade) of spinach

1. Heat a medium soup pot over medium-low heat. Put in the onions and olive oil, shaking the pot to coat the onions. Cover and sweat until the onions are translucent, 3 to 4 minutes. Uncover and stir in the cinnamon, cumin, paprika, turmeric, and cardamom. Allow the spices to bloom until they are fragrant, 2 to 3 minutes, stirring often.

2. Stir in the tomato paste, cover, and cook over low heat for 2 to 3 minutes, stirring now and then.

3. Stir the lentils into the pot. Add the stock, scraping the pot bottom to loosen the browned bits. Bring to a simmer over medium heat, then reduce the heat to medium-low and gently simmer until the lentils are getting soft but still have a bit of crunch, 15 to 20 minutes. Stir in the pumpkin and cook until the lentils are tender, about 5 minutes more.

4. Season the soup with the lemon juice, salt, and pepper. Just before serving, stir in the spinach.

OPTION

- To serve this as a side dish, use 3 cups of stock instead of 5 cups to create a thicker consistency.

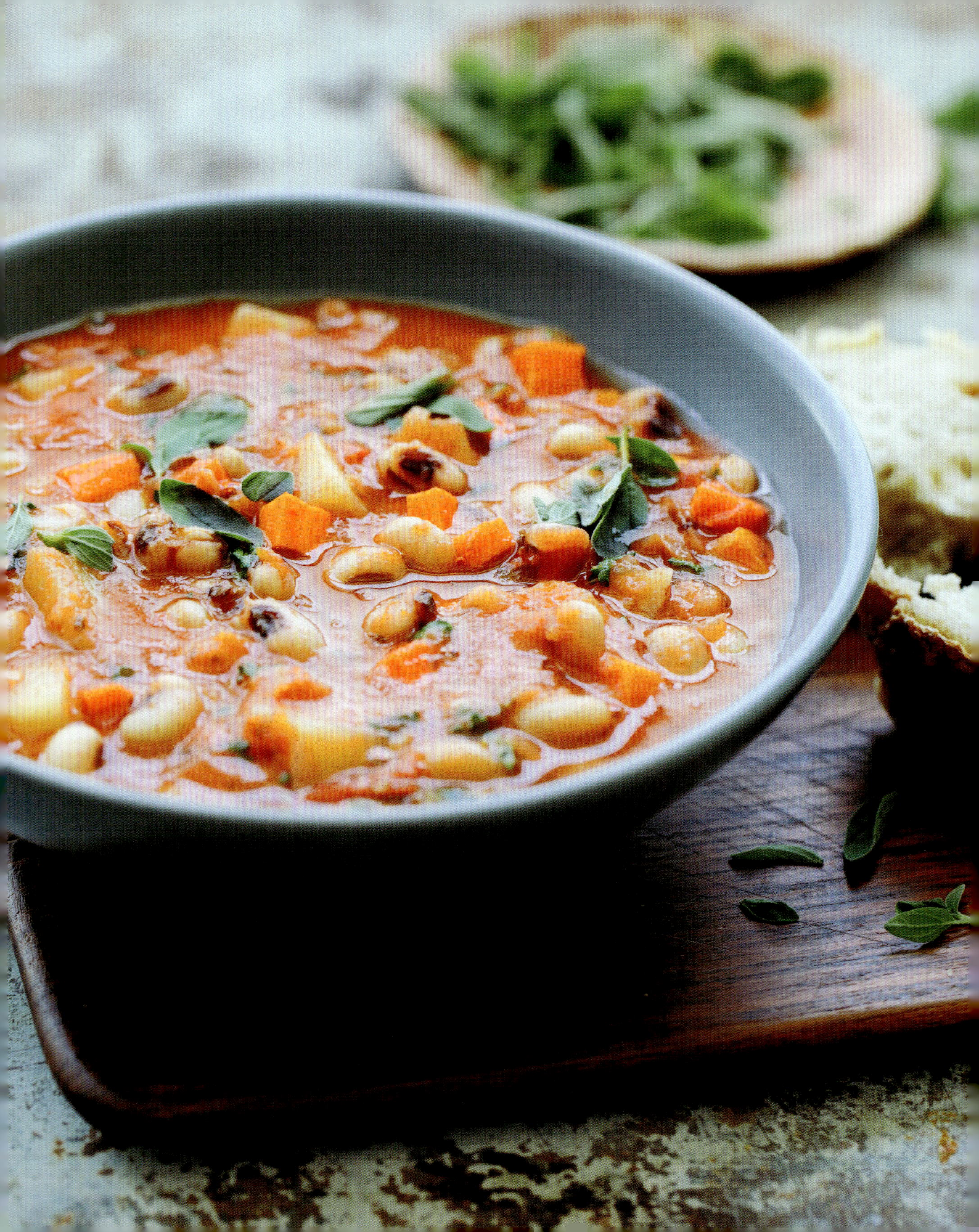

Vegan Black-Eyed Pea Soup

↑V
↓P
↓K

BLACK-EYED PEAS ARE the unsung heroes of the bean world. They cook quickly and take on a variety of flavors. With tomatoes and potatoes, we go toward the American South here but skip the smoky pork products in favor of a little smoked paprika.

Ayurvedic Insight: With beans, potatoes, and warming spices, this hearty soup is balancing for both kapha and pitta.

Serves 4

1/2 cup dried black-eyed peas
1/2 cup 1/4-inch diced onions
1/4 cup 1/4-inch diced carrots
2 tablespoons extra-virgin olive oil
1 tablespoon finely chopped garlic
1/2 teaspoon ground cinnamon
1/2 teaspoon ground cumin
1/2 teaspoon ground coriander
1/4 teaspoon smoked paprika
1/2 cup tomato puree
5 cups Vegetable Stock (page 281)
3/4 cup peeled 1/4-inch diced red potatoes
1/2 teaspoon chopped fresh marjoram
1/2 teaspoon chopped fresh oregano
1 teaspoon fine sea salt
Pinch of freshly ground black pepper

1. Soak the black-eyed peas overnight in water to cover.

2. Heat a medium soup pot over medium heat. Put in the onions, carrots, and oil, shaking the pot to coat the vegetables. Cook until the onions are translucent and just beginning to brown, 4 to 6 minutes. Stir in the garlic, cinnamon, cumin, coriander, and smoked paprika, and let the spices bloom for 2 to 3 minutes. Stir in the tomato puree and let simmer for 2 to 3 minutes.

3. Drain the peas and add them to the pot along with the stock. Bring to a boil over high heat, then reduce the heat to medium-low and simmer until the peas are almost tender, 30 to 35 minutes. Stir in the potatoes, marjoram, and oregano and cook until the potatoes and peas are tender, 10 to 12 minutes more. Season with salt and pepper and serve hot.

OPTIONS

- To substitute canned black-eyed peas, use one 14-ounce can (rinsed and drained) and add the peas along with the potatoes, cooking for 10 to 12 minutes at the end.
- For even more smoky flavor, use smoked salt or mince a slice of turkey bacon or some turkey sausage and cook it with the onions.

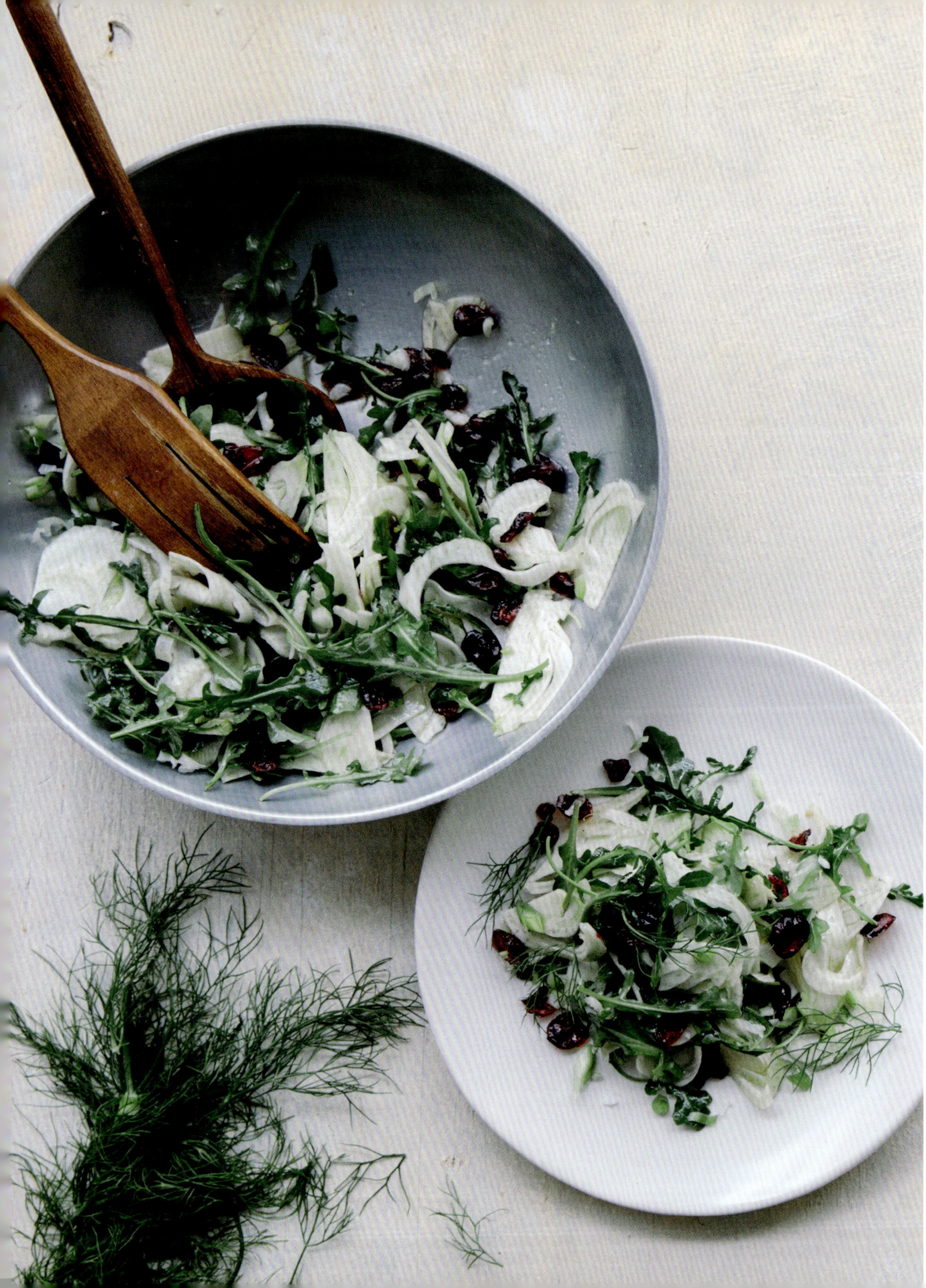

SALADS AND SANDWICHES

In the Kripalu dining room, our buffet line sits front and center. On it, we offer an array of healthy and life-sustaining international dishes, sometimes with unfamiliar names and unusual ingredients. The salad and sandwich bar, on the other hand, is more familiar ground. Twenty different kinds of greens, carrots, tomatoes, vinaigrettes, nuts, and seeds encourage you to enjoy fresh produce every day. Panini makers and breads, wraps, tuna salad, chicken salad, various deli salads, and an assortment of mayos, mustards, spreads, and dips also allow guests to build a recognizable, comforting meal. Especially when you are working hard on your health, fitness, flexibility, spirituality, or psychological wellness, familiar food such as a salad or sandwich can serve to center and ground you when you need it most.

This chapter is a gold mine for vegans and vegetarians. Chickpea of the Sea (page 126) is a classic—an everyday vegan salad that captures the spirit and satisfaction of tuna salad. Mushroom Nut Pâté (page 129) can be spread on toast for a savory snack or formed into patties, roasted, and proudly served with Gluten-Free Vegan Gravy (page 130) as the centerpiece of any vegan holiday celebration. An unsung hero among pestos, Trapenese Sauce (page 152) is equally at home on pasta and slathered on a whole-grain wrap that's rolled up with Mediterranean Chickpea Salad (page 123). Even kids will enjoy a simple bowl of Sesame Noodles with Peanut Sauce (page 131). And creamy Kripalu House Dressing (page 147) amplifies the flavor of any green salad or roasted vegetable platter without stealing the spotlight.

We all know we should be eating more vegetables, as they have been shown to improve our health in multiple ways, from helping to prevent cancer and lowering heart disease risk to improving the immune system. This chapter helps you enjoy a wide variety of fresh vegetables, particularly in warmer weather. If you think about it, summertime is when we tend to crave fresh salads and sandwiches most. That makes sense because, according to Ayurveda, salads and sandwiches are considered cold and dry. For hot pitta types, a cold salad can be exceptionally cooling and refreshing. Salads are also dry enough to absorb the excess moisture of kapha. On the other hand, if you are a cold and dry type in search of a sandwich, try making a cooked panini to add some balancing heat to your system.

Mediterranean Chickpea Salad

WE COULD HAVE called this Greek salad, but fresh fennel, roasted peppers, and artichokes reflect an even broader cross-section of the Mediterranean region. The chickpeas make it substantial and are a delicious source of fiber that can help improve digestion.

Ayurvedic Insight: Like all legumes, chickpeas are astringent in taste. They are also an excellent source of plant-based protein. If you have difficulty digesting chickpeas, soak them overnight before cooking to help make them easier on your system.

Serves 6 (about 4 cups total)

1 red bell pepper

1 teaspoon red wine vinegar

1 tablespoon extra-virgin olive oil

1/2 teaspoon chopped fresh oregano

1/2 teaspoon chopped fresh mint

1/2 teaspoon fine sea salt

1/4 teaspoon freshly ground black pepper

Pinch of crushed red pepper flakes

3 cups cooked or rinsed and drained canned chickpeas

1 cup 1/2-inch diced fresh tomatoes

1/4 cup 1/4-inch diced fresh fennel

1/4 cup crumbled feta cheese

2 teaspoons kalamata olives, quartered lengthwise

2 teaspoons finely chopped canned, jarred, or frozen artichoke hearts

2 teaspoons thin strips (chiffonade) of fresh basil

2 cups baby arugula leaves

↑V
=P
↓K

1. Preheat the oven to 400°F. Place the bell pepper on a small baking sheet and roast until it is lightly charred all over and the skin begins to split and wrinkle. Transfer the roasted pepper to a small bowl, cover with plastic wrap, and let cool for 15 minutes. This process steams the pepper, softening it and making the skin easier to peel. When cool, peel and discard the skin. Pull out and discard the pepper core and seeds. Slice the remaining pepper into thin strips.

2. Put the vinegar in a large bowl. Whisk in the oil in a slow, steady stream until the mixture blends and thickens. Whisk in the oregano, mint, salt, black pepper, and red pepper flakes.

3. Stir in the roasted pepper, reserving a few strips to garnish the salad. Fold in the chickpeas, tomatoes, fennel, feta, olives, artichokes, and basil. Use immediately or, for more flavor, cover and marinate in the refrigerator for 3 to 6 hours.

4. To serve, fold in the arugula and spoon the salad onto a serving platter or individual plates. Garnish with the reserved roasted pepper strips.

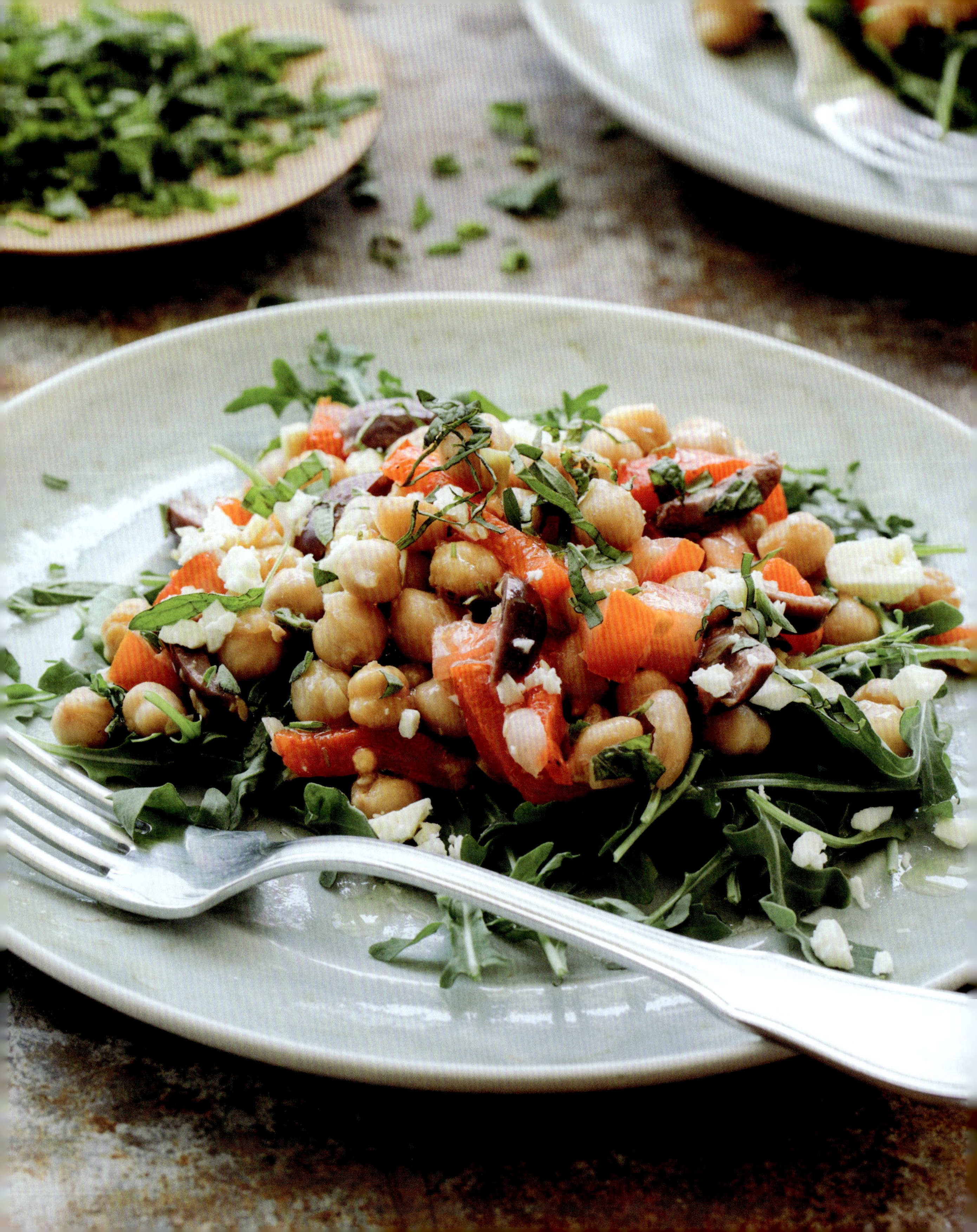

OPTIONS

- To make a sandwich wrap, lightly mash the chickpeas before mixing them into the salad. That will help everything stick together as a sandwich filling.
- To save time, use jarred roasted red peppers instead of roasting and peeling the peppers yourself.
- For a dairy-free or vegan version, omit the feta.

Chickpea of the Sea

↑V
=P
↓K

FROM THE KRIPALU ARCHIVES, this vegetarian mashed chickpea salad doesn't exactly taste like tuna salad but somehow conveys its essence. It has been popular with our guests for decades. Spoon it on whole-grain bread, fold it in a wrap, or spread it on crostini. Either way, it's full of satisfying, savory umami flavor.

Ayurvedic Insight: This is a great recipe for reducing excess kapha, which often manifests as weight gain or congestion. Favor this salad in springtime, and reap the rewards of the energy-boosting B vitamins in nutritional yeast.

Makes about 4 cups

1 tablespoon cider vinegar
2 teaspoons umeboshi vinegar
1/4 cup extra-virgin olive oil
5 teaspoons nutritional yeast
1 teaspoon celery seeds
1 teaspoon fine sea salt
1/4 teaspoon freshly ground black pepper
4 cups cooked or rinsed and drained canned chickpeas
1/2 cup minced celery
1/4 cup minced scallion greens

1. Pour the cider vinegar and umeboshi vinegar into a medium bowl. Whisk in the oil in a slow, steady stream until the mixture blends and thickens. Whisk in the nutritional yeast, celery seeds, salt, and pepper.

2. Add 2 cups of the chickpeas and mash them into the vinaigrette with a fork. The mixture should thicken considerably. Fold in the remaining 2 cups chickpeas, celery, and scallions. Use immediately or refrigerate for up to 3 days.

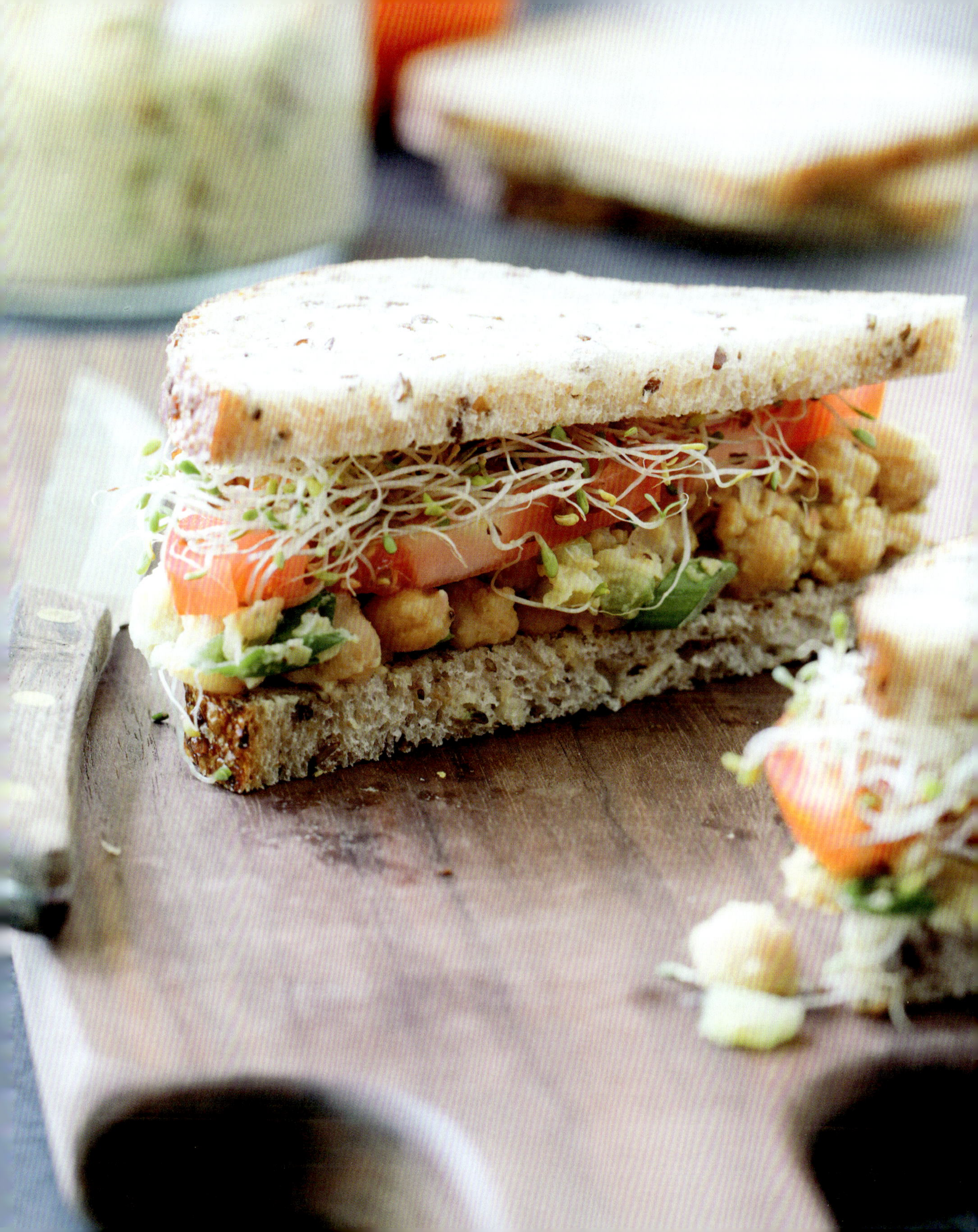

Herbed Tofu Spread

=V

↓P

↑K

SUMMERY AND LIGHT, this spread is essentially a fine vegan pâté. Some people scoop it up with bread. Others crumble it over their salad in place of goat cheese. My kids even like this stuff. The herbs are what really make it, and you could certainly add more basil if you like.

Ayurvedic Insight: Chilled tofu is best in the summer for hot body types. But the warming mustard and black pepper also make this spread suitable for vata on occasion.

Makes about 3 cups

- 1 block (14 to 16 ounces) extra-firm tofu, drained
- 1 tablespoon extra-virgin olive oil
- 1 1/2 teaspoons thinly sliced scallion greens
- 1 1/2 teaspoons chopped fresh flat-leaf parsley
- 1 1/2 teaspoons chopped fresh basil
- 1/2 teaspoon chopped fresh thyme
- 1/2 teaspoon chopped fresh rosemary
- 1/2 teaspoon chopped fresh oregano
- 1 teaspoon stone-ground mustard
- 1/2 teaspoon umeboshi vinegar
- 1/2 teaspoon fine sea salt
- 1/4 teaspoon freshly ground black pepper
- 1 1/2 teaspoons sunflower seeds, toasted

1. Place the block of tofu in a colander in the sink. Place a small bowl on the tofu and put a heavy weight inside the bowl to press excess liquid from the tofu. Let press for at least 30 minutes and up to 60 minutes.

2. For the dressing, combine the oil, scallions, parsley, basil, thyme, rosemary, oregano, mustard, vinegar, salt, and pepper in a medium bowl.

3. Coarsely crumble the pressed tofu into a small food processor. Add the toasted sunflower seeds and pulse until the tofu is very finely chopped but not completely pureed smooth, periodically scraping down the sides with a rubber spatula. The texture should resemble tiny beads and be spreadable like pâté.

4. Transfer the tofu to the bowl with the dressing and mix with a rubber spatula until well combined. Use immediately or cover and refrigerate for up to 3 days.

Mushroom Nut Pâté

HERE'S A MORE ROBUST vegan pâté. It can also be formed into patties and roasted until crisp. Ladled with Gluten-Free Vegan Gravy (recipe follows), these crisp and savory patties have proven to be our most popular Thanksgiving offering. Either way, the critical first step is cooking the onions and mushrooms way down. The mushrooms should shrink in size quite a bit, becoming more dense and meaty.

Ayurvedic Insight: Mushrooms are considered "tamasic" in Ayurveda, meaning they create heaviness and darkness. This dish is good at calming the nervous system and promoting sleep. To make it more friendly for pitta and kapha types, skip the nuts and use only seeds.

Makes 4 to 5 cups

1 tablespoon extra-virgin olive oil
2½ cups sliced button mushrooms
1 cup ½-inch diced onions
3 garlic cloves, chopped
1½ cups walnuts
1 cup raw sunflower seeds
2 tablespoons tamari
1½ tablespoons fresh lemon juice
1½ teaspoons tahini
1 tablespoon fresh oregano leaves
1 teaspoon fresh thyme leaves
Fine sea salt (optional)

1. Preheat the oven to 350°F.

2. Pour the oil onto an 18 x 13-inch sheet pan and add the mushrooms, onions, and garlic. Use your hands to rub the oil all over the vegetables, coating them thoroughly. Spread the vegetables in a single layer and roast until the onions are lightly browned and the mushrooms have lost most of their liquid, 10 to 12 minutes. Remove from the oven and let cool on the pan.

3. Meanwhile, put the walnuts and sunflower seeds in a small food processor and puree until smooth. If the nuts and seeds are too big, the pâté won't hold together, so make sure everything is chopped fine. Add the cooled mushroom mixture, tamari, lemon juice, tahini, oregano, thyme, salt if using, and ½ cup water. Continue to puree until very smooth, periodically scraping down the sides of the bowl. Taste the mixture and add salt if needed. Pack the mixture into an airtight container and refrigerate until cold, at least 2 hours and up to 4 days. Serve cold as a spread.

=V
↑P
↑K

OPTION

- *Vegan Mushroom Nut Patties:* Preheat the oven to 375°F. Press the chilled pâté into twelve 2-ounce patties, each about 3 inches in diameter and ½ inch thick. Bake on an oiled sheet pan until heated through and crusty on the outside yet tender in the center, 10 to 15 minutes. Serve with Gluten-Free Vegan Gravy (recipe follows).

GLUTEN-FREE VEGAN GRAVY

=V

=P

=K

CARAMELIZING YOUR VEGETABLES is the secret to savory vegan gravy. That, and a tincture of nutritional yeast. From there, it's a matter of thickening the broth with some flour (we use brown rice flour) and flavoring the gravy with plenty of aromatic herbs such as thyme, tarragon, and parsley. This one comes together pretty quickly.

Ayurvedic Insight: Compared to the drippings from a Thanksgiving turkey, this gravy is much lighter yet equally delicious. Still, all gravy is heavy in nature, so moderation is key.

Makes about 2 cups

2 tablespoons extra-virgin olive oil

1 1/4 cups chopped onions

3/4 cup sliced mushrooms

1/4 teaspoon dried tarragon

1/4 teaspoon dried thyme

2 tablespoons brown rice flour

1 1/2 cups unsalted Vegetable Stock (page 281) or store-bought stock

2 1/2 teaspoons soy sauce or Bragg liquid aminos

1 teaspoon nutritional yeast

1/2 teaspoon fine sea salt

1 teaspoon chopped fresh flat-leaf parsley

1. Heat a medium saucepan over medium heat. Put in the oil, onions, and mushrooms, shaking the pan to coat the vegetables. Reduce the heat to low, cover, and sweat the vegetables until they are soft and the mushrooms release their liquid, 3 to 4 minutes. Uncover, raise the heat to medium, and cook, stirring occasionally, until the vegetables are lightly caramelized and browned, 5 to 7 minutes.

2. Stir in the tarragon and thyme and cook for 1 minute. Stir in the rice flour and then gradually stir in the stock. Simmer until the mixture is smooth and slightly thickened. Stir in the soy sauce, nutritional yeast, and salt. Simmer gently for 5 minutes.

3. Puree the mixture until smooth with an immersion blender or in an upright blender. If using an upright blender, avoid a blowout by slightly cooling the mixture and partially removing the center lid of the blender.

4. Stir in the parsley and serve hot. Or refrigerate the gravy in an airtight container for up to 3 days and reheat before serving.

Sesame Noodles with Peanut Sauce

ALONG WITH ITALIAN AND MEXICAN, Chinese food always tops the list of favorite meals in America. We serve these noodles alongside fried rice, spring rolls, sautéed bok choy, and steamed edamame topped with Gomasio (page 171). If you're wondering what to serve the kids, this big bowl of creamy, comforting noodles just might do the trick.

Ayurvedic Insight: Sticky and nourishing, wheat noodles help to balance the dry qualities of vata while satisfying the hunger of pitta. For kapha types, use rice noodles instead of wheat.

↓V
=P
↑K

Serves 4 to 6
(about 6 cups total)

- 8 ounces udon noodles
- 2 1/2 tablespoons tamari
- 2 tablespoons fresh lime juice
- 2 tablespoons peanut butter (creamy or chunky)
- 2 teaspoons tahini
- 2 teaspoons honey, brown rice syrup, or agave nectar
- 2 teaspoons toasted sesame oil
- 1 teaspoon chili garlic paste, such as Lan Chi, or red curry paste
- 1 cup matchstick-cut or 1/4-inch diced cucumbers
- 1/2 cup matchstick-cut or 1/4-inch diced red bell peppers
- 1/4 cup thinly sliced scallion greens

1. Bring a large pot of water to a boil. Drop in the noodles and cook until tender, 10 to 12 minutes. Drain and rinse under cold running water to stop the cooking. Let drain and reserve.

2. In a large bowl, whisk together the tamari, lime juice, peanut butter, tahini, honey, sesame oil, and chili paste until smooth. The dressing should be somewhat runny yet thick enough to coat and stick to the noodles. Whisk in 3 to 4 tablespoons water to achieve that consistency.

3. Add the cooled noodles, cucumbers, bell peppers, and scallions. Toss to coat well, then cover and refrigerate until cold, at least 1 hour and up to 6 hours. Serve cold or at room temperature.

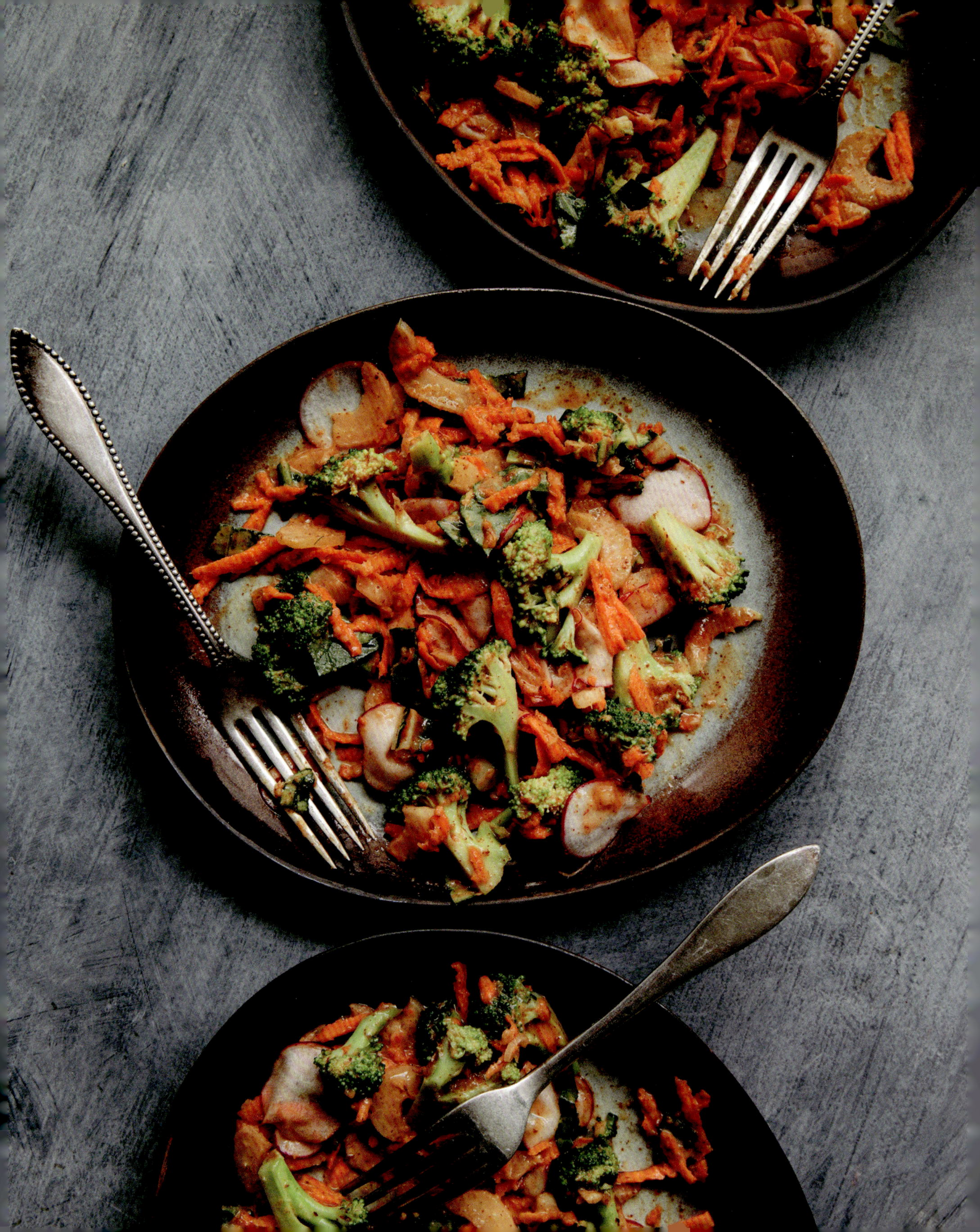

Ginger Almond Broccoli Salad

I'M NOT A BIG FAN of broccoli that's nearly raw, but this salad works. Kripalu guests absolutely love it. The dressing is rich and creamy with almond butter and toasted sesame oil, sweet with golden honey, pungent with minced ginger, and aromatic with fresh cilantro and lime. You could also mix this dressing with noodles, drizzle it over a salad, or spoon it onto leftover Pineapple Purple Rice (page 240).

Ayurvedic Insight: The warmth of the almond ginger dressing makes this salad great for vata, and quick blanching makes the broccoli easier to digest for all.

Makes 4 modest servings (about 4 cups)

↓V
=P
↑K

SALAD

1 1/4 cups small broccoli florets

1 1/4 cups scrubbed and shredded carrots

1 1/4 cups shredded bok choy (leaves and bulbs sliced crosswise superthin)

1/2 cup paper-thin slices red radish (use a mandoline)

ALMOND GINGER DRESSING

3 tablespoons almond butter

Grated zest and juice of 1 lime

2 tablespoons honey, brown rice syrup, or agave nectar

1 tablespoon toasted sesame oil

2 1/2 teaspoons minced fresh ginger

1 teaspoon minced fresh garlic

1/2 teaspoon fine sea salt

Pinch of cayenne pepper

1 1/2 tablespoons chopped fresh cilantro

1. For the salad, bring 6 cups of water to a boil in a medium saucepan. Drop in the broccoli and blanch for 2 minutes. Use a strainer to remove the broccoli and then run cool water over it for a minute or two to stop the cooking. Let drain and reserve.

2. For the dressing, spoon the almond butter into a medium bowl. Whisk in the lime zest and juice, honey, sesame oil, ginger, garlic, salt, cayenne, and cilantro until the dressing is well blended and creamy. If your almond butter is thick and the dressing isn't creamy enough to easily coat the broccoli, whisk in 1 to 2 tablespoons water. Add the blanched broccoli, carrots, bok choy, and radishes.

3. Toss to coat, and serve immediately. You can cover and refrigerate the salad, but as it sits it will get increasingly wet as the salt in the dressing draws moisture from the vegetables.

OPTION

- If you prepped a bunch of broccoli for another purpose and have stems left over, peel the stems then shred them and use the shredded broccoli stems instead of florets in this salad.

Cucumber Kimchi Salad

↓V
=P
↑K

WE GET OUR KIMCHI from Abe Hunrichs and Maddie Elling, who run the local Hosta Hill food company here in Massachusetts. They make fantastic fermented foods. I wanted to offer their kimchi in something approachable for guests who were looking for probiotic foods but not used to eating kimchi. The solution? Cucumbers. Cucumbers are so refreshing and cooling that they tame any funky qualities in the fermented cabbage.

Ayurvedic Insight: There are few salads that can be enjoyed by someone who runs cold in body temperature. If you always need a sweater, enjoy the warmth of kimchi and juiciness of cucumbers here.

Serves 4 to 6

4 cups very thinly sliced cucumbers (a mandoline works best here)

1 tablespoon minced fresh ginger

1/4 cup thinly sliced scallion greens

2 tablespoons toasted sesame oil

2 tablespoons untoasted sesame oil or sunflower oil

1/2 cup mild or spicy kimchi, coarsely chopped

1/4 teaspoon fine sea salt

3 tablespoons sesame seeds, toasted

In a medium bowl, mix the cucumbers, ginger, scallions, toasted sesame oil, and untoasted sesame oil. Stir in the chopped kimchi and salt. Serve within 2 hours or refrigerate for up to 6 hours. Stir in the sesame seeds just before serving.

OPTION

- For a vegan version, look for vegan kimchi made without fish sauce.

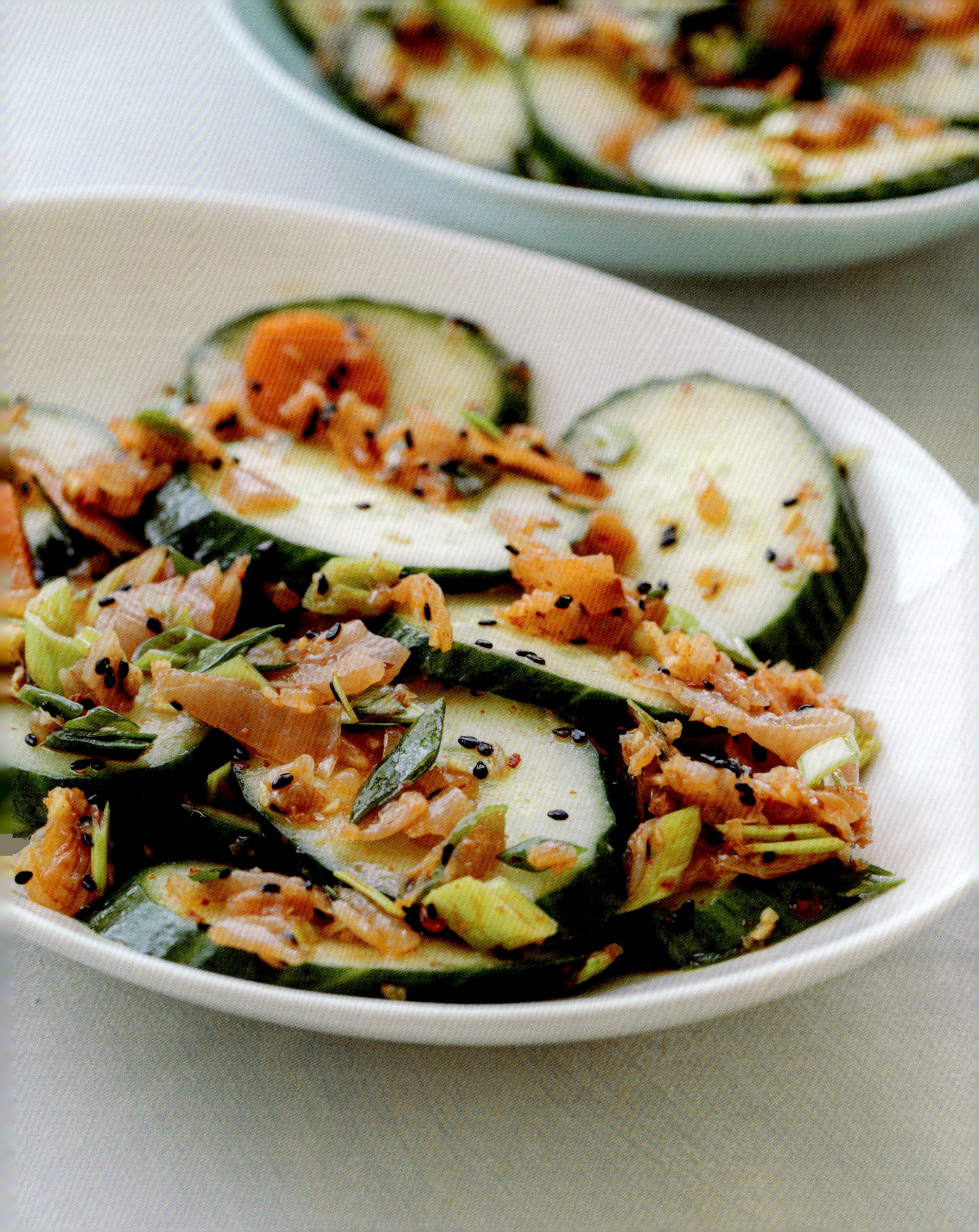

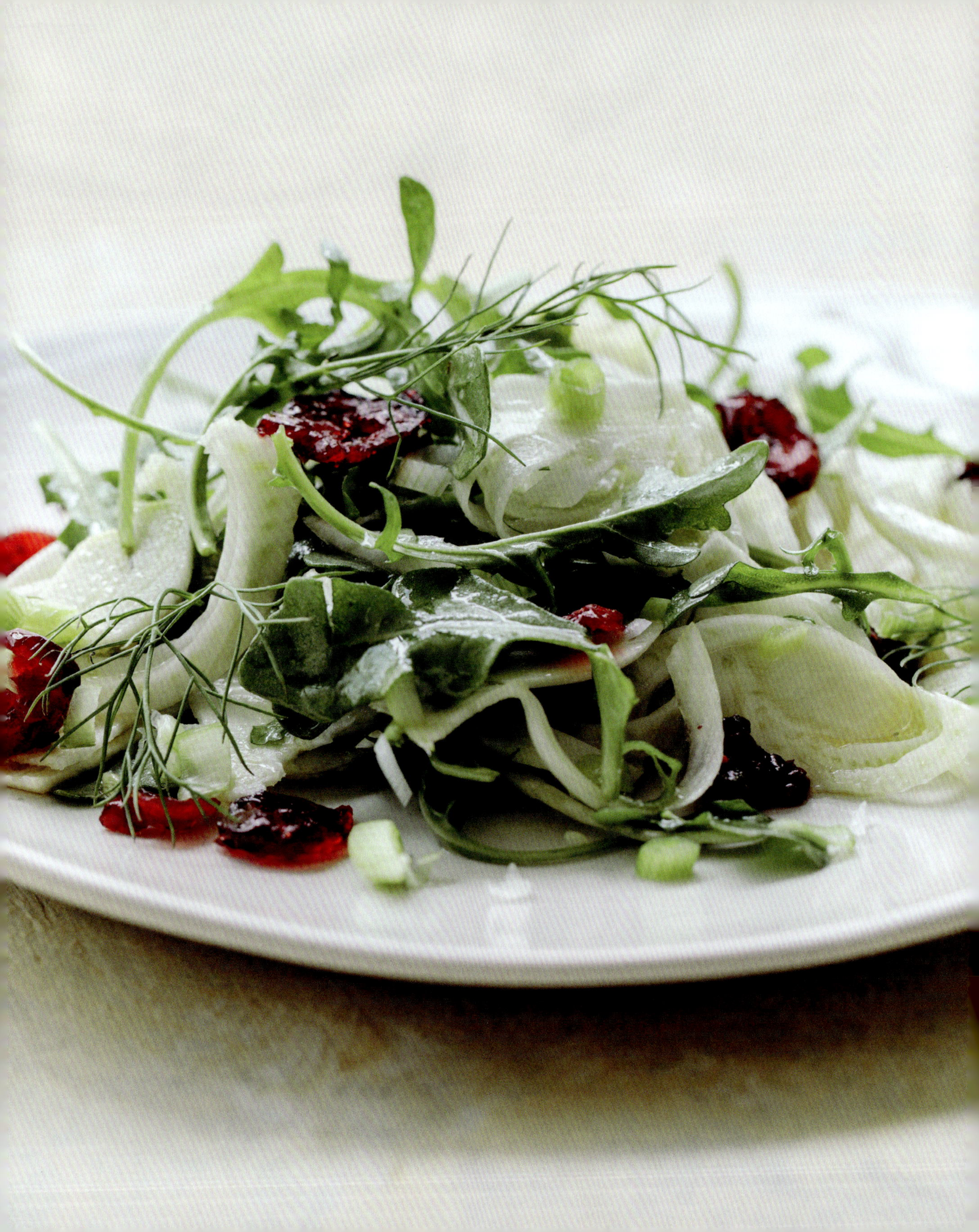

Shaved Fennel and Cranberry Salad

MOST COOKS ROAST FENNEL or cook it some other way because it is such a firm vegetable. But shave it thin, and fresh fennel takes on a completely different character: pleasantly crunchy, juicy, and aromatic. To shave it, just halve or quarter the bulb and run it across a mandoline—even an inexpensive handheld model will suffice. Fennel also helps to aid digestion through the anticramping effect of a phytonutrient called *anethole*.

Ayurvedic Insight: The perfect transition to cooler weather, this salad helps to soothe the body from excess heat buildup during the summer, preparing us to digest the heartier foods of winter.

Serves 4 (about 4 cups total)

1 tablespoon sherry vinegar

3 tablespoons extra-virgin olive oil

1 tablespoon agave nectar or honey

2 cups shaved fresh fennel (use a mandoline)

2 cups (2 ounces) baby arugula leaves

1/4 cup dried cranberries

1/4 cup thinly sliced scallion greens, preferably sliced on an angle

Fine sea salt and freshly ground black pepper

↑V ↓P ↓K

1. Pour the vinegar into a medium bowl. Whisk in the oil in a slow, steady stream until the mixture blends and thickens. Whisk in the agave.

2. Add the fennel, arugula, cranberries, and scallions, and toss to coat. Season with salt and pepper until the salad tastes good to you. Serve immediately.

OPTIONS

- Garnish with toasted walnuts or slivered almonds for more protein.
- Cranberries thrive here in Massachusetts. But you could just as easily use dried cherries or even raisins.
- For a less sweet version, omit the sweetener.

Raw Kale Greek Salad

↑V ↓P ↓K

IN THE KRIPALU KITCHEN, we joke that kale is served for breakfast, lunch, and dinner. But it's true: we try to use it as much as possible. Kale is just that good for you. With iron, vitamin C, chlorophyll, calcium, potassium, vitamin K, and a slew of antioxidants, kale has been shown to help with everything from lowering blood glucose levels and controlling diabetes to lowering cancer risk and reducing blood pressure. Definitely use deep green Tuscan lacinato (aka dinosaur) kale here. Curly kale would be too chewy.

Ayurvedic Insight: Kale is the superfood of spring and summer. Its bitter and astringent profile helps to cool your head and dry excess oil.

Serves 4 to 6

2 tablespoons fresh lemon juice

1/3 cup extra-virgin olive oil

1 tablespoon chopped fresh oregano

Pinch of fine sea salt and freshly ground black pepper

6 cups loosely packed thin strips (chiffonade) of lacinato kale

1 cup 1/4-inch diced cucumbers

1/2 cup halved cherry or grape tomatoes

1/4 cup 1/4-inch diced red bell peppers

1/4 cup raw pine nuts

2 tablespoons very thinly sliced red onions

1. Pour the lemon juice into a medium bowl. Gradually whisk in the oil in a slow, steady stream until blended and thickened. Whisk in the oregano, salt, and pepper.

2. Add the kale to the dressing and mix well, making sure the kale is completely coated. To serve within 1 hour, use your hands to massage the dressing into the leaves, which helps to break down the kale and make it more tender and easier to digest. Or, to serve the salad the next day, let it marinate overnight at room temperature and the lemon juice will tenderize the kale for you.

3. Just before serving, stir in the cucumbers, tomatoes, peppers, pine nuts, and red onions.

OPTIONS

- To make this a true Greek salad, add kalamata olives and crumbled feta cheese. It will not be raw but it will be good. If you don't use olives and feta, you may want a little extra salt in the vinaigrette to balance the flavors.
- The onions should be sliced paper thin. An inexpensive mandoline is a good tool for the job.

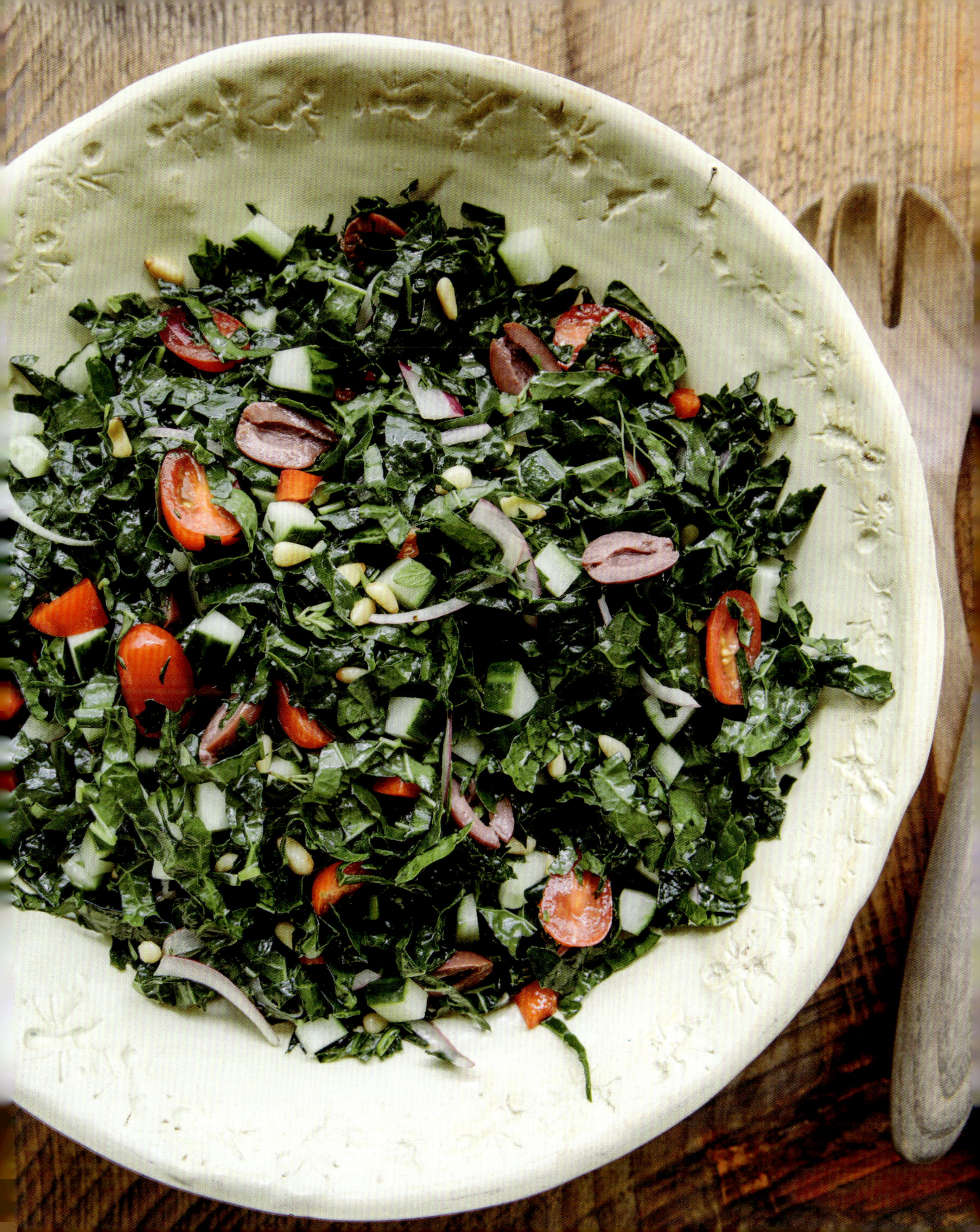

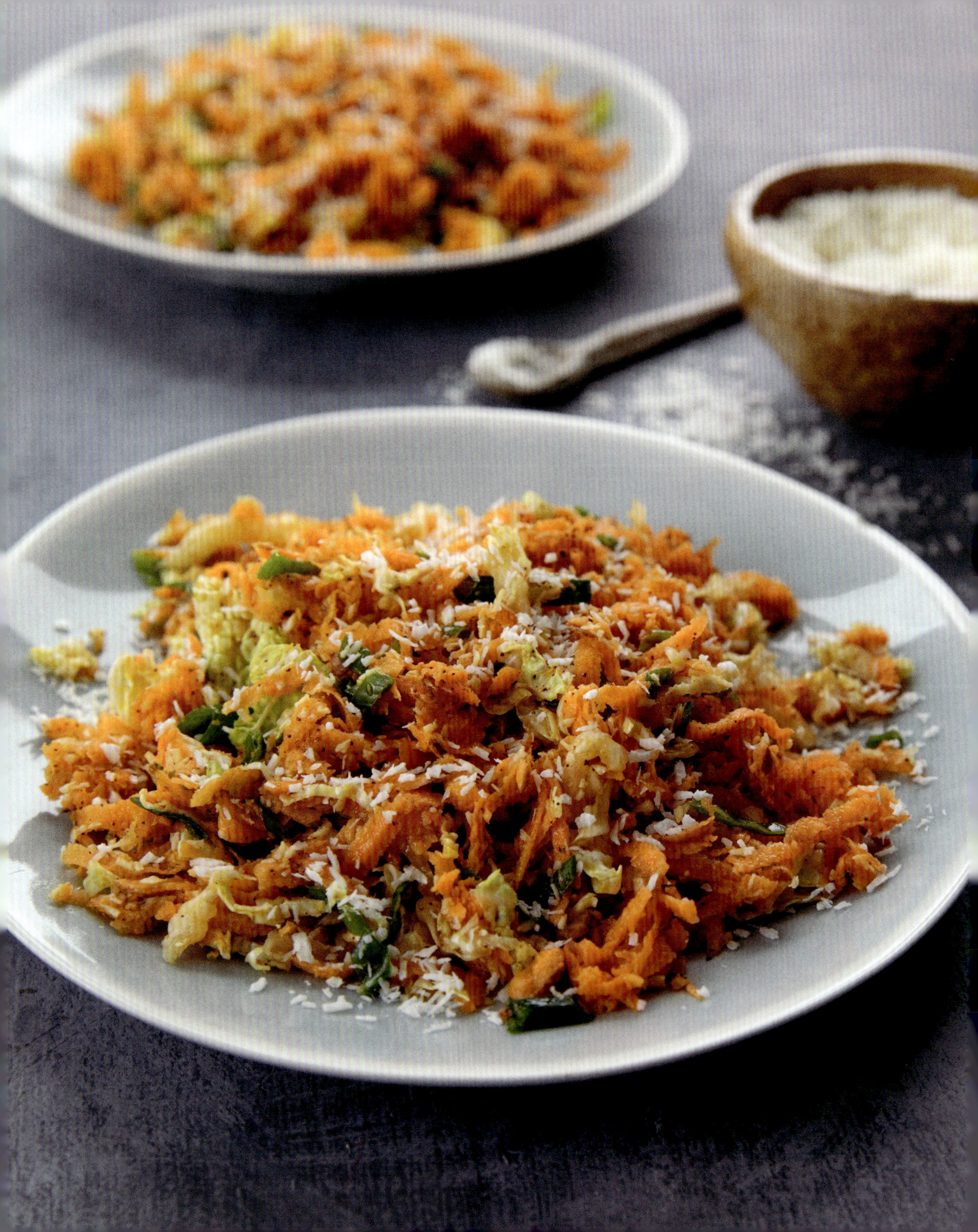

Raw Sweet Potato Slaw

IN THE SUMMER, we offer raw salads daily. One year, I was looking through the Kripalu database (which has over five thousand recipes!) and came across this unique slaw. Sweet potato isn't something most people think to eat raw, but it's very much like shredded carrots. With coconut, lime, and shredded napa cabbage, it makes a deliciously sweet slaw that will be at home in any backyard barbecue.

Ayurvedic Insight: If you have a hearty appetite and strong digestion in the summer months, this dish will definitely satisfy. Take it on a picnic!

Serves 4 to 6 (about 6 cups total)

↑V ↓P ↑K

Grated zest and juice of 2 limes

1/2 cup extra-virgin olive oil

1 teaspoon toasted sesame oil

1 teaspoon chili powder

3/4 teaspoon fine sea salt

4 1/2 cups grated sweet potatoes (about 2 large)

2 cups finely shredded napa cabbage (use a mandoline here)

1 cup thinly sliced scallion greens, preferably sliced on an angle

1/2 cup unsweetened dried shredded coconut

1. To make the dressing, grate the lime zest and set it aside. Squeeze the lime juice into a medium bowl. Whisk in the olive oil in a slow, steady steam until the mixture blends and thickens. Then whisk in the sesame oil, chili powder, lime zest, and salt.

2. Add the sweet potatoes, cabbage, scallions, and coconut to the dressing, and toss until everything is mixed well. Before serving, let the salad stand at room temperature for 30 to 60 minutes to allow the flavors to blend. You can also refrigerate the slaw for up to 8 hours.

OPTIONS

- Use half sweet potatoes and half grated carrots.
- Add ¼ cup raisins for a little more sweetness.

Raw Summer Salad

↑V
↓P
↑K

DICED ZUCCHINI AND YELLOW squash are the stars here. People don't often eat raw squash, but marinating the vegetable in vinaigrette for a few lazy summer hours makes it completely delicious, almost like a light, fresh version of ratatouille.

Ayurvedic Insight: When we eat raw, we need our digestive fire to be up to the task of "cooking" the rawness out. Always balance raw foods with warming foods such as vinegar, oil, and spices, as done here.

Serves 4

1 tablespoon cider vinegar

1 teaspoon Dijon mustard

1/3 cup extra-virgin olive oil

1/2 teaspoon fine sea salt

1/4 teaspoon freshly ground black pepper

1 1/2 cups 1/2-inch diced zucchini

1 1/2 cups 1/2-inch diced yellow squash

3/4 cup 1/2-inch diced red bell peppers

1/4 cup chopped fresh flat-leaf parsley

1/4 cup chopped fresh basil

2 cups mixed salad greens

1. In a medium bowl, whisk together the vinegar and mustard. Slowly whisk in the oil in a steady stream until blended and thickened. Then whisk in the salt and pepper.

2. Add the zucchini, yellow squash, bell peppers, parsley, and basil, then toss gently to coat everything with the vinaigrette. Cover and marinate in the refrigerator for 2 to 3 hours. Just before serving, add the salad greens and toss gently.

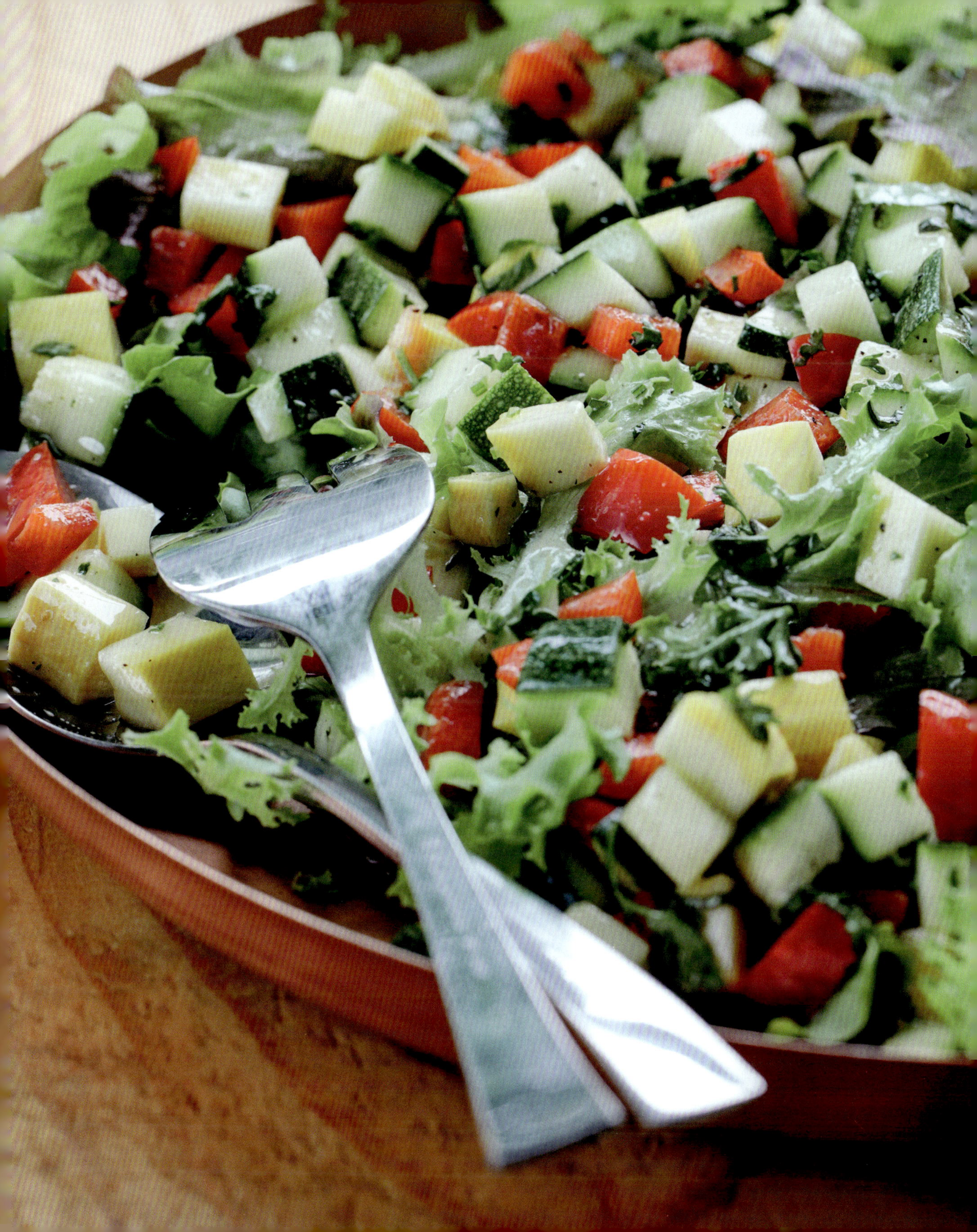

↓V
=P
=K

Chipotle Chicken Salad

OUR SALAD AND SANDWICH BAR has some unusual items like Herbed Tofu Spread (page 128), but this one is likely more familiar. Lime, cumin, and a little chipotle chile give it Tex-Mex flair, but otherwise it is a straight-up mayo-based chicken salad. To make it, grill some boneless, skinless breasts or simply use leftover roasted or rotisserie chicken.

Ayurvedic Insight: The ancient texts of Ayurveda define each animal product by its different qualities, and, in general, the grounding properties of lean animal protein are considered medicinal when used judiciously.

Makes about 4 cups

- 1 pound chicken, cooked
- 1/2 cup mayonnaise
- 2 tablespoons 1/4-inch diced red bell peppers
- 1 tablespoon minced red onions
- 1 1/2 tablespoons chopped fresh cilantro
- 2 teaspoons minced canned chipotle peppers in adobo
- 1 1/2 teaspoons plain yogurt
- 1 tablespoon fresh lime juice
- 1 teaspoon fresh lemon juice
- 1/2 teaspoon ground cumin
- 1/2 teaspoon ground coriander
- 1/2 teaspoon fine sea salt
- 1/4 teaspoon freshly ground black pepper

1. Dice the chicken into bite-size pieces and set aside.

2. In a medium bowl, combine the mayo, bell peppers, onions, cilantro, chipotles, yogurt, lime juice, lemon juice, cumin, coriander, salt, and black pepper. Stir in the chicken. Use immediately or refrigerate for up to 2 days.

OPTIONS

- Add a spoonful of chicken salad to a green salad for more protein. Or make it into a sandwich with whole-grain bread, lettuce, and tomatoes. You can also wrap it up in a whole-wheat tortilla.

Sriracha Chicken

MANY FOODS AT KRIPALU are mildly seasoned so guests can customize their seasonings at the table. This isn't one of those dishes. This one explodes with flavor. Sriracha, coconut sugar, lime zest, and fish sauce really amp up the taste of chicken. After marinating and baking the chicken, it can be served hot or chilled, sliced, and served cold as a sandwich, in a wrap, or on a salad.

Ayurvedic Insight: Enjoy this dish on a cool, rainy day, as the pungency of sriracha helps to circulate heat through a cold, damp body and mind.

↓V
=P
↓K

Serves 4

1/4 cup toasted sesame oil
1 tablespoon sriracha
1 tablespoon coconut sugar
Finely grated zest and juice of 2 limes
1/2 teaspoon fish sauce
1/2 teaspoon fine sea salt
1 pound boneless, skinless chicken breasts

1. For the marinade, mix the sesame oil, sriracha, coconut sugar, lime zest, lime juice, fish sauce, and salt in a shallow dish just large enough to hold the chicken. Lay the chicken in the marinade, turning to coat all over. Cover and marinate in the refrigerator for at least 6 hours or up to 24 hours for more flavor, turning once or twice during that time.

2. Preheat the oven to 350°F.

3. Heat a medium cast-iron or ovenproof skillet over high heat for 3 minutes. Lay the chicken in the pan and slather some leftover marinade over the top of each piece. Sear until nicely browned on the bottom, 2 to 3 minutes. Flip and slather more marinade over the top. Transfer the pan to the oven and bake until the internal temperature of the chicken registers 160°F, 6 to 8 minutes. Serve warm, or let the chicken cool, refrigerate it for up to 2 days, and serve cold. Either way, we like to serve it thinly sliced on an angle.

OPTIONS

- Serve hot with Pineapple Purple Rice (page 240) or cold with Avocado Crème (page 217) or Cucumber Kimchi Salad (page 134). This chicken also makes a great sandwich.
- You could grill the chicken on a medium-hot grill instead of searing and baking it. The grill gives the chicken a nice crust. Just be sure to turn the chicken often to avoid burning.
- For more even cooking, gently pound the chicken breasts until they are evenly thick.
- *Sriracha Tofu:* Place a block of drained tofu (14 to 16 ounces) in a colander in the sink. Place a small bowl on the tofu and put a heavy weight inside the bowl to press excess

liquid from the tofu. Let press for at least 30 minutes and up to 60 minutes. Cut the tofu into slabs (cutlets) and marinate them as described for the chicken. Cook the tofu as described above, then cut the slabs into triangles. For vegans, omit the fish sauce. Or buy vegan fish sauce at 24vegan.com.

Kripalu House Dressing

A FIXTURE ON our salad bar, this creamy dressing has become synonymous with Kripalu Kitchen. It reflects the many culinary styles we touch on, including Indian, Japanese, Chinese, and Israeli. It's a dressing as comfortable drizzled over green salads, roasted vegetables, and cooked grains as it is spooned over pan-seared fish and grilled chicken.

Ayurvedic Insight: Tahini, or sesame seed butter, helps to settle the mind, and this warming dressing can help make all kinds of salads more amenable to vata types and cold, dry bodies.

Makes 2 cups

1 cup sunflower oil or grapeseed oil
1/3 cup tahini
1/4 cup tamari or soy sauce
1/4 cup fresh lemon juice
2 tablespoons toasted sesame oil
2 garlic cloves
1 1/2 teaspoons dry mustard
1 1/4 teaspoons paprika
1/4 teaspoon cayenne pepper
1/2 teaspoon fine sea salt

Blend all the ingredients and ½ cup water with an immersion blender or in an upright blender. Use immediately or refrigerate for up to 5 days.

↓V
↑P
↑K

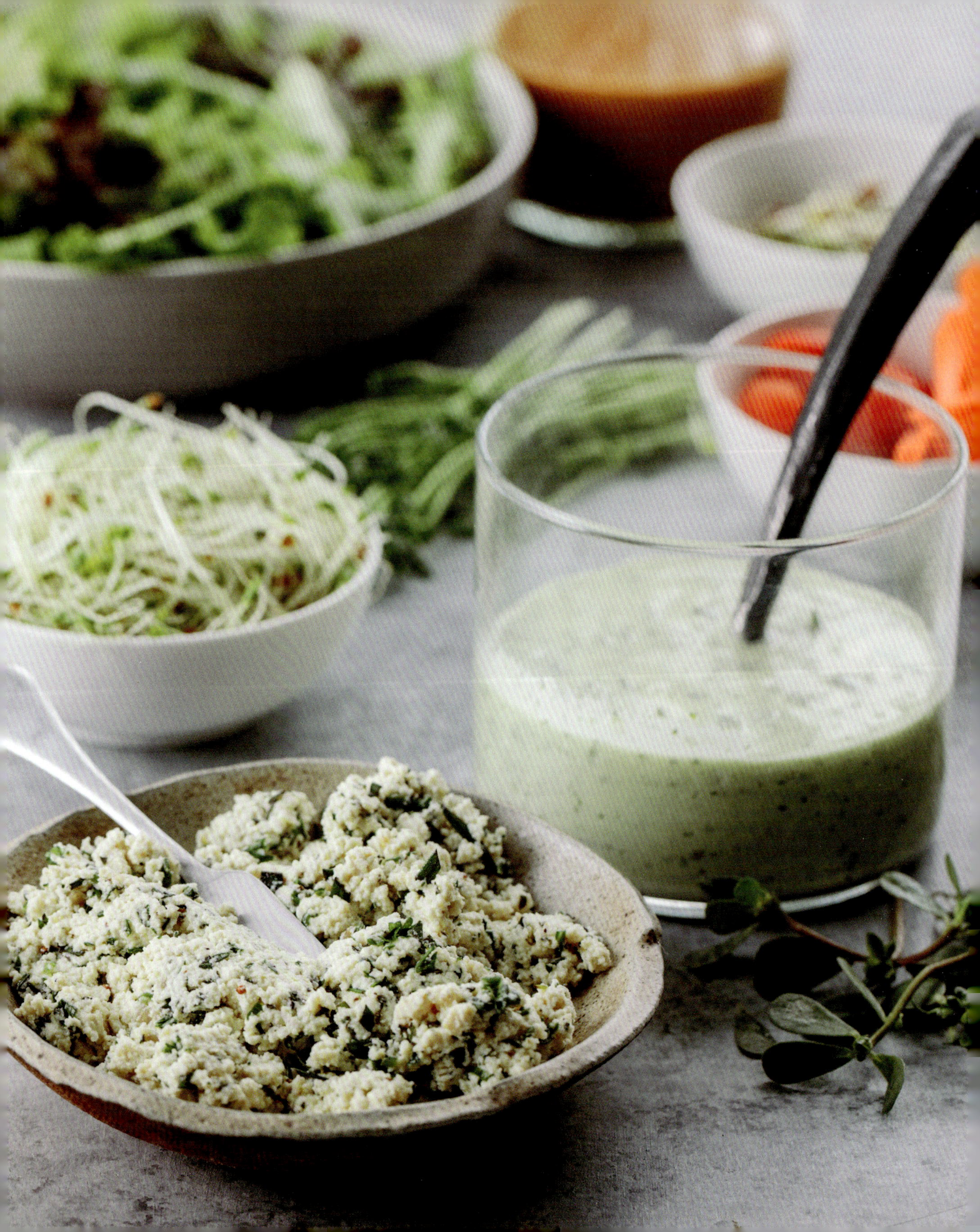

Creamy Parsley Feta Dressing

THIS FRESH SPIN on ranch dressing goes with every green salad imaginable.

Ayurvedic Insight: Salty feta cheese and sour lemon juice mitigate the cold nature of green lettuces.

Makes about 1½ cups

1/4 cup chopped fresh flat-leaf parsley

2/3 cup plant-based mayonnaise, such as Vegenaise

2/3 cup extra-virgin olive oil

1/4 cup fresh lemon juice

1/4 cup crumbled feta cheese

1 tablespoon chopped garlic

1 teaspoon fine sea salt

Put the parsley and ¼ cup water in a small blender or food processor. Blend until the parsley is very finely chopped and the water looks light green. Add the mayo, oil, lemon juice, feta, garlic, and salt. Pulse until lightly blended. Use immediately or refrigerate for up to 2 days.

↓V
↑P
↑K

Umeboshi Scallion Vinaigrette

↓V
=P
↑K

WE GO THROUGH a lot of this vinaigrette. The umeboshi (Japanese pickled plums) taste salty, sour, and savory all at once. Plus, they give you the digestive benefits of lactic acid fermentation. Look for umeboshi paste or umeboshi vinegar in the Asian section of the store.

Ayurvedic Insight: Vinegar in general, and especially umeboshi, increases digestive fire, helping to break down the raw vegetables in a salad.

Makes about 2 cups

1 bunch scallions (about 2 ounces), greens trimmed and coarsely chopped

1½ tablespoons umeboshi paste or 2 to 3 tablespoons umeboshi vinegar

1⅓ cups extra-virgin olive oil

Put the scallion greens, ¾ cup water, and umeboshi paste in a small blender or food processor. Process until mostly smooth. With the machine running, gradually blend in the oil in a slow, steady stream. Use immediately or refrigerate for up to 3 days. If using umeboshi paste, the vinaigrette should stay emulsified and smooth for days. If using vinegar, whisk or blend it briefly to re-emulsify it.

OPTION

- If the scallions are too pungent, rinse them under cold water and drain thoroughly before using.

Cilantro Mint Chutney

WE CALL THIS the ketchup of Kripalu. Guests put it on everything from sandwiches, steamed rice, and Kitchari (page 245) to sautéed vegetables, chicken, and shrimp. We easily make 8 to 10 gallons a week, using over a hundred bunches of herbs. Cilantro has the amazing ability to help remove heavy metals from your system, a detoxification process known as chelation.

Ayurvedic Insight: In this tridoshic chutney, the cooling mint and cilantro help to brighten and balance any spicy dish.

Makes about 1 cup

1/2 teaspoon ground coriander
1/2 teaspoon garam masala
1/4 cup extra-virgin olive oil
1 bunch cilantro (about 4 ounces), chopped, leaving some small stems
1/4 cup coarsely chopped fresh mint
1 tablespoon minced fresh ginger
1 tablespoon minced red onions
1/4 teaspoon minced jalapeño peppers
Grated zest and juice of 1 lemon
1/4 teaspoon honey, preferably raw
1/4 teaspoon fine sea salt

1. In a small saucepan or sauté pan, stir together the coriander, garam masala, and olive oil. Bloom the spices over low heat until they smell fragrant, 2 to 3 minutes.

2. Remove from the heat and let cool.

3. Scrape the pan contents, including the oil, into a small food processor or blender. Add the cilantro, mint, ginger, onions, jalapeños, lemon zest and juice, honey, and salt. Puree until still slightly chunky, stopping periodically to scrape down the sides with a rubber spatula. Refrigerate and serve cold.

↓V
↓P
↓K

OPTIONS

- Spoon the chutney over grilled vegetables or cooked grains. It also goes well with Red Lentil Dal (page 161) and Coconut Chana Saag (page 180).
- If cilantro often tastes soapy or disagreeable to you, soak the herb in a bowl of water for a few hours or until the water appears sudsy. Then rinse it to reduce its alkalinity.
- For a raw version, skip the first step of blooming the spices in oil.
- For a vegan version, omit the honey or replace it with brown rice syrup or agave nectar.

Trapenese Sauce

=V

↑P

=K

IF YOU LIKE PESTO, you'll love this spunky Sicilian sauce. Roasted cherry tomatoes make all the difference. In the summer, our local cherry tomatoes are nature's candy, and roasting them concentrates the flavor. We first served the sauce tossed with pasta, and then put it on the deli bar, where guests started slathering it on everything. It's that good.

Ayurvedic Insight: Along with salt and oil, the warming spice of chiles here will stimulate the mind for bright thinking.

Makes about 1½ cups

1 cup cherry tomatoes (4 to 6 ounces)
1/2 cup unsalted skin-on whole almonds or slivered almonds
1/4 cup plus 1 tablespoon extra-virgin olive oil
1/4 teaspoon plus a pinch of fine sea salt
2 garlic cloves
1/4 teaspoon crushed red pepper flakes
3/4 cup gently packed fresh basil leaves
1/4 cup gently packed fresh mint leaves
Pinch of freshly ground black pepper

1. Preheat the oven to 375°F.

2. Toss the tomatoes, almonds, the 1 tablespoon olive oil, and a pinch of salt on a sheet pan until everything is well coated. Roast until the tomato skins split and the nuts are lightly toasted, 8 to 10 minutes. Remove the pan from the oven and let the tomatoes cool a bit.

3. Scrape the cooled ingredients from the sheet pan into a blender or food processor. Add the remaining ¼ cup oil, remaining ¼ teaspoon salt, garlic, red pepper flakes, basil, mint, and black pepper. Blend until the mixture is a coarse puree. Blend in ¼ cup water a tablespoon or two at a time, just until the mixture reaches the consistency of a spoonable pesto. Taste and add more salt and pepper until it tastes good to you.

OPTIONS

- You can use this sauce like any other pesto. It makes enough to toss with about 12 ounces of pasta. You could also spread the sauce on tofu, spoon it over sautéed fish or chicken, or drizzle it over grilled vegetables.
- For a bit more richness, add 2 tablespoons grated Parmesan along with the herbs.

Arugula Chèvre Pesto

We make a lot of pestos at Kripalu because they are fresh, green, healthy and—let's be honest—easy to make for a ton of people. One spring, during a cooking demonstration, I was roasting sweet potatoes and wanted to incorporate some creamy goat cheese. Pesto to the rescue! It adds just enough richness to the herbs without sacrificing the sauce's hallmarks of lightness and freshness.

Ayurvedic Insight: Spring is typically not the time for the heaviness of cheese, but goat cheese is the exception because it is drier and lighter than cow's milk cheese.

Makes about 1 cup

- 2 teaspoons minced fresh garlic
- 1 cup packed baby arugula or watercress leaves and small stems
- 1 cup packed flat-leaf parsley leaves and small stems
- 1/2 cup extra-virgin olive oil
- 1/4 cup walnuts, toasted
- 3 tablespoons chèvre (soft goat cheese)
- 1/2 teaspoon fine sea salt
- 1/4 teaspoon freshly ground black pepper

Combine everything in a food processor and blend until smooth, scraping down the sides once or twice.

OPTION

- For a dairy-free version, replace the chèvre with nondairy cream cheese. Or for a raw version, simply omit the cheese.

=V
↓P
↓K

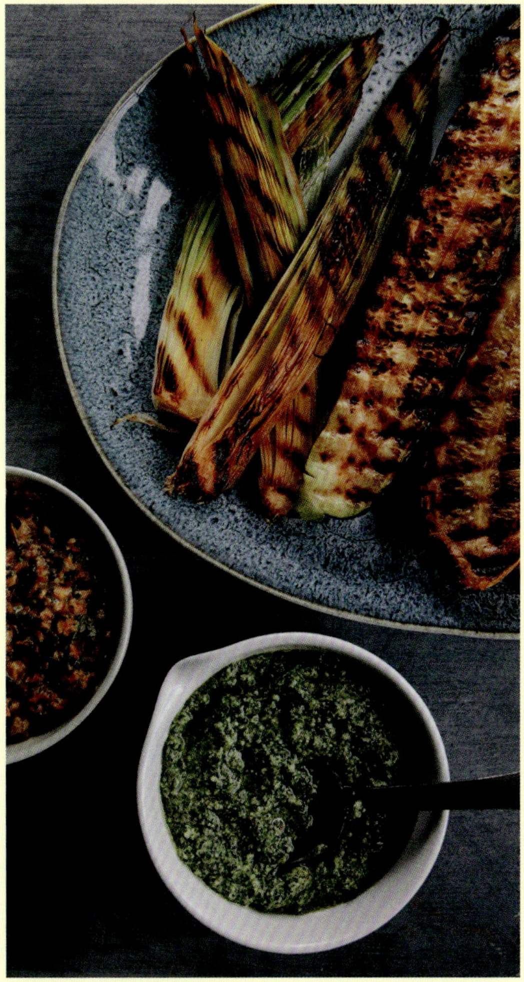

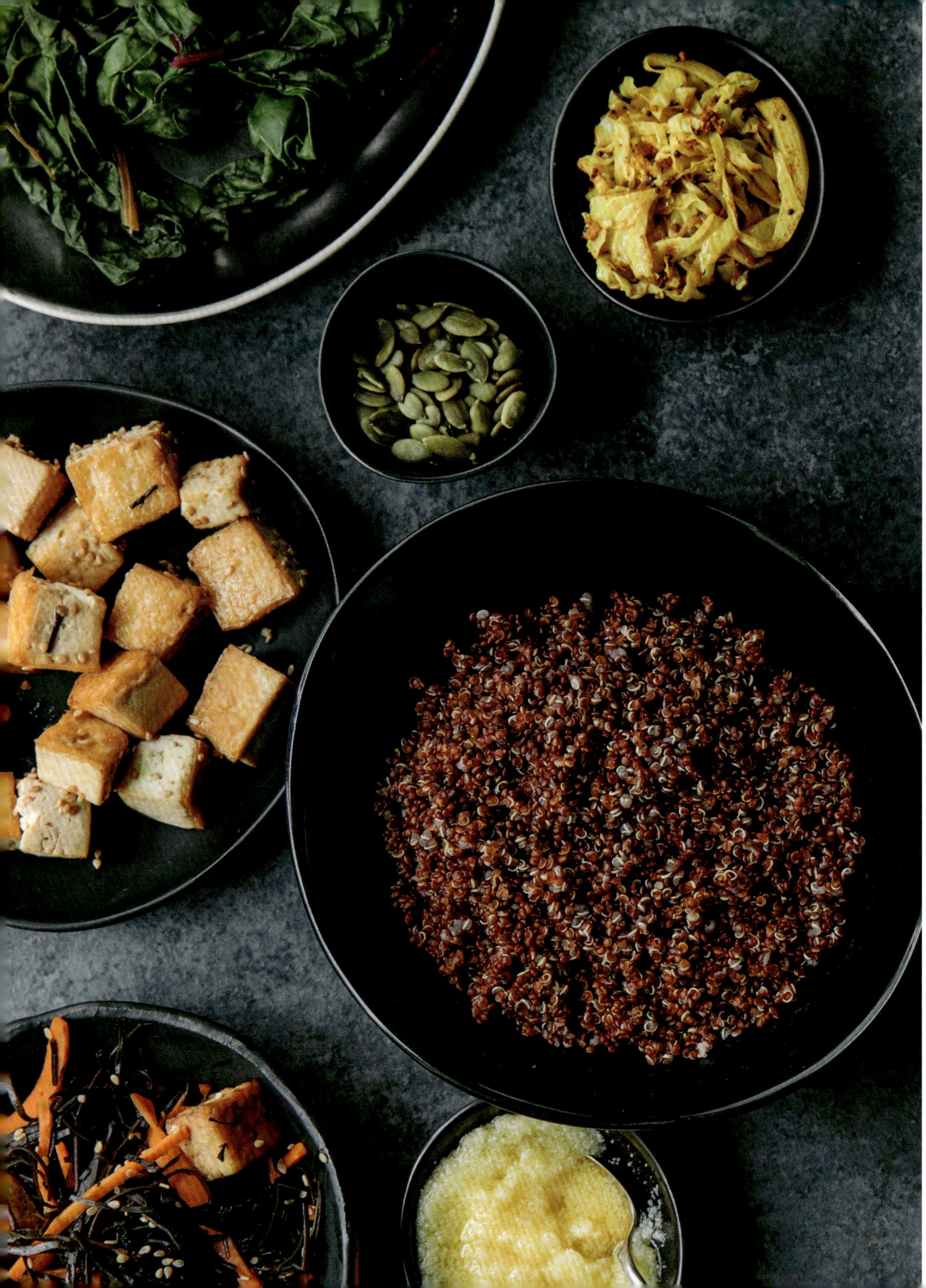

BASICS FROM THE BUDDHA BAR

The Buddha was an enlightened yogi who taught the "middle way" between the extremes of self-deprivation and self-indulgence. At Kripalu, the Buddha Bar is for those who wish to avoid overstimulation. This section of our dining room offers a selection of simply seasoned, vegan dishes with optional condiments. Sauces, pickles, steamed rice, gently cooked vegetables, and seasoning blends on the side allow you to customize meals at your own discretion. Guests often spoon a few items into one of our Buddha Bowls to create a nourishing meal that is just right for them at that particular time on that particular day.

Back in the 1980s, the entire dining room at Kripalu consisted of dishes that are now staples on the Buddha Bar. These dishes adhere to macrobiotic and Ayurvedic principles and almost all are completely free of potential allergens that may show up here and there on our primary buffet. If you have a delicate digestive system, are recovering from illness, or are on a cleanse, the Buddha Bar is a safe haven. These dishes are all vegan, gluten-free, minimally seasoned with herbs, low in sodium, free of nightshade vegetables (such as potatoes, tomatoes, peppers, and eggplant), and free of onions, garlic, and black pepper.

These recipes are also some of the easiest to make in this book. Turmeric Cauliflower and Peas (page 162) and Saag with Spice Trio (page 163) come together in about fifteen minutes. For plant-based protein, we recommend dishes such as Miso-Baked Tofu (page 157), Arame and Tempeh (page 160), and Red Lentil Dal (page 161). Dishes like Umeboshi Pickled Radishes and Greens (page 166) provide the digestive benefits of lactic acid fermentation, while condiments like Tahini Sauce (page 170), Tamarind Sauce (page 169), and Pumpkin Dulse (page 173) add gentle, satisfying flavors. Most of these recipes can be made ahead and kept in your refrigerator so your own personal Buddha Bar is always ready and waiting.

The foods in this chapter are not only deeply nourishing. They are also meant to clear your mind. In Ayurveda, the concept of *sattva* is a gentle yet "woke" mode of existence that epitomizes this sort of clarity. Sattva embodies purity, harmony, serenity, balance, peace, and virtue. Things like yoga, meditation, contemplation, studying sacred texts, slowing down, spending time outside in natural settings, and eating simple, clean, cooked foods all enhance sattva. Foods on the Buddha Bar and in this chapter are intended to diminish agitation in the body, support clarity of mind, and allow those who meditate to reach the deeper, quieter aspects of consciousness.

Miso-Baked Tofu

SIMPLE AND SAVORY, these slabs of tofu have lots of umami flavor from the tamari and miso. For a dinner party, keep the miso glaze fairly thick and spoon it into a piping bag fitted with a star tip, then pipe a star of the miso mixture onto the tofu just before baking.

Ayurvedic Insight: Tofu, or soybean curd, is a great source of plant-based protein but can cause bloating in some digestive systems. The warming aspects of ginger, miso, vinegar, sesame oil, and tamari act as digestive aids and make this tofu dish more enjoyable for all doshas.

=V
=P
=K

Serves 4 to 6

1 pound extra-firm tofu
1/4 cup tamari
1 tablespoon minced fresh ginger
1/4 cup white miso
2 tablespoons brown rice vinegar
2 teaspoons stone-ground mustard
1 tablespoon toasted sesame oil

1. Drain the tofu and place it in a colander in the sink. Place a small bowl on the tofu and then put a large can of tomatoes or beans in the bowl. Let the tofu press for 20 minutes to drain excess water. Cut the drained tofu through the side into cutlets about ½ inch thick.

2. Put the tamari, ginger, and 1½ cups water in a small saucepan and bring to a boil over high heat. Place the pressed tofu cutlets in a wide, shallow baking dish and pour the marinade over them. Let marinate at room temperature for 20 minutes.

3. While the tofu marinates, preheat the oven to 350°F.

4. In a small mixing bowl, whisk together the miso, vinegar, and mustard. The mixture should be thick yet spreadable. If necessary, stir in up to 1 tablespoon water to make it spreadable. Place the marinated cutlets on a sheet pan in a single layer, and coat each side of the cutlets with sesame oil. Use a rubber spatula to slather the miso mixture over the top of each cutlet.

5. Bake until the miso mixture browns lightly, 8 to 10 minutes. Serve warm.

OPTIONS

- For a bit of decadence, replace the vinegar with white wine.
- Instead of baking, you can grill the tofu, searing both sides until nicely browned over medium heat. Spread the miso glaze on the top side toward the end of cooking.
- You can use this miso glaze on salmon or chicken instead of tofu.

Tofu in Tamari Ginger Broth

=V

=P

=K

THIS DISH IS LIKE a healthy version of Chinese takeout and comes together just as fast. My kids love it over rice with an extra spoonful of tamari ginger broth. Keep this one in the fridge for impromptu meals.

Ayurvedic Insight: The sea vegetable kombu makes beans and tofu more digestible. As Western medicine explains it, enzymes in kombu break down the raffinose sugars in beans that cause gas. Once those sugars are broken down, we can more easily enjoy beans and tofu, and reap their nourishing rewards.

Serves 4 to 6

1 pound extra-firm tofu

1/2 cup tamari

1 1/2 tablespoons minced fresh ginger

1 small piece of kombu, about 1/2 inch square

3/4 cup bok choy (white and light green parts only), sliced 1/2-inch thick

2 tablespoons cornstarch

1. Drain the tofu and place it in a colander in the sink. Place a small bowl on the tofu and then put a large can of tomatoes or beans in the bowl. Let the tofu press for 20 minutes to drain excess water. Cut the drained tofu into 1-inch cubes.

2. Place the tofu cubes, tamari, ginger, kombu, and 2½ cups water in a medium saucepan. Cover and bring to a boil over high heat, then reduce the heat and simmer gently for 10 minutes.

3. Uncover, stir in the bok choy, and simmer until it is just barely tender, about 3 minutes. In a small bowl, mix the cornstarch and ¼ cup cold water to make a slurry. Bring the broth mixture back to a boil over high heat and stir in the slurry. Boil until the mixture thickens slightly, 1 to 2 minutes. Serve warm with the broth.

OPTION

- Use the tofu and broth as the basis of a stir-fry. Cook the vegetables of your choice (such as carrots, celery, bok choy, peppers, broccoli, and garlic) in a hot wok or sauté pan. At the very end of cooking, add the cooked tofu and some of the ginger broth.

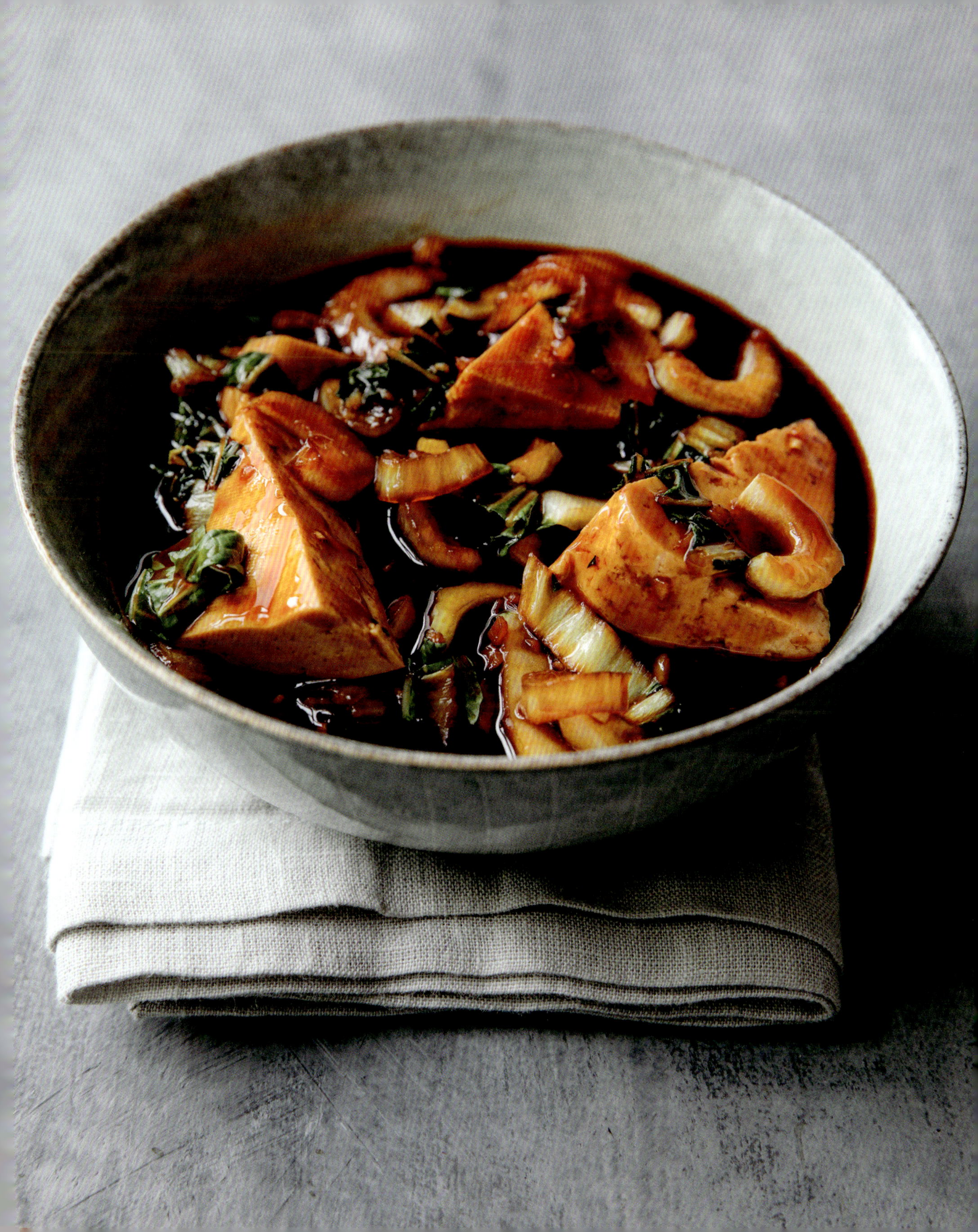

Arame and Tempeh

↑V ↓P ↓K

SEA GREENS LIKE ARAME are underrated powerhouses of nutrition—and flavor! We get our "seaweeds" from Maine Coast Sea Vegetables; they are sustainably harvested, certified organic, and completely delicious. They're also local and seasonal, two fundamental concepts of the Ayurvedic diet.

Ayurvedic Insight: Tempeh, a fermented food traditionally made from soybeans, offers some fantastic probiotic benefits. However, it can be difficult for some to digest. Sea greens and vinegar help to ease the way.

Serves 4 to 6

1½ cups dried arame seaweed or kelp
8 ounces tempeh, cut into ½-inch cubes
2 tablespoons toasted sesame oil
1¼ cups carrot matchsticks
3 tablespoons tamari
1 tablespoon brown rice vinegar
1½ teaspoons sesame seeds

1. In a medium bowl, combine the arame and 2 cups water. Let soak at room temperature until rehydrated, about 20 minutes. Drain and reserve.

2. Place the tempeh in a medium saucepan and add water to cover by 1 inch. Bring to a boil over high heat, then reduce the heat to medium and simmer for 15 minutes. Drain the tempeh.

3. Preheat a large sauté pan over medium-high heat for 2 minutes. Swirl in 1 tablespoon of the sesame oil, add the tempeh, and cook until it is lightly browned all over, 3 to 5 minutes. Add the remaining 1 tablespoon sesame oil and the carrots and cook, stirring often, until they are just beginning to get tender, 2 to 3 minutes. Stir in the rehydrated arame and cook for 2 minutes more, stirring often. Remove from the heat and stir in the tamari and vinegar. Sprinkle on the sesame seeds just before serving.

Red Lentil Dal

↓V ↓P ↓K

AT KRIPALU, WE MAKE all kinds of dal (cooked legumes). Split pea dal is very substantial and filling, while mung bean dal is lighter. Red lentil dal takes the middle ground, and we prepare it simply so guests can add their seasonings of choice.

Ayurvedic Insight: Asafetida is like Ayurvedic Beano. Add this spice to legumes, and it reduces their gassiness. Many swamis and Brahmins use it as a seasoning in place of garlic and onions, which are thought to disturb the mind.

Serves 4 to 6

1/2 cup 1/4-inch diced carrots
1/2 cup 1/4-inch diced celery
2 teaspoons extra-virgin olive oil or ghee
1 1/2 teaspoons brown mustard seeds
1 1/2 teaspoons ground coriander
1/2 teaspoon ground turmeric
Pinch of asafetida (hing)
1 cup red lentils
Seasoning of choice, such as sea salt, tamari, liquid aminos, hot sauce, Gomasio (page 171), Pumpkin Dulse (page 173), Tahini Sauce (page 170), Tamarind Sauce (page 169), or Cilantro Mint Chutney (page 151)

1. Heat a medium saucepan over medium heat. Put in the carrots, celery, and oil, shaking the pan to coat the vegetables. Cover, reduce the heat to low, and sweat the vegetables until tender, 3 to 5 minutes.

2. Uncover and raise the heat to medium. Stir in the mustard seeds, coriander, turmeric, and asafetida. Let the spices bloom until they are fragrant, 1 to 2 minutes. Mix in the lentils and 2½ cups water and bring to a boil over high heat. Cover, reduce the heat to low, and simmer gently until the lentils are soft, about 15 minutes.

3. Partially puree the mixture with an immersion blender or in an upright blender. If using an upright blender, avoid a blowout by cooling the mixture slightly and partially removing the center lid of the blender. The dal should still be somewhat chunky. After pureeing, simmer it over medium heat, stirring often, until the dal reaches your desired consistency; it can be served thick or thin. Season with your seasoning of choice and serve warm.

Turmeric Cauliflower and Peas

=V
↓P
↓K

ONE OF THE KEY steps in this recipe is blooming the spices in hot oil. It releases many aromas and really bumps up the flavor. From there, you simply braise some cauliflower florets in a little liquid, then add peas, lemon juice, and cilantro.

Ayurvedic Insight: Turmeric is an Ayurvedic superfood with anti-inflammatory properties and a pleasant pungency. This dish is perfect as part of a warming meal on cool spring evenings.

Serves 4 to 6

2 tablespoons extra-virgin olive oil or ghee
1 tablespoon ground turmeric
1½ teaspoons brown mustard seeds
1 tablespoon minced fresh ginger
5 cups medium cauliflower florets
1 cup fresh or frozen peas
2 teaspoons fresh lemon juice
3 tablespoons chopped fresh cilantro
Seasoning of choice, such as sea salt, tamari, liquid aminos, hot sauce, Gomasio (page 171), Pumpkin Dulse (page 173), Tahini Sauce (page 170), Tamarind Sauce (page 169), or Cilantro Mint Chutney (page 151)

1. In a medium saucepan, combine the oil, turmeric, and mustard seeds. Cook over medium heat until the spices are fragrant (the mustard seeds may begin to pop), 2 to 3 minutes. Stir in the ginger and cook until fragrant, about 1 minute.

2. Stir in the cauliflower and cook until lightly browned, about 5 minutes, stirring to coat with the spices. Stir in 2 tablespoons water, cover the pan, and cook over low heat, stirring occasionally, until the cauliflower is tender, 8 to 10 minutes.

3. Uncover, stir in the peas, and cook just until they are tender, 2 to 3 minutes. Remove from the heat and stir in the lemon juice and 2 tablespoons of the cilantro. Season with your seasoning of choice and garnish with the remaining 1 tablespoon cilantro.

OPTION

- Use diced sweet potatoes or broccoli instead of cauliflower.

Saag with Spice Trio

A CLASSIC INDIAN DISH, saag consists of spiced and braised greens pureed with heavy cream or coconut milk. We skip the creamy element on our Buddha Bar to keep the dish lighter. With all the greens and cruciferous vegetables here, it's almost like having a hot, green juice. Spoon on some Tamarind Sauce (page 169) to round out the flavors.

Ayurvedic Insight: In the spring, eat all things green. Ayurveda favors cooked foods, and this dish provides your greens in a form preferable to a cold salad.

Serves 4 to 6

1 tablespoon extra-virgin olive oil or ghee
2 teaspoons curry powder
1½ teaspoons ground cumin
Pinch of ground nutmeg
1½ tablespoons minced fresh ginger
1¾ cups halved Brussels sprouts
1¾ cups small or chopped broccoli florets
4½ cups gently packed mustard greens
4 cups gently packed fresh spinach leaves
¼ cup chopped fresh cilantro
Seasoning of choice, such as sea salt, tamari, liquid aminos, hot sauce, Gomasio (page 171), Pumpkin Dulse (page 173), Tahini Sauce (page 170), Tamarind Sauce (page 169), or Cilantro Mint Chutney (page 151)

=V
↓P
↓K

1. In a large saucepan over medium heat, combine the oil, curry powder, cumin, and nutmeg. Bloom the spices until they smell fragrant, 2 to 3 minutes. Stir in the ginger and cook for 1 minute.

2. Stir in the halved sprouts, broccoli, mustard greens, and spinach, and cook, stirring occasionally, until the greens are wilted, about 3 minutes. Stir in ¾ cup water, cover, and cook until the vegetables are fork-tender, 10 to 12 minutes, stirring occasionally.

3. Remove from the heat and stir in the cilantro. Puree the mixture until relatively smooth with an immersion blender or in an upright blender. If using an upright blender, avoid a blowout by cooling the mixture slightly and partially removing the center lid of the blender. Saag should be thick rather than watery so it flattens out only slightly on the plate. If it is too watery, cook it over low heat, uncovered, until it thickens up a bit. Season with your seasoning of choice and serve warm.

OPTION

- Tri-Spice Mix: Replace the curry powder, cumin, and nutmeg here with a mixture of equal parts (1 teaspoon each) ground cumin, coriander, and turmeric. We keep this tri-spice mix on the Kripalu dining tables at all times. It acts as a great digestive aid (especially for digesting proteins) and helps to improve your metabolism.

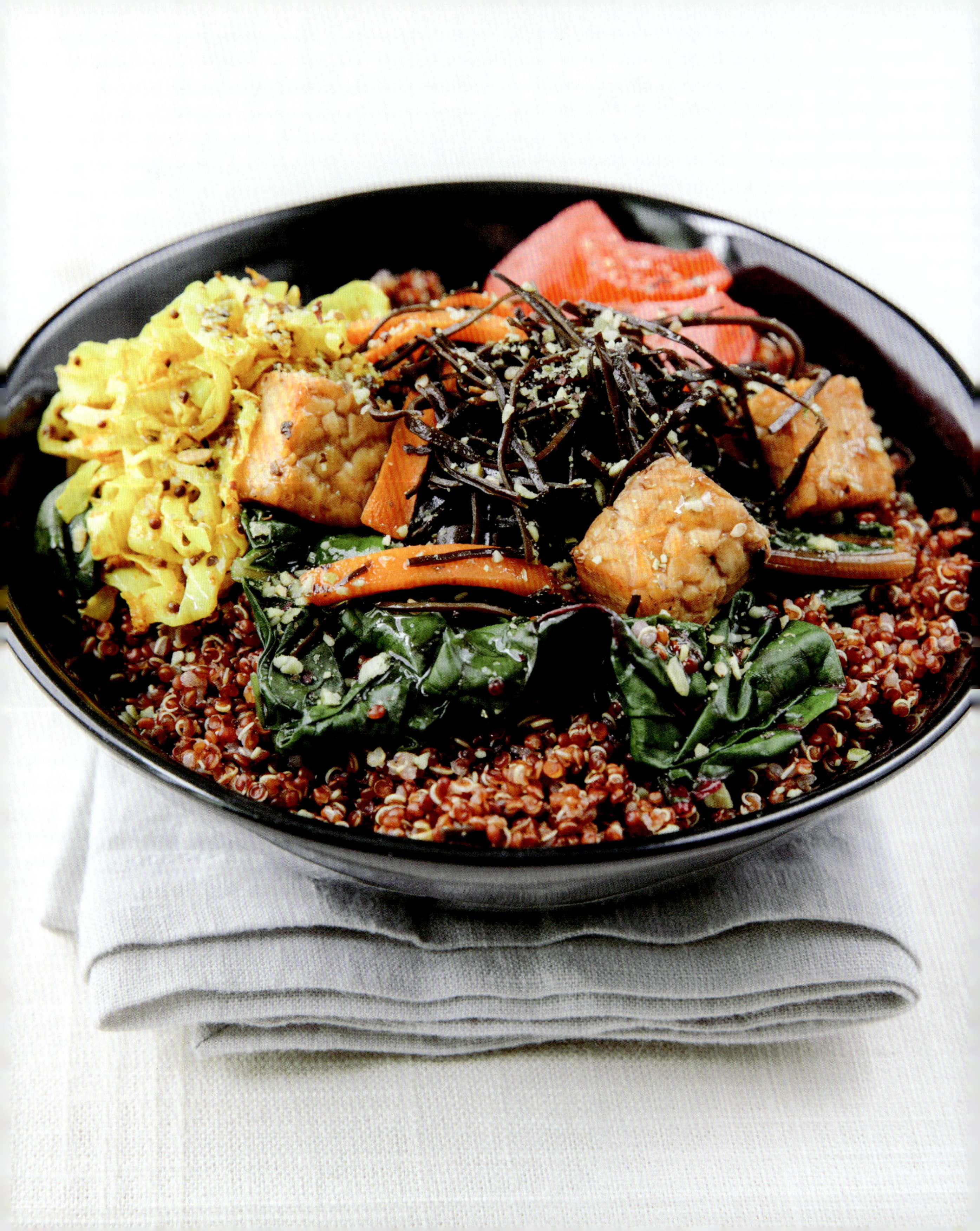

Buddha Bowl

The Buddha Bar at Kripalu offers a variety of foods simply prepared along with various spices, sauces, and condiments. Guests love to build their own Buddha Bowls according to their dietary needs for that day. The bowls themselves are sized to provide enough food to sustain you but not so much that you feel sluggish. Our Buddha Bowls sell like hotcakes in the gift shop, but any 3-cup bowl will do. It's most important to fill your bowl with a balance of colorful greens, grains, vegetables, protein-rich foods, and some nuts, seeds, seasonings, or sauces for color, pop, spice, and crunch.

GRAINS: brown rice, quinoa, or millet

VEGETABLES: steamed, sautéed, roasted, or grilled

SEA GREENS: arame, wakame, or kelp

PICKLES: kimchi, sauerkraut, Umeboshi Pickled Radishes and Greens (page 166)

PROTEIN: cooked beans or legumes, tofu or tempeh

SAUCES: tamari, hot sauce, Tamarind Sauce (page 169), Tahini Sauce (page 170), Cilantro Mint Chutney (page 151)

SEEDS: roasted almonds, roasted pumpkin seeds, Pumpkin Dulse (page 173), Gomasio (page 171)

SPICES: cayenne, turmeric, cumin, coriander, kelp powder, cardamom, ginger, garam masala

OILS: ghee, extra-virgin olive oil, toasted sesame oil

Umeboshi Pickled Radishes and Greens

↑V
=P
↓K

IF YOU'VE NEVER tasted umeboshi (pickled plums), grab a bottle of umeboshi vinegar on your next grocery store run. This unique vinegar tastes salty, sour, fruity, and savory all at once. Plus, it gives pickled radishes a beautiful pale pink color.

Ayurvedic Insight: Kale is bitter and astringent, making it best to enjoy in spring, summer, and late fall.

Serves 4 to 6

1½ cups thinly sliced red radishes
3 tablespoons umeboshi vinegar
3 cups coarsely chopped kale, preferably lacinato
3 cups shredded napa cabbage

1. In a medium sauté pan, combine the radishes and vinegar with just enough water to cover the radishes. Bring to a simmer over medium heat and simmer until the radishes are fork-tender, about 5 minutes.

2. Stir in the kale, cabbage, and ¼ cup water. Return to a simmer, cover, and cook until the greens are just tender, 3 to 4 minutes. Serve.

OPTION

- You can pickle only the radishes in the umeboshi vinegar as described, and then keep the pickles in the refrigerator for about a week. Don't be alarmed if the radishes begin to smell pungent. That is the aroma of beneficial lactic acid bacteria developing as the radishes ferment.

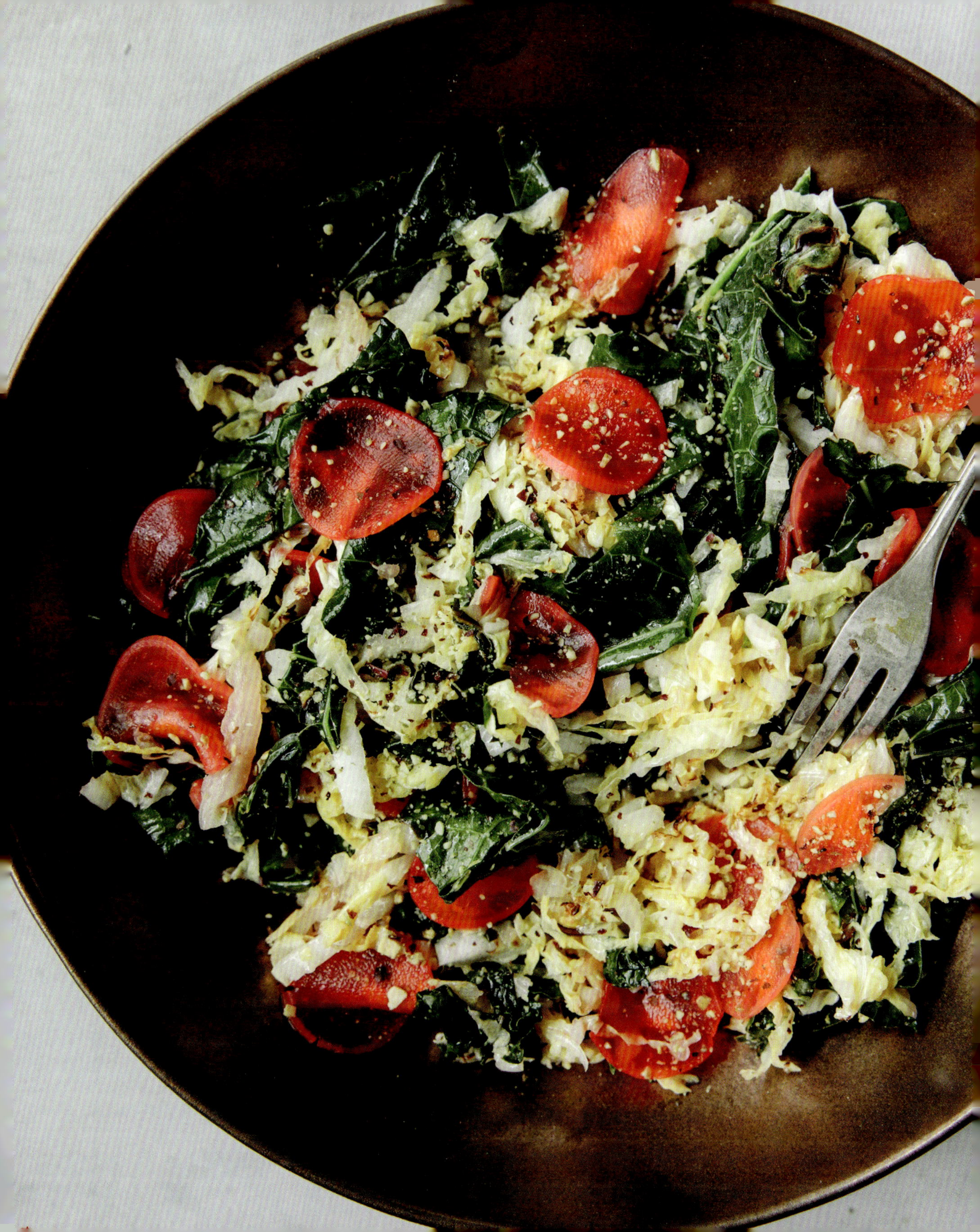

Spiced Braised Cabbage

=V

↓P

↓K

CABBAGE AND MUSTARD are popular in German cooking, and this bright yellow dish takes that combo closer to India. Turmeric, coriander, and ginger round out the spices, while gentle braising mellows the sulfurous aromas of cooked cabbage.

Ayurvedic Insight: The dry qualities of cabbage help to absorb excess dampness, and the warming spices here mitigate the vegetable's natural cooling properties.

Serves 4 to 6

1 tablespoon extra-virgin olive oil or ghee
1 teaspoon ground turmeric
1 teaspoon ground coriander
1 teaspoon brown mustard seeds
1/2 teaspoon paprika
1 teaspoon minced fresh ginger
1 small head of green cabbage, shredded
2 teaspoons fresh lemon juice
Seasoning of choice, such as sea salt, tamari, liquid aminos, hot sauce, Gomasio (page 171), Pumpkin Dulse (page 173), Tahini Sauce (page 170), Tamarind Sauce (page 169), or Cilantro Mint Chutney (page 151)

1. Combine the oil, turmeric, coriander, mustard seeds, and paprika in a large soup pot. Bloom the spices over medium heat until fragrant (the mustard may begin to pop), 2 to 3 minutes. Stir in the ginger and cook for 1 minute.

2. Stir in the cabbage and ½ cup water, then cover the pot and gently braise the cabbage, stirring occasionally, until tender, 12 to 15 minutes.

3. Uncover and simmer to evaporate any residual liquid left in the pan. Just before serving, stir in the lemon juice and season with your seasoning of choice.

OPTION

- Replace the green cabbage with almost any other cabbage, such as bok choy or napa cabbage.

Tamarind Sauce

YOU COULD THINK of this as Ayurvedic BBQ sauce. It's sweet, sour, and just a little spicy. You also get a little crunch from the cumin seeds. Drizzle this sauce over rice, beans, and vegetables. It works great when drizzled side by side with creamy Tahini Sauce (page 170).

Ayurvedic Insight: Tamarind is the pod-like fruit of a leguminous tree. It tastes both sweet and sour, making it perfect for vata types. Spoon this sauce over bean dishes to improve their digestibility.

Makes about 2 cups

1 tablespoon sunflower oil
2 teaspoons cumin seeds
1/8 teaspoon crushed red pepper flakes
3/4 cup tamarind paste
3/4 cup rapadura (panela) or packed dark brown sugar
1/2 teaspoon fine sea salt

1. Combine the oil, cumin seeds, and red pepper flakes in a small saucepan over medium heat. Let the spices bloom until they are fragrant, 1 to 2 minutes.

2. Stir in the tamarind, rapadura, salt, and 1½ cups water. Bring to a boil over high heat and boil until the liquid reduces in volume by about half, 3 to 5 minutes. The sauce should cool to a thick yet pourable consistency similar to thin pancake batter. Let cool before serving. Use immediately or refrigerate for up to 1 week. Return to room temperature before serving.

↓V
↑P
↑K

Tahini Sauce

↓V

↑P

↑K

YOU'VE PROBABLY HAD some version of this creamy sesame sauce drizzled on falafel or another Middle Eastern dish. Our version is supersimple: just tahini, lemon, and salt. Spoon it over steamed vegetables, rice, beans, or pan-seared fish.

Ayurvedic Insight: Sesame seeds are considered too heating for pitta types and too heavy for kapha. But vata types will enjoy this sauce.

Makes about 2 cups

1 cup tahini

1/4 cup fresh lemon juice

1/4 teaspoon fine sea salt

Put the tahini, lemon juice, and salt in a medium bowl. Using a fork or whisk, gradually stir in ⅔ cup water until the mixture is smooth. Use immediately or refrigerate for up to 1 week. Return to room temperature before serving.

Gomasio

MADE WITH GROUND sesame seeds and salt, this seasoning is deceptively compelling. Roasting the sesame and salt brings out lots of flavors. Make this blend a kitchen staple and you'll find yourself sprinkling it on vegetables, soups, and other dishes instead of plain salt.

Ayurvedic Insight: Seeds carry within them the potential for future life, so enjoy their deeply nourishing properties. This seasoning blend is particularly high in bone-strengthening calcium.

Makes about 1 cup

1 cup sesame seeds

3/4 teaspoon sea salt

1. Preheat the oven to 350°F.

2. Combine the sesame seeds and salt on a sheet pan and bake until the seeds are lightly toasted and beginning to brown, 4 to 6 minutes. Let cool completely. You want the sesame seeds to be cool when you chop everything.

3. Transfer the mixture to a food processor or spice grinder and pulse until the seeds resemble coarse meal. To store, cover and refrigerate the gomasio for up to 4 weeks.

↓V
↑P
↑K

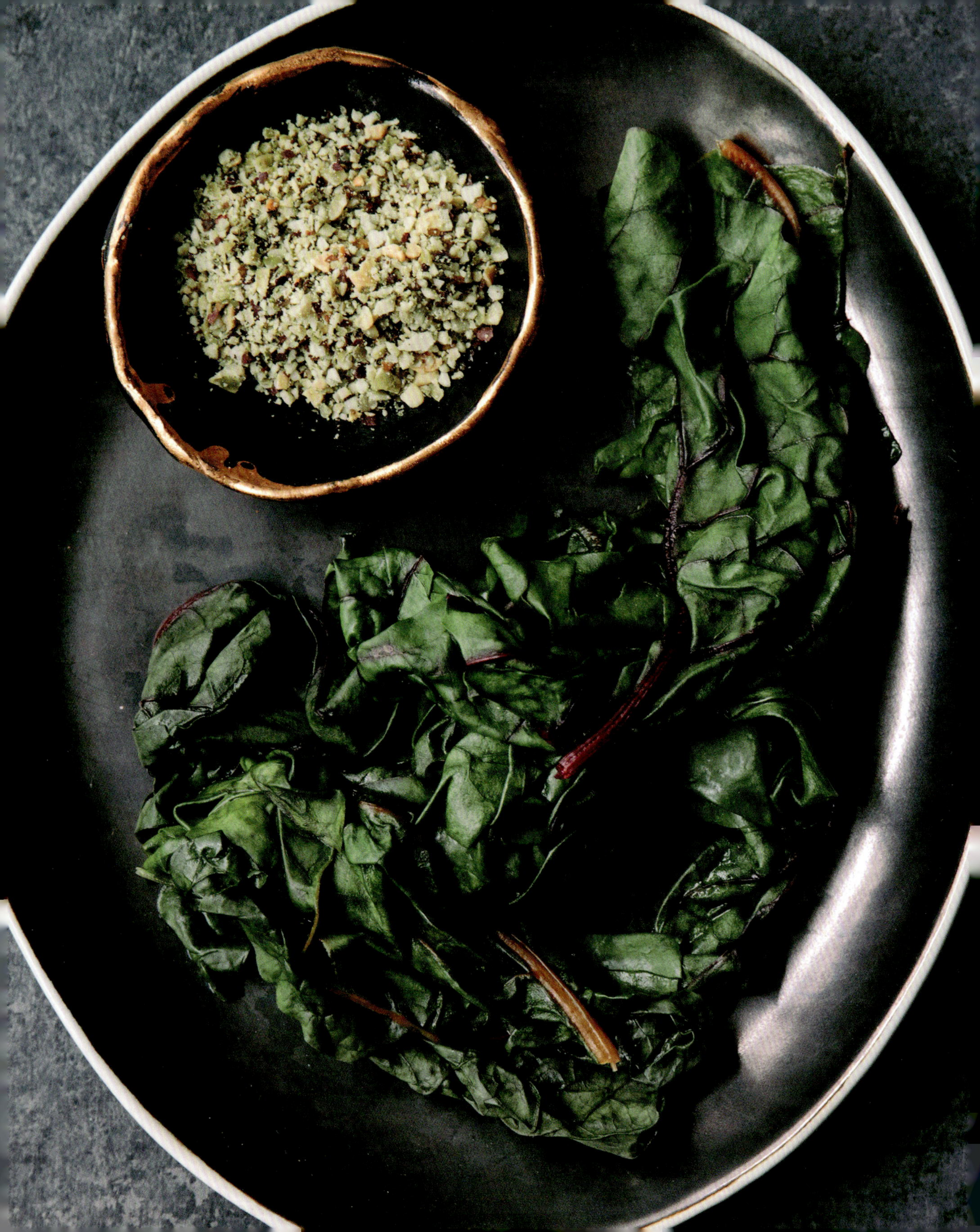

Pumpkin Dulse

HERE'S ONE FROM the macrobiotic archives. The minerals in pumpkin seeds and in the sea vegetable called dulse make this a seasoning blend with numerous health benefits. You also get some good crunch from the ground pumpkin seeds.

Ayurvedic Insight: Seeds are balancing for all doshas, but this condiment is best enjoyed by those with colder, drier constitutions.

Makes about 1½ cups

2 cups hulled raw pumpkin seeds

1/2 cup dulse flakes

1/2 teaspoon umeboshi vinegar

1. Preheat the oven to 350°F.

2. Combine the pumpkin seeds, dulse, and vinegar on a rimmed baking sheet until evenly mixed. Bake until the pumpkin seeds are lightly toasted and fragrant, 6 to 8 minutes. Let cool completely. You want the pumpkin seeds to be cool when you chop everything.

3. Transfer the cooled mixture to a food processor or spice grinder and pulse until the seeds are finely chopped to the size of grains of rice. Use immediately or refrigerate for up to 4 weeks.

↓V
=P
=K

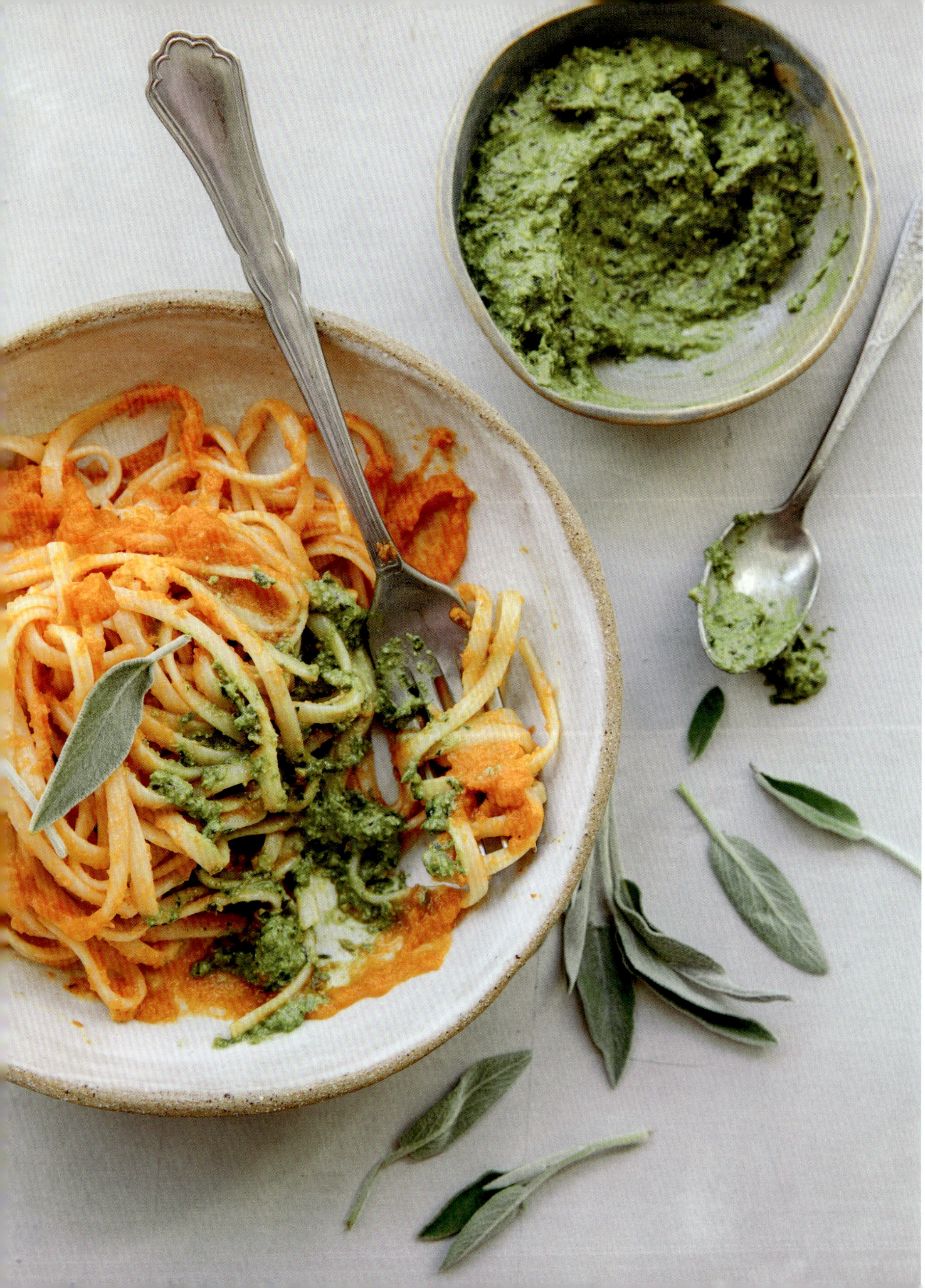

MAIN DISHES

While India remains at the heart of Ayurvedic health principles, Kripalu embraces culinary traditions from around the globe. After all, healing foods are ubiquitous. From Chinese stir-fries and Thai curries to Italian pastas and Israeli sauces, this chapter reflects the diversity of flavors to be enjoyed on a diet of balance and moderation.

On the whole, these dishes are more substantial than those in other chapters. But that does not mean this is the dinner chapter. Many of the dishes here, such as Garden Pea, Leek, and Potato Cakes with Avocado Mint Raita (page 177), can be easily made ahead and enjoyed for lunch—even at your place of work. Likewise, dishes like Coconut Chana Saag (page 180) keep for days in the fridge and can be reheated at a moment's notice for a midday meal.

If you are looking for healthy main dishes for a dinner party, recipes like Pan-Seared Shrimp with Spicy Cilantro Pesto and Butternut Squash (page 209) and Adobo-Rubbed Chicken with Avocado Crème (page 217) will fill the bill. Likewise, Roasted Chicken with Sesame Cider Glaze (page 220) and Braised Sumac Chicken and Lentils with Za'atar Yogurt Sauce (page 222) will satisfy a hungry family for Sunday dinner.

Many of these recipes are easily adaptable for different dietary needs and restrictions. We pay close attention to gluten-free, grain-free, nut-free, dairy-free, soy-free, sugar-free, vegan, vegetarian, paleo, no salt, no oil, clean, and low-FODMAP (easily digestible) diets. We respect everyone's individual restrictions and choice, and the recipes here include several options for adapting the dish to your needs, whether that means using tofu instead of chicken to make Adobo-Rubbed Tofu with Avocado Crème (page 217) or making gluten-free Sweet Potato, Kale, and Parsley Pesto Pizza (page 189) with our Gluten-Free Pizza Dough (page 91). We even include suggestions for adapting half the recipe for those times when you have mixed company at the table.

Keep in mind that Ayurveda recommends eating your largest meal of the day at lunchtime. That is when the sun is highest in the sky and feels the warmest to our bodies. Since we are reflections and components of the living universe around us, our *agni*, or digestive fire, is also at its warmest and strongest at that time of day. Of course, American culture does not always promote a leisurely lunch—especially during the workweek. If that is the case for you, take time on the weekend to enjoy a long, relaxing lunch. In the evenings, favor smaller meals to match the body's lower activity during the sunset hours. A lighter evening meal can do wonders for your health. Going to bed with a full belly can slow digestion, lead to weight gain, and leave you feeling lethargic upon waking. On the other hand, entering sleep after fully digesting a nourishing meal can help you feel refreshed and energetic the following morning.

Garden Pea, Leek, and Potato Cakes with Avocado Mint Raita

↑V
↓P
↓K

WITH MINT, NEW POTATOES, and English peas, this dish is all about the refreshing flavors of spring. It's based on *aloo tikki*, the classic Indian street snack. Instead of deep-frying the cakes to make fritters, I form cakes and bake them in the oven. I work some fresh green avocado into the creamy raita, which is usually made with yogurt alone.

Ayurvedic Insight: The dryness of peas and potatoes makes an excellent antidote to the dampness of the spring season. A light touch with spices gives these cakes a little warmth without making them too spicy.

Serves 6 to 8

CAKES

1½ pounds new potatoes, coarsely chopped (about 5 cups)

2 tablespoons ghee or extra-virgin olive oil

1½ cups finely chopped cleaned leeks

¼ cup minced shallots

1½ teaspoons curry powder

½ teaspoon ground cumin

½ teaspoon ground coriander

1½ teaspoons garam masala

1 teaspoon minced fresh garlic

1 teaspoon minced fresh ginger

¼ cup fine corn flour

1 large egg

1 teaspoon fine sea salt

½ teaspoon freshly ground black pepper

2 cups fresh English peas, steamed until tender, or frozen and thawed petite peas

AVOCADO MINT RAITA

1 avocado, pitted and peeled

½ cup plain yogurt (not Greek yogurt)

2 teaspoons fresh lemon juice

½ cup ¼-inch diced red bell peppers, plus extra for garnish

¼ cup chopped fresh mint

¼ teaspoon fine sea salt

¼ teaspoon freshly ground black pepper

4 ounces fresh arugula leaves, for serving

1. For the cakes, place the potatoes in a small saucepan with water to cover by about 1 inch. Cover and bring to a gentle simmer over medium heat, then simmer uncovered until a knife slides in and out of a potato easily, about 15 minutes.

2. Meanwhile, heat a large ovenproof sauté pan over medium-low heat. When hot, put 1 tablespoon of the ghee and the leeks and shallots in the pan, tossing to coat. Cook gently until the vegetables are very soft and translucent, about 12 minutes.

3. Stir in the curry powder, cumin, coriander, and garam masala and cook until fragrant, 1 to

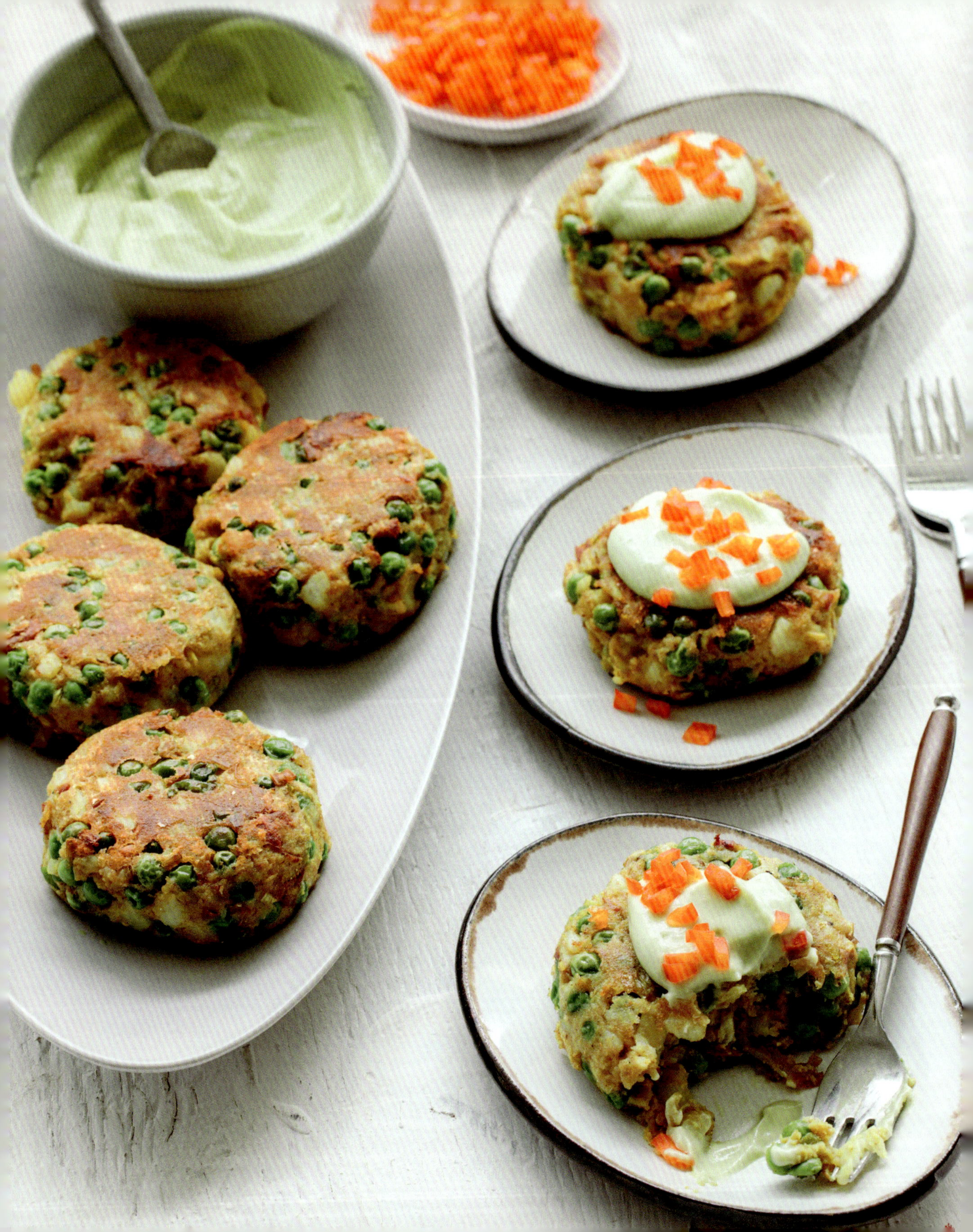

2 minutes. Stir in the garlic and ginger and cook for 1 minute. Remove from the heat and let cool.

4. Preheat the oven to 350°F.

5. Drain the potatoes, spread out on a sheet pan, and let cool until just warm and fairly dry looking, 15 minutes or so. Mash the potatoes right on the sheet pan with a potato masher or sturdy fork until they are mostly smooth with a few small potato chunks remaining. Stir in the leek mixture along with the corn flour, egg, salt, and pepper. Mix well, then fold in the peas. Scrape the mixture to one side of the sheet pan and form it into eight to nine 4-ounce patties about 3 inches across and 1 inch thick.

6. Heat the large sauté pan over medium heat. When hot, heat the remaining 1 tablespoon of the ghee and add as many patties as you can fit in the pan. If your pan won't hold all the patties, heat another sauté pan as well with some of the ghee. Cook the patties until golden brown on the bottom, 3 to 5 minutes. Flip the patties and transfer the pan(s) to the oven until the cakes are crispy on the edges but soft inside, 10 to 12 minutes.

7. For the raita, place the avocado, yogurt, and lemon juice in a food processor and puree until smooth. Fold in the peppers and mint and then taste the mixture, adding more lemon juice, salt, and/or black pepper until it tastes good to you.

8. Divide the arugula among 6 to 8 plates or a platter. Arrange the patties over the arugula and spoon on the raita. Garnish with the reserved diced bell pepper.

OPTIONS

- For the most fiber and minerals, leave the skins on the new potatoes.
- If you can't find corn flour (fine cornmeal), you can use chickpea flour instead.
- For a vegan version, replace the egg with a mixture of 3 tablespoons flax meal, 3 tablespoons water, and 1 tablespoon olive oil. For the raita, replace the yogurt with nondairy yogurt or ½ cup mashed avocado.
- To serve these as hors d'oeuvres, form smaller patties about 1½ inches wide and ½ inch thick.

Coconut Chana Saag

=V

↓P

↓K

EVEN MEAT EATERS LOVE this quick and easy vegetarian dish because it is approachable, satisfying food. The flavor comes mostly from fresh ginger, minced garlic, ground coriander, cumin, and garam masala (a warm Indian spice mix). Many Indian restaurants enrich their saag with heavy cream, but we use coconut milk so those who don't eat dairy products can also enjoy it. Vegetable Biryani (page 246) makes the ideal accompaniment.

Ayurvedic Insight: Sweet, bitter, and astringent, this dish is perfect for absorbing excess moisture in the spring and summer. The spices here warm the naturally cool spinach and coconut milk.

Serves 4 (about 5 cups total)

1/2 large onion, diced

1 tablespoon coconut oil

1 1/2 teaspoons finely chopped fresh garlic

1 1/2 teaspoons minced fresh ginger

1 1/2 teaspoons ground coriander

1 1/2 teaspoons ground cumin

1 1/2 teaspoons garam masala

1 1/2 teaspoons chili powder

2 cups crushed tomatoes

1 1/2 cups canned full-fat 100% coconut milk

1 1/2 cups chopped fresh spinach

2 cups cooked or rinsed and drained canned chickpeas

1 teaspoon fine sea salt

2 tablespoons chopped fresh cilantro

1. Heat a large, deep sauté pan over medium-low heat. Put the onions and oil in the pan, shaking it to coat the onions. Cook gently until the onions are translucent, 5 to 8 minutes. Stir in the garlic, ginger, coriander, cumin, garam masala, and chili powder, and cook until the spices are fragrant, 1 to 2 minutes. Stir in the tomatoes and bring to a simmer over medium heat, then reduce the heat to medium-low and simmer gently until the flavors blend, 8 to 10 minutes.

2. Stir in the coconut milk, spinach, and chickpeas, and simmer over medium heat until the spinach wilts, about 5 minutes. Stir in the salt and cilantro, reserving some cilantro to garnish the plates. Serve hot, garnished with cilantro.

OPTIONS

- To cook dried chickpeas, soak about ⅔ cup dried chickpeas in water to cover for 8 to 24 hours. Drain, cover with 1 inch fresh water, and cook until the chickpeas are tender, about 1 hour. You should get about 2 cups cooked.
- You can replace the fresh spinach with ½ cup thawed frozen spinach. Or use 1½ cups

chopped kale, chard, or whatever sturdy greens you have on hand.

- You could make a double batch of this dish and freeze it. Prepare it as directed, but leave out the spinach and coconut milk. Freeze it, then reheat it in a sauté pan with the coconut milk and spinach until the spinach wilts.
- To add meat to half the dish, season 8 ounces chicken or peeled and deveined shrimp with salt and pepper. Sauté the chicken or shrimp in a separate sauté pan in a little coconut oil over medium heat until the chicken is no longer pink in the center and reaches 160°F internal temperature or the shrimp is firm and no longer pink. Add to the dish just before serving. For a paleo version, replace all of the chickpeas with chicken or shrimp.

Sweet and Spicy Vegetable Stir-Fry

↓V
↑P
↓K

EVERY COOK NEEDS a reliable vegetable stir-fry in her or his cooking repertoire. This is it: an ideal last-minute, kitchen-sink meal. Toss in all those bits and pieces from your produce drawer, whether they be carrots, bell peppers, celery . . . whatever. Just cut everything small and have your sauce ready to go. The actual cooking takes less than 5 minutes. Serve over cooked rice or noodles.

Ayurvedic Insight: The warming spices in this dish balance the cold qualities of both vata and kapha, and overall, the dish is not too heavy to bother kapha. Enjoy it in the winter when the sweet, sour, and salty combo is most welcome.

Serves 4

- 1/4 cup tamari
- 2 teaspoons coconut sugar or pure maple syrup
- 2 teaspoons brown rice vinegar
- 2 tablespoons toasted sesame oil
- 1/2 cup carrot coins, cut on an angle
- 1/2 cup small broccoli florets
- 1/2 cup 1/2-inch diced red bell peppers
- 1/2 cup sliced bok choy
- 1/2 cup 1/2-inch diced sugar snap peas
- 1/2 cup 1/2-inch diced pineapple
- 1 tablespoon finely chopped garlic
- 2 teaspoons minced fresh ginger
- 2 scallions (whites minced and greens sliced crosswise)
- 1/4 teaspoon crushed red pepper flakes
- 2 teaspoons cornstarch
- 1/2 cup roasted peanuts
- 2 teaspoons toasted sesame seeds

1. In a small measuring cup or bowl, combine the tamari, coconut sugar, and vinegar. Set aside. Have all the other ingredients prepped and ready to go.

2. Heat a wok or large sauté pan over high heat for 3 minutes. Swirl 1 tablespoon of the sesame oil around the pan, then add the carrots, broccoli, peppers, bok choy, snap peas, and pineapple all at once. Stir-fry over high heat until the vegetables are crisp-tender, 1 to 2 minutes.

3. Stir in the garlic, ginger, minced scallion whites, and red pepper flakes, and cook until fragrant, 30 seconds. Stir in the tamari mixture.

4. Quickly mix ½ cup cold water and the cornstarch with a fork, then add to the vegetables, stirring to coat. Cook, stirring, until the sauce comes to a boil, thickens, and coats the vegetables. Remove from the heat.

5. Fold in the nuts. Serve garnished with the sliced scallion greens and sesame seeds.

OPTION

- To add some protein, use 1 pound finely sliced chicken or peeled and deveined shrimp. Cook the chicken or shrimp in the wok first over medium-high heat until the chicken is no longer pink in the center and reaches 160°F internal temperature or the shrimp is firm and no longer pink, then remove and reserve. Proceed with the recipe, adding the protein at the very end. For a mixed crowd of diners, cook the protein separately.

Harissa Cauliflower Steaks with Castelvetrano Olive, Raisin, and Caper Tapenade

=V
↓P
↓K

TUNISIA'S MOST POPULAR CONDIMENT, harissa is a hot chili paste redolent with aromas of ground caraway and coriander. Look for dried versions in the spice aisle of markets like Whole Foods. I like to mix in just a little oil and spread the fragrant paste over slabs, or "steaks," of cauliflower. With the tapenade, you taste sweet, tart, salty, pungent, crunchy, and aromatic all in a single bite.

Ayurvedic Insight: Cauliflower is substantial enough to feel like a meal in itself, and this dish makes an excellent dinner option that won't weigh you down before sleep.

Serves 4

CAULIFLOWER STEAKS

1 tablespoon dry harissa spice mix (Frontier brand is good)

1/2 teaspoon fine sea salt

3 tablespoons grapeseed oil or sunflower oil

1 head of cauliflower, cut lengthwise into steaks about 1 inch thick

TAPENADE

1/2 cup pitted and finely chopped Castelvetrano or other green olives

1/2 cup golden raisins

1/4 cup almonds, toasted and chopped

Grated zest and juice of 1 lemon

1 tablespoon extra-virgin olive oil

1 1/2 teaspoons chopped fresh cilantro

1 teaspoon chopped fresh flat-leaf parsley

1 teaspoon minced scallion greens

1/2 teaspoon small drained capers

1/8 teaspoon freshly ground black pepper

1. Preheat the oven to 350°F.

2. For the cauliflower steaks, mix the harissa, salt, and oil in a cup to make a paste. Spread the paste all over both sides of the cauliflower steaks.

3. For the tapenade, combine all of the ingredients in a small bowl.

4. Heat a very large ovenproof sauté pan (or 2 large ones) over high heat for 1 minute. You'll need enough space for all the steaks. Lay the steaks in the pan(s) in a single layer, reduce the heat to medium-high, and sear the steaks until the undersides are golden brown and caramelized, 1 to 2 minutes. Flip the steaks and place the pan(s) in the oven. Cook until the cauliflower is fork-tender in the center, 10 to 15 minutes.

5. Remove from the oven and transfer the steaks to a serving platter or individual plates. Spoon on the tapenade.

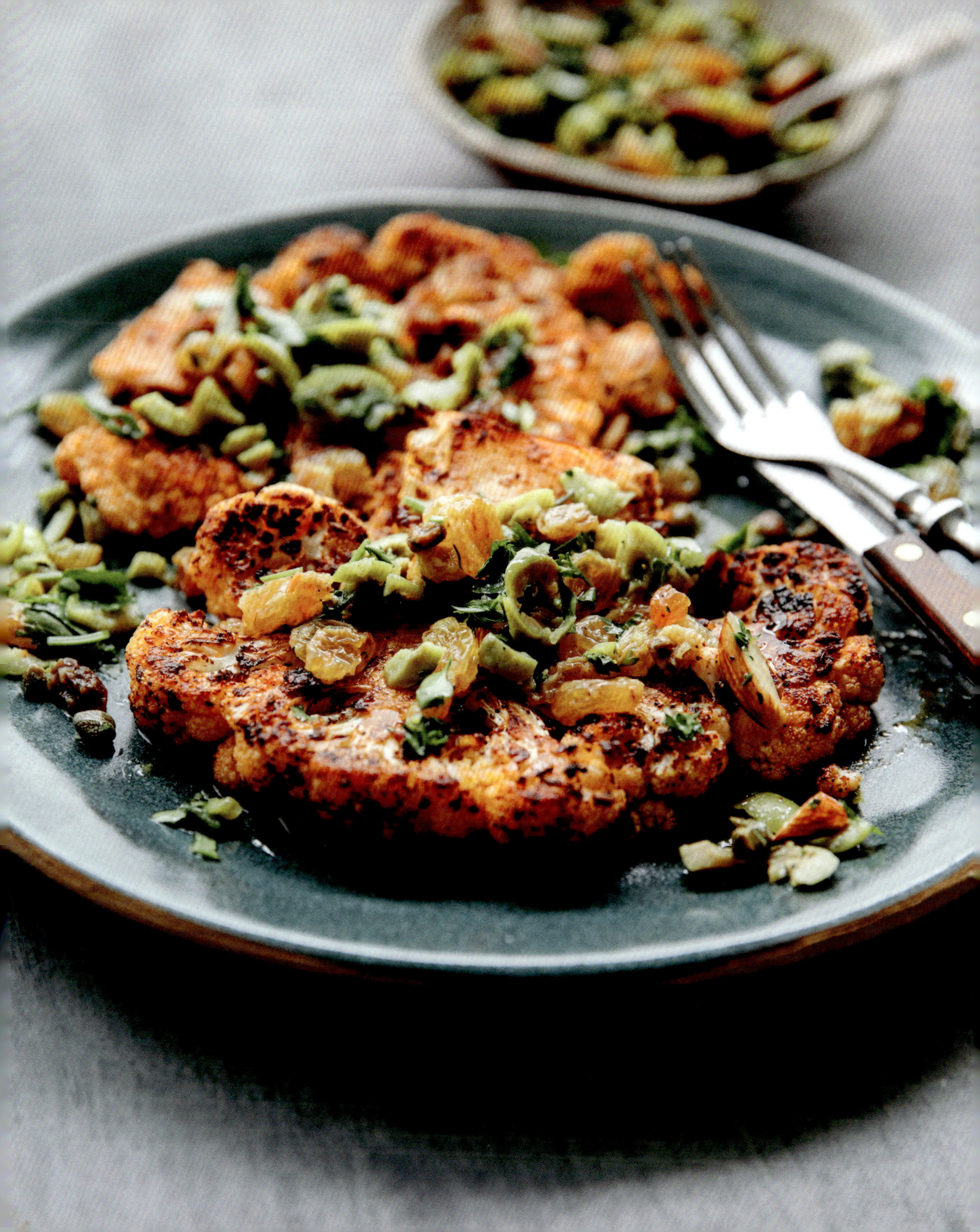

OPTION

- Instead of making steaks to serve as a light main dish, you could make a side dish by breaking the cauliflower into florets. Toss the florets with the harissa paste and roast on a sheet pan in a 425°F oven until golden brown, about 20 minutes. Serve over the tapenade. Even if you do make steaks, you can roast any leftover cauliflower florets this way.

Summer Vegetable Tian with Chèvre and Smoked Sea Salt

=V
=P
=K

TIAN IS A CLASSIC southern French dish from the Provencal region. It is similar to lasagna but with layers of sliced vegetables instead of pasta. Sweet potatoes make this one more contemporary and perfectly balance the saltiness of olives and the richness of goat cheese. Smoked salt lends just the right head-swirling aroma.

Ayurvedic Insight: With so many summer vegetables in it, this nourishing dish can be enjoyed in moderation by all doshas.

Serves 6 to 8

1 small eggplant (12 ounces), sliced into rounds 1/4 inch thick

1 zucchini (8 ounces), sliced lengthwise 1/4 inch thick

1 yellow squash (8 ounces), sliced lengthwise 1/4 inch thick

1/2 teaspoon fine sea salt

5 teaspoons extra-virgin olive oil, plus more for the pan and for drizzling

2 cups thinly sliced cleaned leeks

1/4 cup fresh thyme leaves or 2 tablespoons dried

1 sweet potato (12 ounces), sliced into rounds 1/8 inch thick

1 teaspoon smoked sea salt, such as Maldon

1/4 teaspoon freshly ground black pepper

6 ounces chèvre (soft goat cheese), crumbled (about 1 1/2 cups)

1/4 cup pitted kalamata olives, coarsely chopped

3 large tomatoes, sliced lengthwise 1/4 inch thick

6 ounces fresh arugula leaves (about 6 cups), for serving

1. Toss the eggplant, zucchini, and yellow squash with sea salt and place in a colander in the sink to drain for at least 30 minutes and up to 1 hour.

2. Preheat the oven to 450°F. Oil a shallow 2-quart baking dish.

3. Heat a large sauté pan over medium heat. Put in the leeks and 2 teaspoons of the olive oil, shaking the pan to coat the leeks. Cook gently until they are tender, 5 to 6 minutes. Stir in 1 tablespoon of the fresh thyme or ½ tablespoon dried, then spread the leeks evenly across the bottom of the prepared baking dish.

4. Use your hands to rub the sweet potatoes and the drained eggplant, zucchini, and yellow squash with the remaining 3 teaspoons olive oil. Toss with the smoked salt, pepper, and remaining 3 tablespoons fresh thyme or 1½ tablespoons dried.

5. Next, layer the vegetables over the leeks in the baking dish, dividing the goat cheese be-

tween each layer and pressing down to compact the vegetables as you build the tian. Use the following order: sweet potatoes, goat cheese, eggplant, goat cheese, zucchini, goat cheese, yellow squash, goat cheese, olives, and tomatoes.

6. Press a piece of parchment paper on top of the vegetables across the entire surface, then cover the dish with foil. Bake until the sweet potatoes are tender but not mushy, 25 to 30 minutes. Remove the foil and parchment paper and continue baking until the tomatoes are lightly browned, about 10 minutes.

7. Let the tian cool for 10 minutes and slice into 6 to 8 portions. Serve warm over a bed of arugula and drizzle a little olive oil over each portion. You can also serve this dish at room temperature.

OPTIONS

- For a smoother texture, peel the eggplant.
- For a dairy-free, vegan, or paleo version, omit the goat cheese or replace it with vegan cream cheese such as Kite Hill or Follow Your Heart.

Sweet Potato, Kale, and Parsley Pesto Pizza

EVERY OTHER THURSDAY, we offer pizza for lunch at Kripalu. After seeing less familiar foods throughout the week, guests are happy to have a slice or two. The "sauce" is a puree of sweet potatoes topped with fontina cheese, kale, red peppers, and a drizzle of parsley pesto. To simplify things, this pizza is baked in a rectangular sheet pan, but you could shape it into two rounds if you'd like.

Ayurvedic Insight: Cold winter days are the best time to enjoy this warming, oily, nourishing pizza. The sourdough crust makes it a great choice for vata. Pittas with strong digestion will enjoy this pizza in winter but should avoid it in the summer.

↓V
=P
↑K

Makes one rectangular sheet pan pizza (18 x 13 inches)

2 pounds Sourdough Whole-Grain Pizza Dough (page 90)
2 cups peeled and chopped sweet potatoes
2 teaspoons finely chopped garlic
1/4 teaspoon ground cinnamon
1/2 teaspoon fine sea salt
1/4 teaspoon freshly ground black pepper
1/2 cup chopped fresh flat-leaf parsley
3 tablespoons roasted cashews
1/4 cup extra-virgin olive oil
1 1/2 teaspoons nutritional yeast
Oil spray
All-purpose flour, for dusting
2 cups shredded kale, preferably lacinato
2 cups shredded fontina cheese
1/2 cup 1/2-inch diced red bell peppers

1. Preheat the oven to 450°F. If you have a baking stone, preheat the stone on the center rack of the oven for at least 45 minutes.

2. Let the dough rest at room temperature while the oven preheats. Have all your toppings prepped and ready to go.

3. For the sweet potato puree, put the sweet potatoes in a medium saucepan and add water to cover. Bring to a gentle simmer over medium heat and simmer until the potatoes are just fork-tender, 6 to 8 minutes. Drain in a colander, then transfer to a food processor. Add the garlic, cinnamon, ¼ teaspoon of the salt, and ⅛ teaspoon of the pepper. Process to a smooth, spreadable puree, scraping down the sides once or twice. Use immediately or cover and keep at room temperature for a few hours.

4. For the pesto, combine the parsley, cashews, oil, nutritional yeast, remaining ¼ teaspoon salt, and remaining ⅛ teaspoon pepper in a small food processor or blender. Blend to a rough puree, scraping down the sides once or twice. If the pesto is too thick to drizzle, stir in a little water. Use immediately or keep at room temperature for a few hours.

5. Lightly spray an 18 x 13-inch sheet pan with oil. Lightly flour a work surface and place the

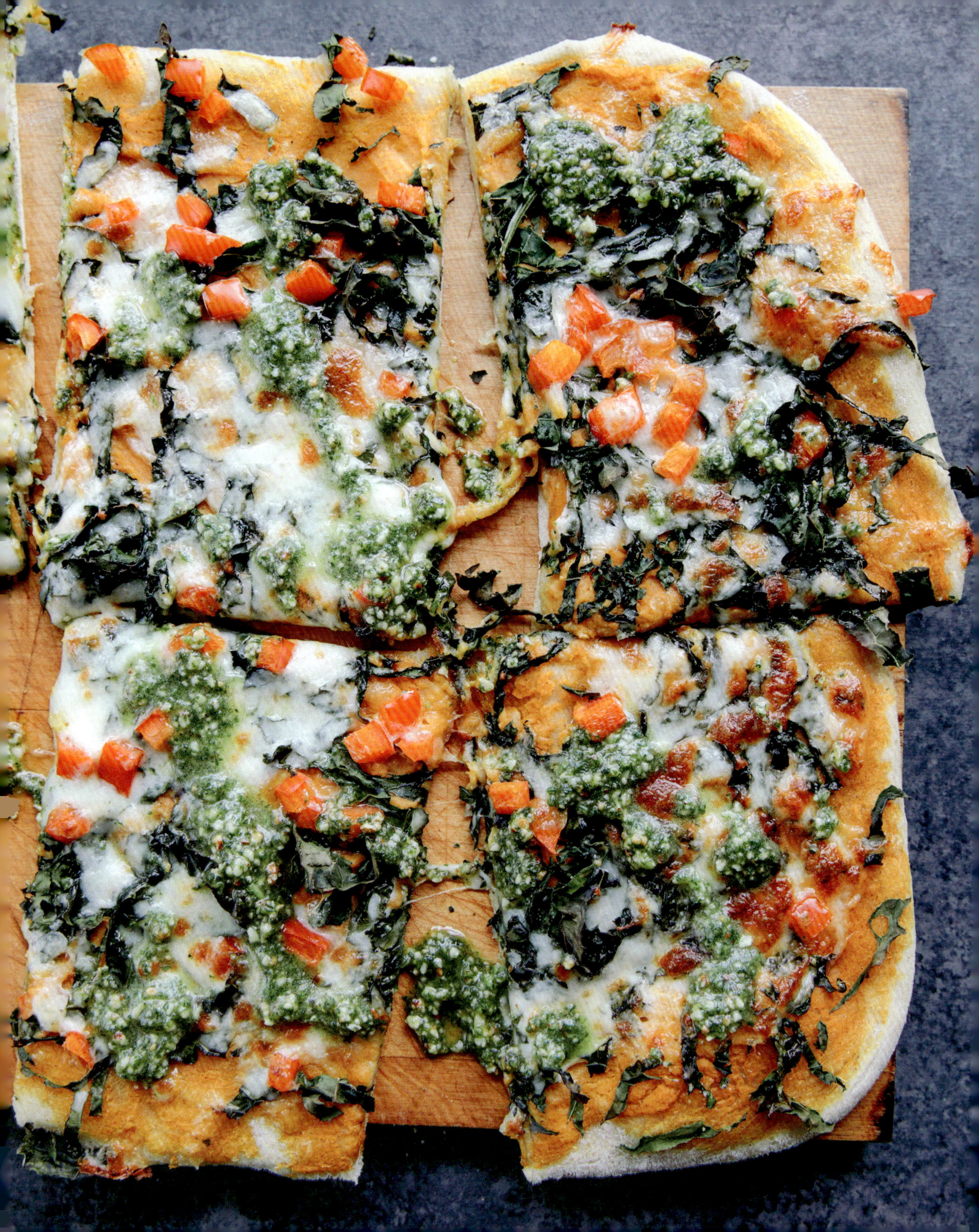

dough on it. Dust the dough with flour and roll it out to a thick rectangle slightly smaller than the pan dimensions. Carefully transfer the dough to the pan, then press it into the pan all the way to the edges.

6. Spread the sweet potato puree evenly over the dough, covering the entire surface with no rim. You should have only a thin layer of the puree. Evenly scatter on the kale, fontina, and bell peppers. Place the sheet pan on the rack or the stone, and bake until the pizza is puffed and well browned on the edges and the cheese melts, 10 to 15 minutes. Drizzle on the pesto, cut into 12 rectangles, and serve.

OPTIONS

- You could use butternut squash instead of sweet potatoes here. Or, if you have leftover roasted squash, puree it with the cinnamon and garlic. You could also bake the potatoes instead of steaming them.
- For a vegan version, you could use vegan cheese. At Kripalu, we simply skip the cheese and double the pesto.
- To make round pizzas, divide the dough in half and press each half on a floured work surface into a circle 12 to 14 inches in diameter. Increase the oven heat to 500°F and bake the pizzas directly on a preheated baking stone. Turn on the broiler just before loading the pizza into the oven to help brown the top.
- For gluten-free pizza, replace the sourdough with Gluten-Free Pizza Dough (page 91). Parbake the dough as directed there, then add the toppings listed here, and bake until they are heated through.
- For a final flourish, make balsamic syrup: Simmer 2 tablespoons balsamic vinegar in a small saucepan until slightly thickened and reduced to about 1 tablespoon. Let cool, then drizzle the balsamic syrup over the pizza just before serving.

Linguine with Pumpkin Sage "Alfredo" and Kale Pesto

=V

↓P

↓K

ONE YEAR, WE SERVED pumpkin gnocchi with sage brown butter sauce in the fall, and our guests loved it. To lighten the dish, I replaced the butter with oil, turned the pumpkin and sage into a creamy sauce, and tossed it with linguine. Now, our guests love it even more. The pumpkin provides a healthy serving of beta-carotene to help boost your immune system, strengthen your eyes, and ward off cancer and heart disease.

Ayurvedic Insight: Kale and butternut squash help to dry out excess fluids in the body. To make the dish more kapha balancing, use gluten-free pasta.

Serves 6

- 4 cups 1/2-inch diced peeled pumpkin or butternut squash
- 1 1/2 teaspoons ground cinnamon
- 4 teaspoons extra-virgin olive oil
- 1/2 cup 1/4-inch diced onions
- 1 tablespoon finely chopped garlic
- 1/8 teaspoon crushed red pepper flakes
- 2 tablespoons dry white wine or lemon juice
- 2 cups Vegetable Stock (page 281) or store-bought stock
- 1/2 teaspoon fine sea salt
- 1/8 teaspoon freshly ground black pepper
- 1 1/2 teaspoons chopped fresh sage
- 1 pound linguine, bucatini, or another strand pasta
- 1 cup Kale Pesto (recipe follows)

1. Preheat the oven to 350°F.

2. Toss the pumpkin, cinnamon, and 2 teaspoons of the oil on a sheet pan. Rub the pumpkin by hand until evenly coated with oil. Spread it in a single layer and roast until fork-tender, about 25 minutes.

3. Meanwhile, heat a large saucepan over medium-low heat. Put in the onions and remaining 2 teaspoons oil, shaking the pan to coat the onions. Cook gently until the onions are translucent but not browned, 4 to 6 minutes. Stir in the garlic and red pepper flakes and cook for 1 minute. Stir in the roasted pumpkin and cook over low heat for 5 minutes.

4. Add the wine, stirring to deglaze the pan and capture all the flavors. When the liquid is mostly evaporated, stir in the stock. Cover and bring to a boil over high heat. Uncover, reduce the heat to medium, and simmer for 5 to 10 minutes.

5. Puree the mixture until smooth with an immersion blender or in an upright blender. If using an upright blender, avoid a blowout by slightly cooling the mixture and partially removing the center lid of the blender.

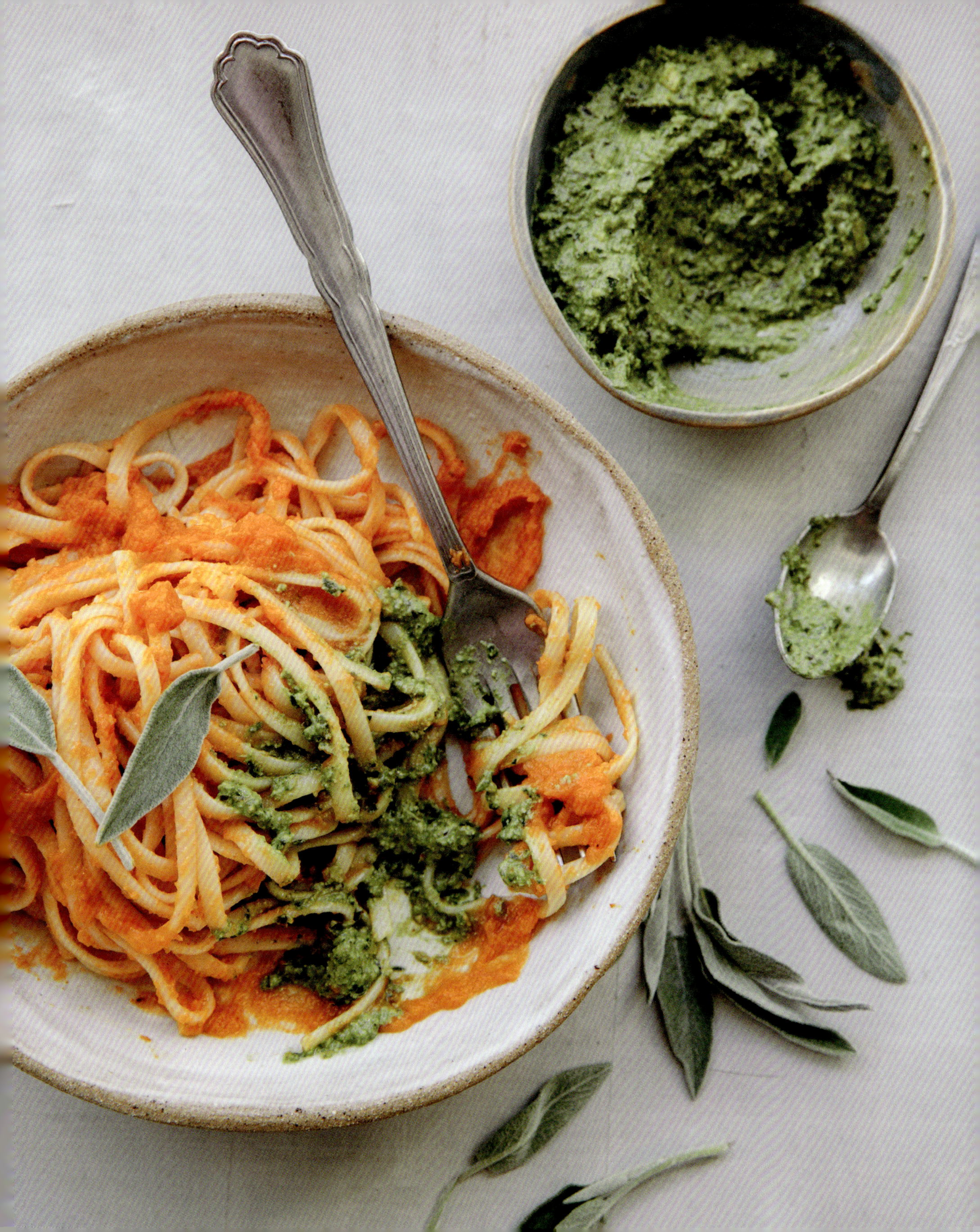

6. Return the mixture to the saucepan (if you used an upright blender) and reheat gently, seasoning with the salt, pepper, and sage.

7. Meanwhile, bring a pot of salted water to a boil. Stir in the pasta and cover the pot to quickly return the water to a boil. Partially cover and boil the pasta until it is slightly underdone, 5 to 8 minutes. You will finish cooking the pasta in the sauce.

8. Use tongs or a small strainer to transfer the pasta to the sauce, reserving the pasta water. Toss the pasta and sauce over medium heat until everything is creamy and the pasta is tender yet firm in the center, about 2 minutes. If the sauce gets too thick, add a splash of pasta water. Divide among 6 plates and serve with dollops of kale pesto.

OPTIONS

- Small "sugar" or "pie" pumpkins such as Baby Bear work best in cooking. Some large varieties of pumpkin, such as Fairytale and Cinderella, will also work well, but it's generally best to save the big orange pumpkins for jack o' lanterns. You can also use butternut squash instead. In a pinch, use frozen diced pumpkin or butternut squash.
- You can double this sauce and freeze it for up to 4 months.
- For a gluten-free version, use gluten-free pasta such as Barilla, Jovial, or Tinkyada.
- For a grain-free or paleo version, use zucchini noodles and blanch the zoodles in the boiling water for 30 seconds.

KALE PESTO

=V
=P
=K

LACINATO (AKA DINOSAUR or Tuscan) kale makes the creamiest pesto due to its tender texture. Use this pesto anywhere you want freshness and creaminess—on a sandwich, in scrambled eggs, tossed with brown rice or pasta, drizzled over roasted root vegetables or boiled potatoes, or even mixed into some oil and vinegar to make a vinaigrette.

Ayurvedic Insight: Kale is the ideal food for balancing pitta and kapha. If you have trouble digesting kale, the nuts, oils, and spices in this sauce may help to reduce bloating.

Makes 1 cup

3 cups chopped lacinato or curly kale
1 lemon
1/4 cup walnuts, toasted
2 teaspoons minced fresh garlic
1/4 teaspoon fine sea salt
1/8 teaspoon freshly ground black pepper
Pinch of crushed red pepper flakes
6 tablespoons extra-virgin olive oil

1. Bring a medium saucepan of water to a boil over high heat. Set up a bowl of ice water.

2. Blanch the kale in the boiling water until bright green, about 1 minute. With a slotted spoon or spider strainer, transfer the kale to the ice water to stop the cooking. When cooled, drain the kale and transfer it to a small food processor or blender. Finely grate the lemon zest into the processor or blender, and squeeze in 1 tablespoon of lemon juice (catch and remove any seeds). Add the walnuts, garlic, salt, black pepper, red pepper flakes, and oil, and process or blend the mixture until very finely minced, scraping down the sides once or twice with a rubber spatula. The pesto should be thin enough to pour off a spoon. If necessary, add a little water to thin it. Use immediately, refrigerate for 3 to 4 days, or freeze for up to a month.

Farfalle with Asparagus, Mushrooms, and Creamed Leeks

=V
=P
↑K

THIS EARLY SPRING pasta dish manages to be light and rich all at once. With savory mushrooms, tender asparagus, and creamy cashew sauce perked up with sautéed leeks, it's like a vegan alternative to Alfredo.

Ayurvedic Insight: Enjoy this meal at lunchtime so you have all day to fully digest its substantial richness.

Serves 6 to 8

SAUCE

1½ cups raw cashews
1 cup finely chopped onions
1 tablespoon extra-virgin olive oil
1 teaspoon finely chopped garlic
1¼ teaspoons chopped fresh sage
¼ cup chopped fresh flat-leaf parsley
¾ teaspoon fine sea salt

PASTA

1 pound farfalle (butterfly) pasta
3 cups thinly sliced cleaned leeks
3 tablespoons extra-virgin olive oil
4 cups sliced cremini or shiitake mushrooms
1 bunch (about 1 pound) asparagus, trimmed and cut into 1-inch pieces
½ cup ½-inch diced red bell peppers
1 cup arugula
1 tablespoon fresh lemon juice
¾ teaspoon fine sea salt
¼ teaspoon freshly ground black pepper

1. For the sauce, combine the cashews and 1½ cups water in a small saucepan. Cover and bring to a boil over high heat. Uncover, reduce the heat to medium-low, and simmer until the nuts are softened, 12 to 15 minutes.

2. Meanwhile, heat a medium saucepan over medium-low heat for 2 minutes. Put in the onions and oil, shaking the pan to coat the onions. Sauté until the onions are lightly browned, about 5 minutes. Stir in the garlic and sage and cook for 1 minute.

3. Pour the nuts and their simmering water over the onions. Add another ½ cup water and simmer everything for 5 minutes. Transfer the pan contents to a food processor or blender. Add the parsley and salt and puree until very smooth. The sauce should be creamy like Alfredo sauce, so that it is pourable but thick enough to coat a spoon. If it is too thick, blend in a bit more water.

4. For the pasta, bring a large pot of salted water to a boil. Add the farfalle and boil until it is tender yet chewy in the center, 10 to 12 minutes.

5. While the pasta cooks, heat a large sauté pan over medium heat for 2 minutes. Put in the leeks and oil, shaking the pan to coat the leeks. Sauté until the leeks just begin to get tender, about 3 minutes. Stir in the mushrooms and cook, stirring occasionally, until they give up their liquid and are lightly browned, 3 to 4 minutes. Stir in

the asparagus and bell peppers and cook until the asparagus is crisp-tender, 2 to 3 minutes. Remove from the heat and stir in the arugula, lemon juice, salt, and pepper. Set aside about one-third of this vegetable mixture.

6. Drain the pasta and mix with the blended sauce and remaining vegetable mixture. Taste it and add more salt, pepper, or lemon juice until it tastes good to you.

7. Divide the pasta among 6 to 8 shallow bowls and top with the reserved vegetable mixture. Serve hot.

OPTIONS

- The cashew sauce can be made ahead and refrigerated for up to 2 days. If it thickens, thin it out with some of the hot pasta water.
- For a gluten-free version, use gluten-free pasta such as Barilla, Jovial, or Tinkyada.
- For a grain-free or paleo version, replace the pasta with zucchini noodles and blanch the zoodles in the boiling water for 30 seconds.

Rigatoni with Vegetable Bolognese

↓V
↑P
↓K

THIS SOUL-SATISFYING WINTER dish has been on the Kripalu menu for many years. It's vegan comfort food. Although the sauce is not a "true" Bolognese, caramelizing the vegetables and mushrooms is a key step in developing the signature flavor and dark red color.

Ayurvedic Insight: You won't miss the meat in this Bolognese. Use gluten-free pasta to make it more kapha balancing.

Serves 4 (about 1 quart sauce)

2 onions, diced
1 large carrot, peeled and diced
2 celery stalks, diced
1/4 cup extra-virgin olive oil
1/2 teaspoon fine sea salt
5 large white mushrooms, diced
3 garlic cloves, finely chopped
1/2 cup burgundy wine
2 tablespoons fresh rosemary leaves
3/4 cup plus 2 teaspoons chopped fresh flat-leaf parsley
3 cups Vegetable Stock (page 281) or store-bought stock
1 1/2 cups canned plain tomato sauce
1/4 teaspoon freshly ground black pepper
1 pound rigatoni

1. Heat a medium saucepan over medium-low heat. Put in the onions, carrots, celery, oil, and ¼ teaspoon of the salt, shaking the pan to coat the vegetables. Cover and sauté over low heat until the onions are translucent, 6 to 8 minutes.

2. Uncover, raise the heat to medium-high, and cook the vegetables until nicely browned and caramelized, 6 to 8 minutes, stirring frequently to prevent burning. Stir in the mushrooms and continue sautéing until they become lightly caramelized, 4 to 6 minutes more. Stir in the garlic and cook until fragrant, 2 to 3 minutes.

3. Pour in the wine and scrape the pan bottom to capture all the flavors. Stir in the rosemary and the ¾ cup parsley. Bring to a simmer and simmer vigorously until the liquid in the pan evaporates, 2 to 3 minutes. At this point, the vegetables should be very soft and browned.

4. Stir in the stock and tomato sauce and bring to a boil. Then reduce the heat and simmer until the flavors are blended and deep, at least 30 minutes and up to 2 hours. Adjust the heat according to your schedule: you can cook the sauce at a high simmer for 30 minutes, at a medium simmer for 1 hour, or at a lazy simmer for 2 hours for the most flavor. If you intend to simmer it for a longer time, add an extra ½ cup stock and keep an eye on it, as the sauce will cook down over time. When done, the sauce should be thick. We always puree it but leave it a little chunky. It's easiest to use a stick blender, but you could also pulse it in a food processor so it thickens up some but remains chunky. Or

you could mash it in the pan with a potato masher. Either way, when the sauce is thick and chunky, yet saucy enough to coat the pasta, season it with the remaining ¼ teaspoon salt and the pepper.

5. Meanwhile, bring a pot of salted water to a boil. Stir in the pasta and cover the pot to quickly return the water to a boil. Partially cover and boil the pasta until it is slightly underdone, 5 to 8 minutes. You will finish cooking the pasta in the sauce.

6. Use tongs or a small strainer to transfer the pasta to the sauce, reserving the pasta water. Toss the pasta and sauce over medium heat until everything is creamy and the pasta is tender yet firm in the center, about 2 minutes. If the sauce gets too thick, add a splash of pasta water. Divide among 4 plates, saving a little sauce to spoon over the top of the pasta if you like. Garnish with the remaining 2 teaspoons chopped parsley.

OPTIONS

- You could serve the Bolognese over rice or quinoa, or as a sauce for chicken.
- For a gluten-free version, use gluten-free pasta such as Barilla, Jovial, or Tinkyada.
- For a grain-free version, replace the pasta with zucchini noodles and blanch the zoodles in the boiling water for 30 seconds. The same goes for a paleo version, but also omit the wine.
- If you are craving carne, brown 1 pound ground turkey in the saucepan before sautéing the vegetables. Remove the browned meat from the pan, sauté the vegetables, then add it back along with the tomato sauce.
- Make the sauce ahead by preparing a double batch and freezing it.
- The cooking time for this sauce is flexible. If you have less time, puree the sauce early and let it simmer for less time. If you have more time, let it simmer slowly on low heat, then puree it at the end of cooking.

Creamy Polenta with Vegan Mushroom Cream Sauce

↑V
=P
↓K

IF YOU LIKE SMOOTH, creamy, and luxuriously rich foods, you'll love this main dish. Coconut milk lends a full body to the sauce while sautéed and dried mushrooms bring a deep, savory flavor. To make the polenta extra creamy, I add a little baking soda, which helps to break down the cornmeal.

Ayurvedic Insight: Due to the dry qualities of cornmeal and mushrooms, even kapha types can enjoy this indulgent dish. To make it lighter, replace the coconut milk with almond milk.

Serves 4

POLENTA

1/2 teaspoon fine sea salt
Pinch of baking soda
1 tablespoon extra-virgin olive oil
3/4 cup coarse cornmeal for polenta

MUSHROOM CREAM SAUCE

1 cup sliced shiitake mushrooms
1 cup sliced portobello mushrooms
2 tablespoons 1/4-inch diced onions
2 teaspoons extra-virgin olive oil
1/4 teaspoon fine sea salt, plus a pinch
2 teaspoons porcini mushroom powder or shiitake powder
1 teaspoon finely chopped garlic
1/4 cup drained petite diced canned tomatoes
1 teaspoon Dijon mustard
1 cup canned full-fat 100% coconut milk
1 teaspoon fresh thyme leaves
Pinch of freshly ground black pepper
2 teaspoons chopped fresh flat-leaf parsley

1. For the polenta, bring 4 cups water, the salt, and the baking soda to a boil in a medium saucepan. Add the oil, then slowly add the cornmeal to the pot while whisking constantly. Once the polenta begins to simmer and thicken, reduce the heat to bring the mixture to a gentle simmer. Cover and cook, stirring every few minutes, until the polenta is thick like loose porridge, 10 to 12 minutes. If the polenta seems too wet, uncover it and simmer until it resembles loose porridge.

2. For the mushroom cream sauce, heat a medium saucepan over medium-low heat for 2 minutes. Put in the shiitakes, portobellos, onions, oil, and a pinch of salt, shaking the pan to coat the vegetables. Reduce the heat to low, cover, and cook until the mushrooms are wilted and release their juices, 5 to 6 minutes. Uncover, raise the heat to high, and cook until the pan is dry, then reduce the heat to medium and cook the mushrooms until lightly browned, stirring now and then.

3. Stir in the porcini powder and cook for 1 minute. Stir in the garlic, diced tomatoes, mustard, and coconut milk. Bring the mixture to a simmer, scraping the pan bottom, then cover and simmer until slightly thickened, about 10 minutes. Uncover and stir in the

thyme, ¼ teaspoon salt, and a pinch of pepper. Taste the sauce, adding more seasonings if you think it needs them.

4. Divide the polenta among 4 bowls and spoon the sauce over the top. Garnish with the parsley.

OPTIONS

- For a grain-free or paleo version, you could serve the sauce over chicken. Or for vegetarians, serve it over tofu.

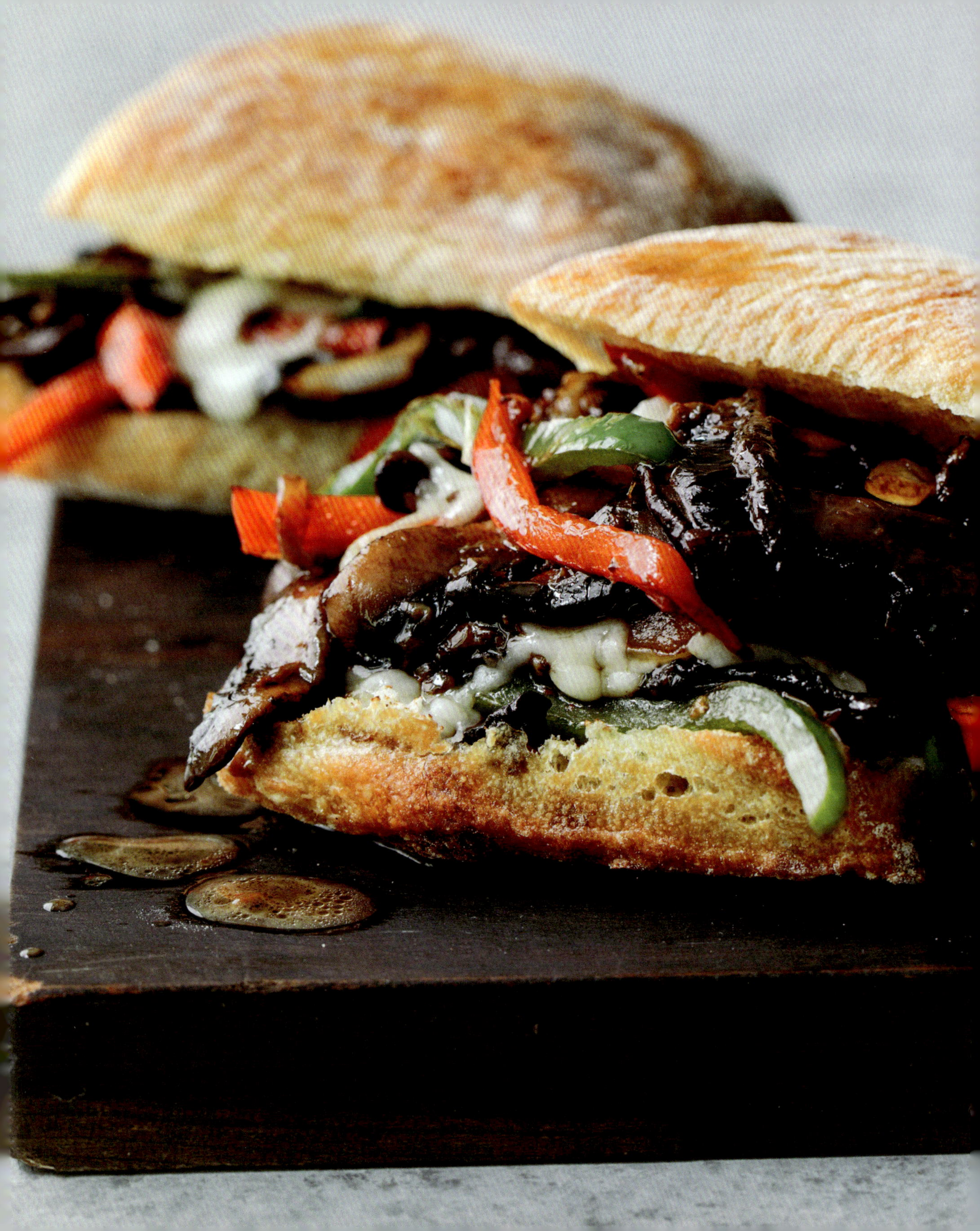

Mushroom Cheesesteaks

↑V

=P

=K

BE PREPARED FOR a big burst of juicy, satisfying, savory flavor in these sandwiches. Caramelized portobello mushrooms, dried mushroom powder, soy sauce, Worcestershire sauce, and provolone cheese are all rich sources of umami, the Japanese word for "delicious."

Ayurvedic Insight: Enjoy these sandwiches in the fall and spring when the dry quality of mushrooms will help to absorb dampness in the body. Kapha types should go light on the cheese.

Makes 4 sandwiches

- 1 cup julienned Spanish onion
- 2 tablespoons extra-virgin olive oil
- 8 cups sliced portobello mushrooms
- 1 teaspoon porcini mushroom powder
- 1/2 teaspoon dried oregano
- 2 teaspoons finely chopped garlic
- 2 tablespoons tamari or soy sauce
- 1/2 teaspoon Worcestershire sauce
- 2 cups julienned red and/or green bell peppers
- 1/4 cup grated provolone cheese
- 4 Sourdough Ciabatta Rolls (page 88) or sub rolls

1. Heat a large sauté pan over medium-low heat. Put in the onions and oil, shaking the pan to coat the onions. Cook until the onions are translucent, 3 to 5 minutes. Raise the heat to medium and cook, stirring occasionally, until the onions are lightly caramelized, 3 to 5 minutes more.

2. Stir in 6 cups of the mushrooms, cover, and sweat the mushrooms until they are tender and release their juices, about 5 minutes.

3. Stir in the porcini powder and oregano and raise the heat to high. Cook, uncovered, until the pan goes dry and the mushrooms caramelize, 2 to 3 minutes, stirring to prevent burning. When the mushrooms are nicely browned, stir in the garlic and cook for 1 minute.

4. Stir in the tamari and Worcestershire, scraping the pan bottom to capture all the flavors. Reduce the heat to medium-low and stir in the peppers and remaining 2 cups mushrooms. Cover and sweat until the peppers are just tender, 2 to 3 minutes. Remove from the heat and fold in the provolone. Serve on the rolls.

OPTIONS

- You can buy porcini mushroom powder or make it yourself by buzzing dried porcini mushrooms to a powder in a clean coffee grinder. Try buzzing a mix of dried mushrooms, such as shiitake, porcini, and matsutake, to make your own signature blend.
- For a vegan version, use vegan Worcestershire and omit the cheese. Or use vegan cheese such as Follow Your Heart pepper jack.
- For a gluten-free version, use gluten-free rolls. Or for a grain-free version, skip the rolls.

Hoisin BBQ Jackfruit Sandwich with Creamy Vegan Slaw

↓V
=P
↑K

HERE'S OUR VEGAN VERSION of pulled pork BBQ. Jackfruit is a large tree fruit native to southwest India. When green, the fruit has a savory taste and meaty texture, and it can be pulled apart in shreds like pulled chicken or pork. Cooked with BBQ sauce, it makes a very satisfying sandwich.

Ayurvedic Insight: The sweet pungency of the sauce here adds to the vata balancing qualities of jackfruit. With the vegan slaw, this sandwich can be enjoyed by all doshas during the summer.

Serves 4

BBQ JACKFRUIT

3/4 cup organic ketchup
1/2 cup hoisin sauce
2 tablespoons molasses
2 tablespoons tamari
2 teaspoons rice vinegar, preferably brown
2 teaspoons minced fresh ginger
2 cups drained jackfruit, from a bag or can

↑V
↑P
=K

CREAMY VEGAN SLAW

1/4 cup plant-based mayo such as Vegenaise
1 1/2 teaspoons cider vinegar
1 1/2 teaspoons dry mustard
1/4 teaspoon fine sea salt
1/4 teaspoon freshly ground black pepper
1 1/2 cups thinly sliced green cabbage
3/4 cup shredded or julienned carrots
2 tablespoons thinly sliced scallion greens
1 tablespoon chopped fresh flat-leaf parsley
4 ciabatta, Kaiser, or other sturdy rolls

1. For the jackfruit, whisk together the ketchup, hoisin, molasses, tamari, vinegar, and ginger in a medium saucepan. Bring to a simmer over medium-low heat.

2. Shred the jackfruit by hand and add it to the sauce in the pan. Bring the mixture to a gentle simmer and cook, uncovered, until the flavors blend and the sauce thickens enough to stay on a bun, 15 to 20 minutes.

3. Meanwhile, for the slaw, whisk together the mayo, vinegar, mustard, salt, and pepper in a medium bowl. Fold in the cabbage, carrots, scallions, and parsley, mixing thoroughly.

4. To serve, spoon the jackfruit onto the rolls and top with the slaw.

OPTIONS

- For a meat version, replace the jackfruit with 12 ounces boneless, skinless chicken breast and simmer the chicken in the sauce over low heat until it can be shredded with a fork, 30 to 40 minutes.

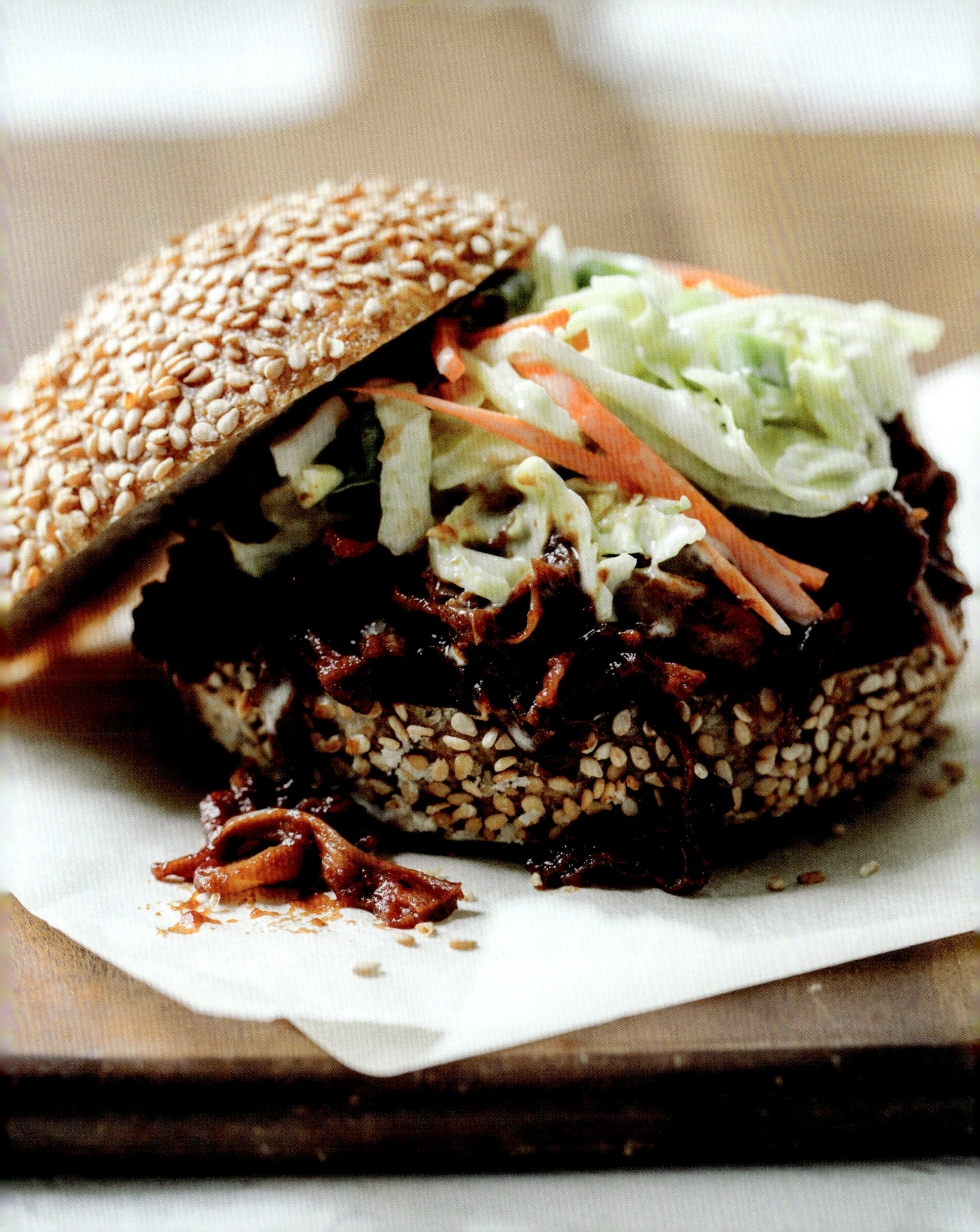

- For a gluten-free version, use gluten-free rolls. Or for a grain-free version, skip the rolls.
- Slow Cooker Method: Mix the sauce in a slow cooker, add the jackfruit or chicken, and cook on low for 4 hours.
- To make tacos, skip the rolls and serve the jackfruit BBQ and slaw in warmed corn tortillas with fresh cilantro and lime wedges for squeezing.

Coconut-Crusted Tempeh with Mango Ginger Salsa

I WAS NEVER a big fan of tempeh until I tasted this dish. The coconut walnut crust makes it rich and crunchy, while the mango ginger salsa gives it a tropical touch of sweetness and spice. Perfect for a light summer meal.

Ayurvedic Insight: The protein in tempeh satisfies the hunger of pitta types and dries out the oiliness of kapha types. It's a little too airy for vatas, but vatas will love the mango salsa.

Serves 4

TEMPEH

Oil spray

12 ounces tempeh, about 1/2 inch thick

2 teaspoons tamari

1/4 cup Dijon mustard

1 tablespoon brown rice syrup, honey, or agave nectar

1 1/2 cups walnuts, toasted and coarsely chopped

1 3/4 cups unsweetened dried shredded coconut

3/4 teaspoon fine sea salt

1/2 teaspoon freshly ground black pepper

MANGO GINGER SAUCE

↓V ↓P =K

2 1/2 cups finely chopped mango (fresh or thawed frozen)

Grated zest and juice of 2 limes

1 tablespoon minced fresh ginger

1 teaspoon minced red onions

1 teaspoon minced fresh garlic

1 teaspoon toasted ground cumin

1 teaspoon honey, brown rice syrup, or agave nectar

1 teaspoon minced jalapeño peppers

1/2 teaspoon hot sauce, preferably Cholula

1/2 teaspoon fine sea salt

4 ounces arugula leaves, for serving

↑V ↓P ↓K

1. Preheat the oven to 400°F. Lightly spray a baking sheet with oil.

2. Cut the tempeh into 3-inch squares, then cut each square on a diagonal into triangles. To remove any bitterness from the tempeh, place the triangles in a small sauté pan with the tamari and just enough water to cover. Bring to a simmer over medium heat and simmer gently for 10 minutes. Drain and set aside to cool.

3. Combine the mustard and brown rice syrup in a wide, shallow bowl and set aside.

4. Place the walnuts in a food processor and pulse until finely ground but not powdery. Very briefly pulse in the coconut, salt, and pepper. Transfer to another wide, shallow bowl.

5. Dip each piece of tempeh into the mustard mixture, coating both sides, then into the coconut mixture, coating both sides. Place the coated pieces on the oiled baking sheet and spritz the pieces with oil spray. Bake until the tempeh is golden brown, 15 to 17 minutes.

6. For the mango sauce, combine everything in a medium bowl. Transfer 1 cup of the mixture to a small food processor or blender and puree until smooth. Spoon the puree back into the chopped mixture and stir to combine.

7. Place the arugula on a serving platter or 4 individual plates. Arrange the tempeh over the arugula and top with the sauce.

OPTIONS

- Coconut-Crusted Chicken: Replace the tempeh with 2 boneless, skinless chicken breasts. Omit the first step of simmering with tamari and water, which is only to remove bitterness from the tempeh. Simply coat the chicken breasts with the mustard and coconut mixture, then bake the coated chicken until it reaches an internal temperature of 160°F, 20 to 25 minutes.
- Refrigerate any leftover tempeh or chicken and serve it cold on a salad.

Pan-Seared Shrimp with Spicy Cilantro Pesto and Butternut Squash

↓V ↓P ↓K

WHEN I STARTED at Kripalu in the fall of 2010, this is the first dish I added to the menu. I was inspired by the red-orange colors of the New England leaves and the earthy flavors of autumn. It was my first foray into satisfying various dietary preferences in a single dish, and our guests now look forward to it every autumn. Make the pesto ahead of time, and this one-pan meal comes together in less than thirty minutes.

Ayurvedic Insight: Cooling cilantro, warming spices, drying squash, and slightly oily shrimp make this dish suitable for all body types.

Serves 4

SPICY CILANTRO PESTO

1/4 cup raw pumpkin seeds

Grated zest and juice of 1 small lime

2 cups fresh cilantro leaves and small stems

1/2 cup extra-virgin olive oil

2 garlic cloves

3/4 teaspoon fine sea salt

Pinch of crushed red pepper flakes

1/4 cup grated Parmesan cheese (optional)

SHRIMP AND SQUASH

2 tablespoons extra-virgin olive oil

3 cups 1/2-inch diced peeled butternut squash

1/4 cup 1/4-inch diced red bell peppers

1 pound wild American extra-jumbo shrimp (U20 or 16/20 per pound), peeled and deveined

1/4 teaspoon fine sea salt

1/8 teaspoon freshly ground black pepper

1 tablespoon grapeseed oil or other vegetable oil for searing

1. For the pesto, toast the pumpkin seeds in a large sauté pan (with a heatproof handle) over medium heat until fragrant, 2 to 3 minutes, shaking the pan now and then. Transfer the toasted seeds to a food processor. You'll be using the sauté pan again, so just set it aside. Add all of the remaining pesto ingredients to the food processor and process until the mixture is still a little chunky, a minute or two. Set aside.

2. For the shrimp and squash, preheat the oven to 350°F. Heat the same sauté pan over medium heat for 2 minutes. When good and hot, pour in the oil and add the squash, tossing to coat with the oil. Shake the squash into a single layer and cook undisturbed until it begins to brown on the bottom, about 2 minutes. Scatter on the bell peppers and transfer the pan to the oven. Bake until the squash is barely fork-tender, another 5 to 7 minutes. Transfer the squash-pepper mix to a bowl, toss with about ¼ cup of the pesto, and then cover loosely to keep it warm.

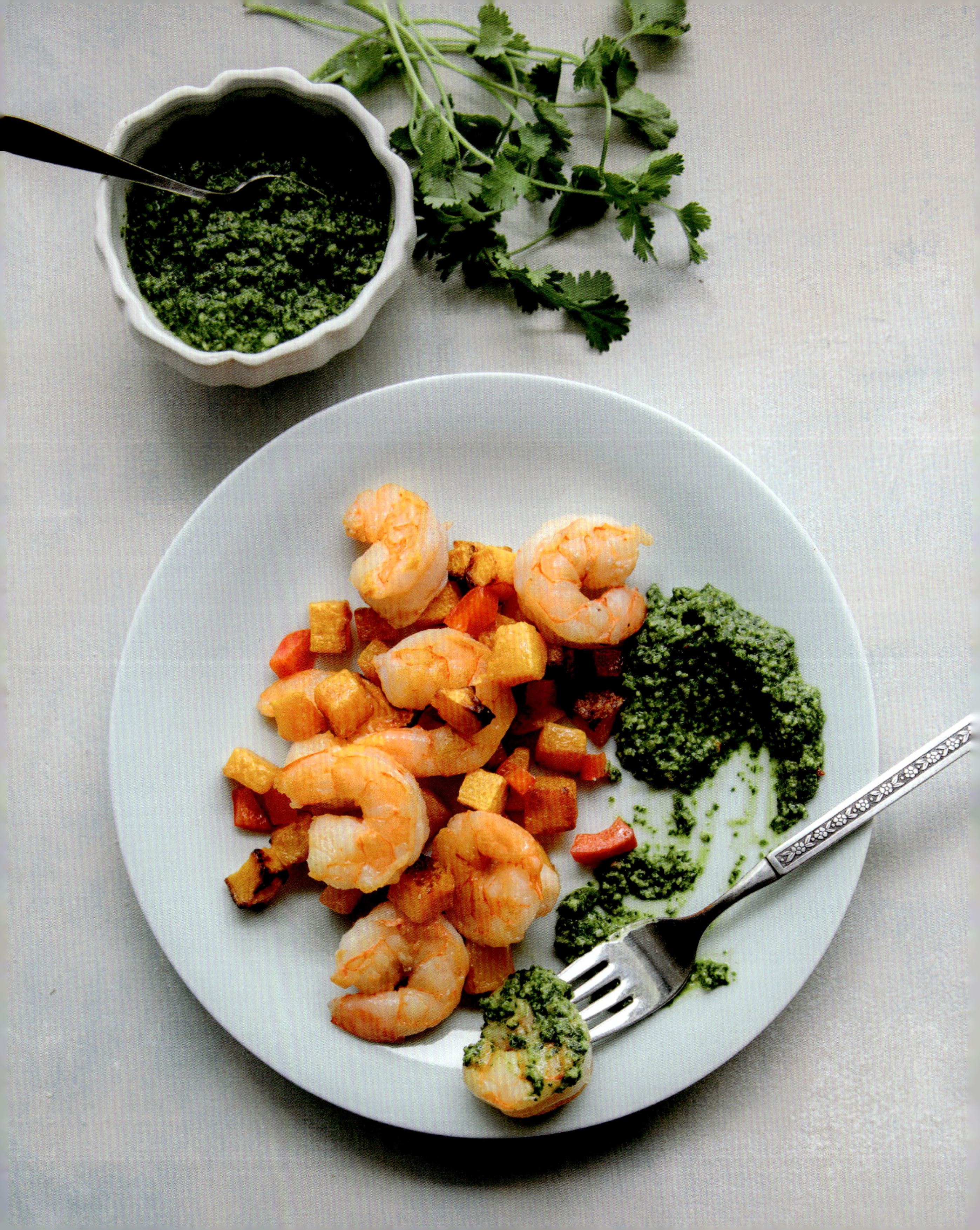

3. Put the same pan over high heat. Season the shrimp with the salt and pepper as the pan heats up. Pour the grapeseed oil into the pan, swirling to coat the pan bottom. Add the shrimp, quickly shaking them into a single layer. Reduce the heat to medium-high and cook undisturbed until the shrimp are lightly browned on the bottom, about 1 minute. Flip the shrimp with tongs and cook until the other side is lightly browned and the shrimp are pink, about another minute.

4. Remove from the heat and toss with the remaining ¾ cup pesto. Serve over the squash-pepper mix or alongside it.

OPTIONS

- If you like, serve the dish over jasmine rice with a little coconut milk stirred into the rice after cooking to give it some creaminess.
- *Pan-Seared Tofu with Spicy Cilantro Pesto and Butternut Squash:* Replace the shrimp with 1 pound extra-firm tofu. Drain the tofu and place it in a colander in the sink. Place a small bowl on the tofu and put a large can of tomatoes or beans in the bowl. Let the tofu press for 20 minutes to 1 hour to drain excess water. When drained, cut the tofu through the side into 4 thinner slabs. Season both sides of the tofu with a little salt and pepper, then sear as directed for the shrimp, allowing a little extra cooking time to brown the tofu on both sides.
- You can cook half tofu and half shrimp in separate pans if you have mixed company at the table.
- You can leave out the Parmesan to make the pesto vegan or paleo, or serve it at the table for vegetarians.

Sautéed Barramundi with Harissa, Toasted Almonds, and Honey

=V

↑P

=K

THIS ENTRÉE WAS INSPIRED by trout almondine, the classic French plate of sautéed trout with toasted almonds, butter, and lemon. At the time I made it, we were on a harissa kick and we decided to make this spicy sauce the focal point of the dish. With homemade harissa, the dish is special enough for guests, but if you follow the shortcuts, you could also whip it up on a busy weeknight. For a table with mixed dietary needs, cook half fish and half tofu in separate pans.

Ayurvedic Insight: Ayurveda advises against cooking honey because it is already "cooked" in the hive. Be sure to add the honey to the almonds after the pan has been removed from the heat.

Serves 4

HARISSA

2 plum tomatoes

3 1/2 tablespoons extra-virgin olive oil

1 1/2 teaspoons minced jalapeño peppers, preferably red

1 teaspoon minced fresh garlic

1 tablespoon tomato paste

1 tablespoon ground cumin

1 teaspoon curry powder

1 teaspoon garam masala

1 teaspoon ground caraway seeds

1/4 teaspoon white wine vinegar

1/4 teaspoon fine sea salt

ALMONDS AND HONEY

1/4 cup slivered almonds

1 tablespoon extra-virgin olive oil

2 teaspoons finely chopped garlic

1 teaspoon honey

1 tablespoon chopped fresh flat-leaf parsley

Pinch of sea salt

SAUTÉED BARRAMUNDI

4 skin-on barramundi fillets, about 1 pound total

1/8 teaspoon fine sea salt

1 tablespoon grapeseed oil or other vegetable oil for searing

1. For the harissa, heat the oven to 350°F.

2. Toss the whole plum tomatoes with ½ tablespoon oil on a sheet pan. Roast the tomatoes until they are soft and the skins start to peel back, 12 to 15 minutes. Let cool. When cool enough to handle, peel off the skins and place the tomatoes in a food processor or blender. Add the remaining 3 tablespoons oil and the remaining harissa ingredients, and puree the mixture until relatively smooth.

3. For the almonds and honey, heat a small sauté pan over medium-low heat. Spread the almonds in the pan and toast until fragrant, 3 to 5 minutes, shaking the pan once or twice. Remove the almonds and pour in the olive oil. When hot, stir in the garlic and cook until it

barely starts to brown, 2 to 3 minutes. Remove from the heat and stir in the honey, parsley, salt, and toasted almonds.

4. For the barramundi, heat a large sauté pan over medium heat until very hot, about 2 minutes. Pat the barramundi dry with a paper towel and season the flesh side with salt. Test the heat of the pan by sprinkling a bit of water on it. The water droplets should evaporate quickly but not skitter across the pan. If they skitter, remove the pan from the heat for a minute to cool it down a bit.

5. Raise the heat to high and swirl in the oil to cover the pan bottom. Lay each seasoned fillet in the pan, flesh side down. After about 20 seconds, reduce the heat to medium. Continue cooking for 2 minutes. Use a spatula to carefully flip each fillet. Cook until the skin is crisp, 2 to 3 minutes.

6. Serve the fish with the harissa and almond honey sauce. For a nice presentation, spoon the harissa on the plate, arrange the fish on top, and spoon the almond sauce over the fish.

OPTIONS

- Look for fresh or even frozen barramundi at Whole Foods Market. If you can't find it, use skin-on sea bass fillets or skinless halibut fillets. If your fish fillets are more than ½ inch thick, use a pan with a heatproof handle and finish cooking the fish in a 350°F oven after flipping the fillets skin side down. Bake until the fish registers an internal temperature of about 130°F, 4 to 6 minutes.
- You can replace the plum tomatoes with 1 cup canned diced tomatoes. Fire-roasted canned tomatoes work especially well.
- If you're short on time, make a quick harissa by mixing 1 cup crushed tomatoes with 3 tablespoons extra-virgin olive oil and 2 tablespoons dry harissa spice mix. In a real pinch, replace the harissa with good-quality store-bought harissa, such as Mina brand.
- Vegan Sautéed Tofu with Harissa and Toasted Almonds: Replace the honey with agave nectar and the barramundi with 1 pound extra-firm tofu. Drain the tofu and place it in a colander in the sink. Place a small bowl on the tofu and put a large can of tomatoes or beans in the bowl. Let the tofu press for 20 minutes to drain excess water. Cut the drained tofu through the side into 4 thinner slabs. Proceed with seasoning and searing the tofu as directed for the fish, allowing a little extra cooking time to lightly brown the tofu on both sides.

Pan-Roasted Pollock with Purple Potatoes and Chimichurri Sauce

=V
=P
=K

USE WHATEVER FIRM white fish is freshest in your market. Haddock, Pacific halibut, and barramundi all work great. Either way, fish, potatoes, and fresh herb sauce make for a very satisfying meal. Purple potatoes also provide anthocyanins, powerful antioxidants that can help to reduce inflammation and lower cancer risk. Plus, they add a cool pop of color to the plate.

Ayurvedic Insight: The pungency of fresh and herbal chimichurri makes this dish best for summer meals. To enjoy the health benefits of herbs all summer long, keep a small herb garden in your kitchen.

Serves 4

POTATOES AND FISH

1 pound fingerling potatoes (preferably purple), halved lengthwise

1/4 cup grapeseed oil or sunflower seed oil

1/2 teaspoon fine sea salt

1 pound pollock or other white fish fillets

Extra-virgin olive oil, for drizzling

CHIMICHURRI

↓V
=P
↓K

2 cups firmly packed fresh flat-leaf parsley leaves

1/4 cup picked fresh oregano leaves

3 garlic cloves, crushed

2 tablespoons 1/4-inch diced red onions

1/2 cup extra-virgin olive oil, plus more for drizzling

Grated zest and juice of 1 lime

2 tablespoons red wine vinegar

Pinch of crushed red pepper flakes

1/2 teaspoon fine sea salt

1. Preheat the oven to 350°F.

2. On a sheet pan, toss the potatoes with 2 tablespoons of the grapeseed oil and ¼ teaspoon of the salt. Arrange them cut sides down in an even layer on the pan and roast until the potatoes are tender, the skins are slightly wrinkled, and the bottoms are golden brown, 40 to 45 minutes. Remove from the oven and set aside.

3. About 20 minutes before the potatoes will be ready, pat the fish dry with a dish towel to remove excess moisture. Sprinkle all over with salt and set aside.

4. For the chimichurri, combine everything in a small food processor or blender and blend until very finely chopped but not completely pureed. Place in a small bowl and reserve.

5. To cook the fish, heat a large ovenproof sauté pan over high heat for 2 to 3 minutes. Swirl in the remaining 2 tablespoons grapeseed oil, covering the pan bottom. Lay each seasoned fillet in the pan, flesh side down. After about 20 seconds of cooking, reduce the heat to medium-high. Continue cooking for 2 minutes. Use a spatula to carefully flip each fillet, then transfer the pan to the oven and cook until the fish reg-

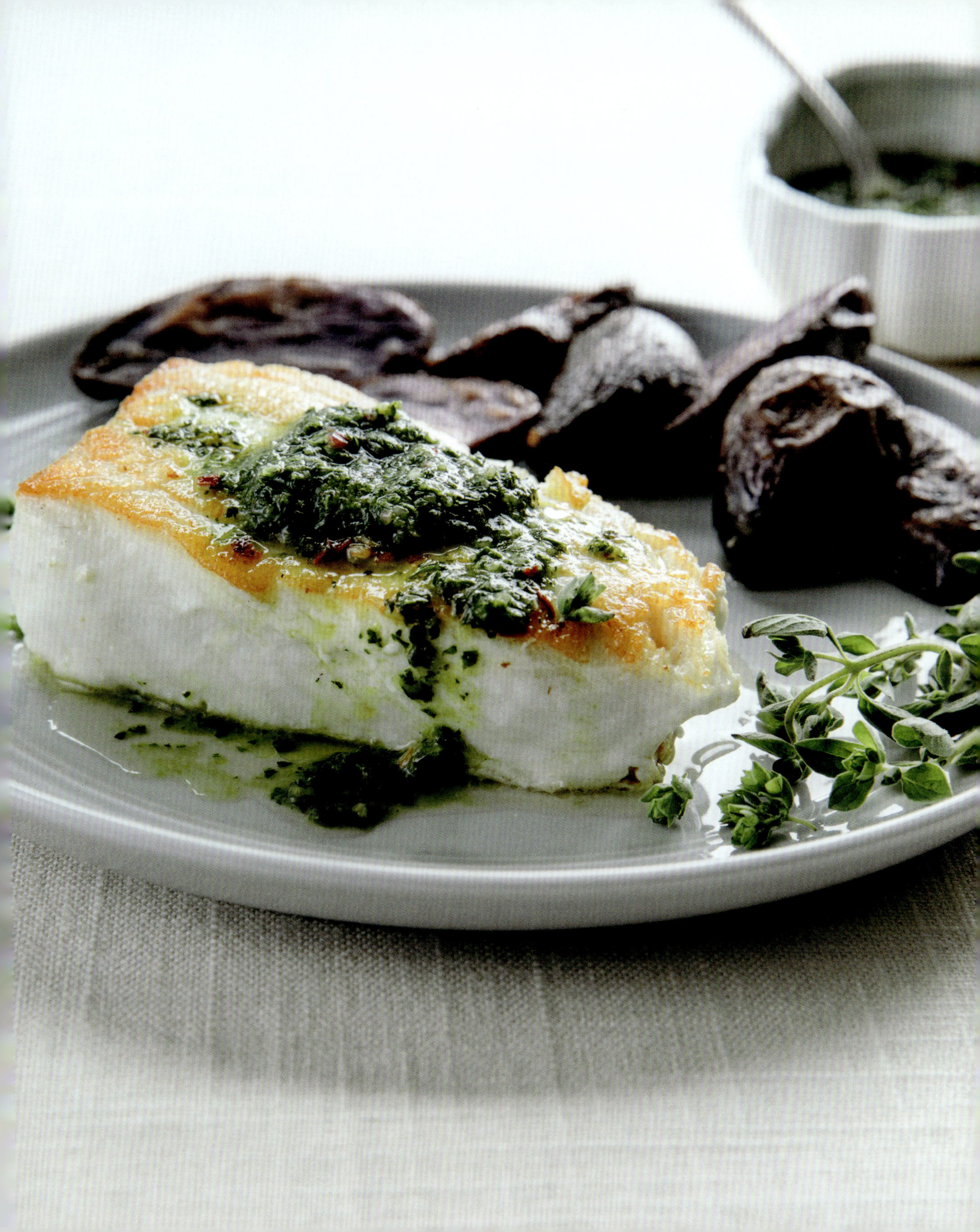

isters an internal temperature of about 135°F, 5 to 6 minutes.

6. To serve, place the potatoes on one side of each plate and drizzle with a little extra-virgin olive oil. Place the fish on the other side and spoon some chimichurri on top.

OPTIONS

- *Pan-Roasted Tofu (or Chicken) with Purple Potatoes and Chimichurri Sauce:* You could replace the fish with pressed tofu or organic boneless skinless chicken breasts. For tofu, drain a 14- to 16-ounce block of tofu and place it in a colander in the sink. Place a small bowl on the tofu and put a large can of tomatoes or beans in the bowl. Let the tofu press for 20 minutes to drain excess water. When drained, cut the tofu horizontally into 4 thinner slabs. Cook the pressed slabs of tofu or the chicken as directed in the recipe, but cook the chicken to an internal temperature of 160°F.
- You may have some chimichurri left over. You can freeze it. Or spoon it onto grilled vegetables or shrimp. Or use it as a sandwich spread.

Adobo-Rubbed Chicken with Avocado Crème

When you puree avocado, it gets fluffy like whipped cream and makes a terrific topping for marinated chicken. In the dog days of summer, here's your go-to weeknight meal. You can marinate the chicken in the morning, then grill it at dinnertime. Serve it hot with basmati rice, and enjoy any leftovers cold.

Ayurvedic Insight: Limes are less warming than lemons and perfect for hot-weather meals. The spices here also help to make this dish suitable for all three doshas.

Serves 4

CHICKEN

2 tablespoons fresh lime juice

2 teaspoons finely grated lime zest

2 teaspoons finely chopped garlic

2 tablespoons coconut sugar or packed light brown sugar

1 tablespoon chili powder

1 teaspoon ground coriander

1 tablespoon grapeseed oil or sunflower oil

1 pound organic boneless, skinless chicken breasts

1/4 teaspoon fine sea salt

AVOCADO CRÈME

↓V ↓P ↑K

2 avocados, peeled and sliced

1 tablespoon fresh lime juice

1/4 teaspoon hot sauce, preferably Cholula

1 teaspoon ground cumin

1/4 teaspoon fine sea salt

1/4 cup 1/4-inch diced tomatoes, plus 2 teaspoons for garnish

1 teaspoon chopped fresh cilantro, plus a few sprigs for garnish

↓V ↓P ↓K

1. Preheat the oven to 350°F.

2. For the chicken marinade, combine the lime juice and zest, garlic, sugar, chili powder, coriander, and 1 teaspoon of the oil in a medium bowl. Mix the ingredients to form a smooth paste. Add the chicken, turning to coat all over with the marinade. Let marinate at room temperature for 20 to 30 minutes or in the refrigerator for 8 to 10 hours.

3. For the avocado crème, combine the avocados, lime juice, hot sauce, cumin, and salt in a small food processor and puree until very smooth and lightly whipped. Remove from the processor and fold in the tomatoes and cilantro.

4. Heat a large ovenproof sauté pan over medium heat for 3 minutes. Swirl in the remaining 2 teaspoons oil. Sprinkle ¼ teaspoon salt all over the chicken, then add the chicken to the pan. Cook until it is lightly browned on the bottom, 2 to 3 minutes. If the pan seems too hot or is smoking, reduce the heat a bit. When nicely browned, use a spatula to flip the chicken, then spoon any remaining marinade over the top.

5. Transfer the sauté pan to the oven and bake until the chicken reaches an internal temperature of 160°F, 6 to 8 minutes.

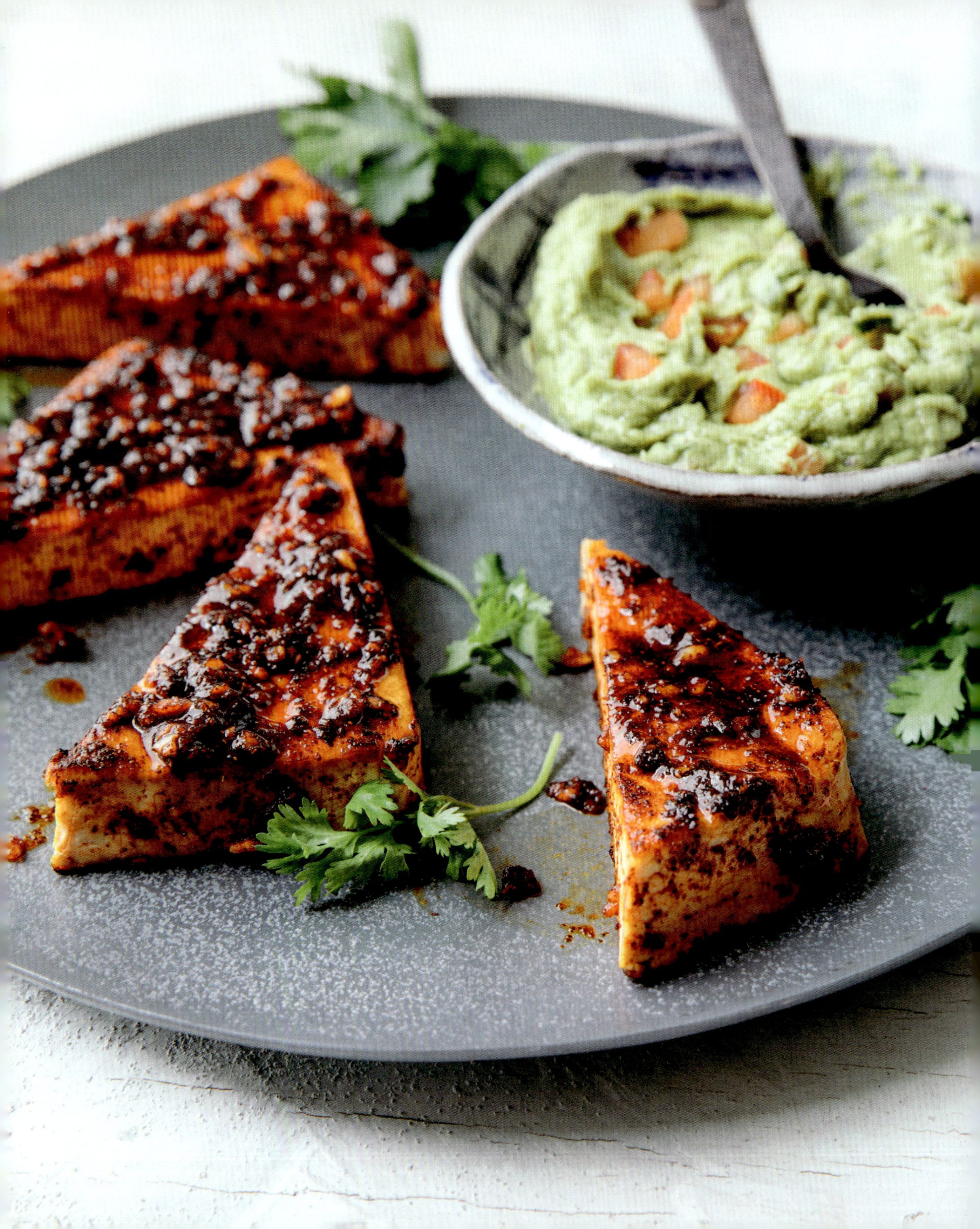

6. Remove the chicken from the oven and let it cool for 3 minutes or so. To serve, thinly slice the chicken and fan it out on 4 plates. Spoon a dollop of avocado crème on top and garnish with the reserved cilantro sprigs and chopped tomatoes.

OPTIONS

- *Adobo-Rubbed Tofu with Avocado Crème:* For a vegan version, replace the chicken with a block (14 to 16 ounces) of extra-firm tofu. Place the tofu in a colander in the sink. Place a small bowl on the tofu and set a can of tomatoes or beans inside the bowl. Press for 30 to 60 minutes to remove excess water. Cut the pressed tofu horizontally into 2 thinner slabs; then cut the slabs diagonally into 4 triangles and proceed with the recipe.
- For a paleo or sugar-free version, omit the sugar.
- For a cold summer sandwich, grill the chicken over medium heat until it reaches an internal temperature of 160°F, then let it cool. You can refrigerate it for up to 2 days. Slice the cooled chicken into thin slabs and serve it on crusty rolls with the avocado crème.
- You may have some avocado crème left over. Use it as a dip, in wraps, or on grilled fish. It keeps refrigerated for several days.

Roasted Chicken with Sesame Cider Glaze

↓V
↑P
↑K

A RECENT ADDITION to the Kripalu menu, this dish has become an instant classic. It's simple and approachable, and blends traditional New England ingredients like apple cider with timeless Indian flavors like ginger and star anise. We source our cider from a local orchard and serve this dish on Berkshire community nights, when we offer meal passes to area residents who might not otherwise eat at Kripalu.

Ayurvedic Insight: Chicken leg and thigh meat is somewhat oily and is best enjoyed in the winter or by dry body types such as vata. Chicken breast meat, on the other hand, is drier and best suited to oily body types such as kapha and pitta.

Serves 4 to 6

2 tablespoons minced fresh ginger

2 tablespoons toasted sesame oil

Pinch of crushed red pepper flakes

1/4 cup cider vinegar

2 teaspoons tamari

1 piece of star anise or 1/2 teaspoon ground fennel seed

2 cups apple cider

1 pound organic bone-in, skin-on chicken thighs, drumsticks, or breasts

2 teaspoons sesame seeds

2 scallions, greens thinly sliced on an angle

1. Preheat the oven to 350°F.

2. Heat a small saucepan over medium heat. Put in the ginger and 1 tablespoon of the oil, shaking the pan to coat the ginger. Sauté just until the ginger is fragrant, about a minute.

3. Add the red pepper flakes, vinegar, tamari, and star anise, and simmer until the liquid reduces by about one-fourth (reduced to about 1 tablespoon), 5 to 7 minutes. Pour in the cider and bring the mixture to a boil over high heat. Boil until the liquid reduces in volume by about half or until it is just thick enough to coat a spoon, scraping the sides once or twice, 30 to 40 minutes total. Check the consistency in a spoonful of the sauce. Drag your finger through the sauce in the spoon, and if it leaves a trail that fills in slowly, it's thick enough. If it fills in quickly, reduce it a bit more.

4. Heat a large ovenproof sauté pan over high heat for 2 to 3 minutes. Swirl in the remaining 1 tablespoon oil, then set the chicken, skin side down, in the pan. Let the chicken cook, without disturbing it, until the skin is golden brown, 4 to 6 minutes. Flip the chicken and brush each piece with the glaze mixture. Transfer to the oven and bake until the chicken registers an internal temperature of 165°F, 10 to 15 minutes.

5. Remove the chicken from the pan and divide among 4 to 6 plates. Pour the pan juices and the remaining sauce through a fine-mesh strainer over each piece of chicken. Garnish with the sesame seeds and scallions.

OPTION

- *Roasted Tempeh with Sesame Cider Glaze:* Replace the chicken with 1 pound tempeh, cut into 4 to 6 portions. To remove any bitterness in the tempeh, steam it for 20 minutes or simmer it in enough water to cover for 20 minutes. Drain the tempeh, then marinate it overnight in a mixture of 1 cup apple cider and 3 tablespoons cider vinegar. The next day, drain the tempeh, then sear it in a pan as described for the chicken. Finish the tempeh in the oven and serve as described above.

Braised Sumac Chicken and Lentils with Za'atar Yogurt Sauce

↓V

↑P

↑K

SUMAC IS A BRILLIANT red herb widely used in Middle Eastern cooking for its sour flavor. Bloomed in a little oil and cooked with lentils, it lends amazing flavor and color to bone-in chicken. This dish makes the perfect Sunday supper in cold weather. Serve it with basmati rice.

Ayurvedic Insight: With sweet chicken, salty olives, and a balance of warming spices, this dish will nourish your spirits even during the coldest winter.

Serves 4 to 6

BRAISED CHICKEN

3 tablespoons coconut oil

1 pound organic bone-in, skin-on chicken legs and thighs

Sea salt and freshly ground black pepper

1 cup 1/4-inch diced onions

1/2 cup 1/4-inch diced celery

1/2 cup 1/4-inch diced carrots

2 tablespoons ground sumac

1 teaspoon smoked paprika

1 tablespoon finely chopped garlic

1/4 cup dry red wine

2 tablespoons tomato paste

1 cup French green lentils

1/4 cup thinly sliced green olives, such as Castelvetrano

4 cups Vegetable Stock (page 281) or chicken stock, or store-bought stock

ZA'ATAR YOGURT SAUCE

3/4 cup plain yogurt

1 tablespoon za'atar spice blend

1 teaspoon finely grated fresh ginger

Sea salt and freshly ground black pepper

1 tablespoon chopped fresh cilantro, plus more for garnish

1. Preheat the oven to 350°F.

2. Heat a large ovenproof braising pan over high heat. Swirl the coconut oil across the pan bottom. Season the chicken with salt and pepper to taste, and sear it until it is golden brown all over, 2 to 3 minutes per side. Transfer the chicken to a plate and reserve.

3. Stir the onions, celery, and carrots into the same pan, scraping the pan bottom to capture all the flavor. Reduce the heat to low, cover, and sweat the vegetables until they are tender, 5 to 6 minutes. Stir in the sumac and smoked paprika and allow the spices to bloom for 1 to 2 minutes. Stir in the garlic and cook for 30 seconds, then raise the heat to medium and stir in the wine. Let the wine simmer for a minute or so. Stir in the tomato paste and cook over low heat for 2 minutes.

4. Stir in the lentils and spread the mixture evenly across the bottom of the pan.

5. Sprinkle the olives evenly over the mixture and place the chicken on top. Pour in the stock

and bring the mixture to a simmer over high heat. Cover and transfer the pan to the oven. Braise until the lentils are tender and the chicken is fall-apart tender (about 180°F internal temperature in the thickest part of a thigh), 45 to 55 minutes.

6. To make the sauce, whisk all the ingredients in a small bowl until well combined.

7. When the chicken is done, transfer it to a plate. Boil the lentil mixture over high heat until it has the consistency of risotto. Taste the mixture, adding salt and pepper until it tastes good to you. To serve, spoon the lentil mixture onto a serving platter or 4 to 6 individual plates, then place the chicken on top and spoon on the za'atar sauce. Garnish with chopped cilantro.

OPTIONS

- *Slow Cooker Pulled Chicken Stew:* Brown the chicken in a sauté pan as described, then transfer it to a slow cooker. Cook the vegetables in the same pan as described. After adding the lentils, bring the mixture to a boil, then pour everything in the pan over the chicken in the slow cooker. Cook for 6 hours on low. At that point, most of the liquid will be gone. Shred the chicken, add 2 cups chicken or vegetable stock to the cooker, then return the chicken to the cooker and mix everything together.
- *Braised Sumac Tempeh and Lentils with Za'atar Yogurt Sauce:* Replace the chicken with 1 pound tempeh. As a first step, place the tempeh in the braising pan with enough water to cover. Bring to a boil over high heat, then reduce the heat and gently simmer the tempeh for 10 minutes to remove any bitterness. Drain and wipe out the pan. Proceed with the recipe as directed, using the tempeh in place of the chicken.
- It's most economical to buy a whole organic chicken (3½ to 4 pounds) and cut it up yourself. Use the legs/thighs in this recipe, and save the breasts for Roasted Chicken with Sesame Cider Glaze (page 220). The wings can be roasted and served as an appetizer or with a salad. You can make chicken stock with the remaining carcass, adding it to the Vegetable Stock (page 281).
- You can freeze any leftovers, then reheat them, shred the chicken, and serve it as a soup by stirring in additional stock.
- To make this dairy-free or vegan, use nondairy yogurt in the sauce or replace the yogurt sauce with Chermoula (page 236).

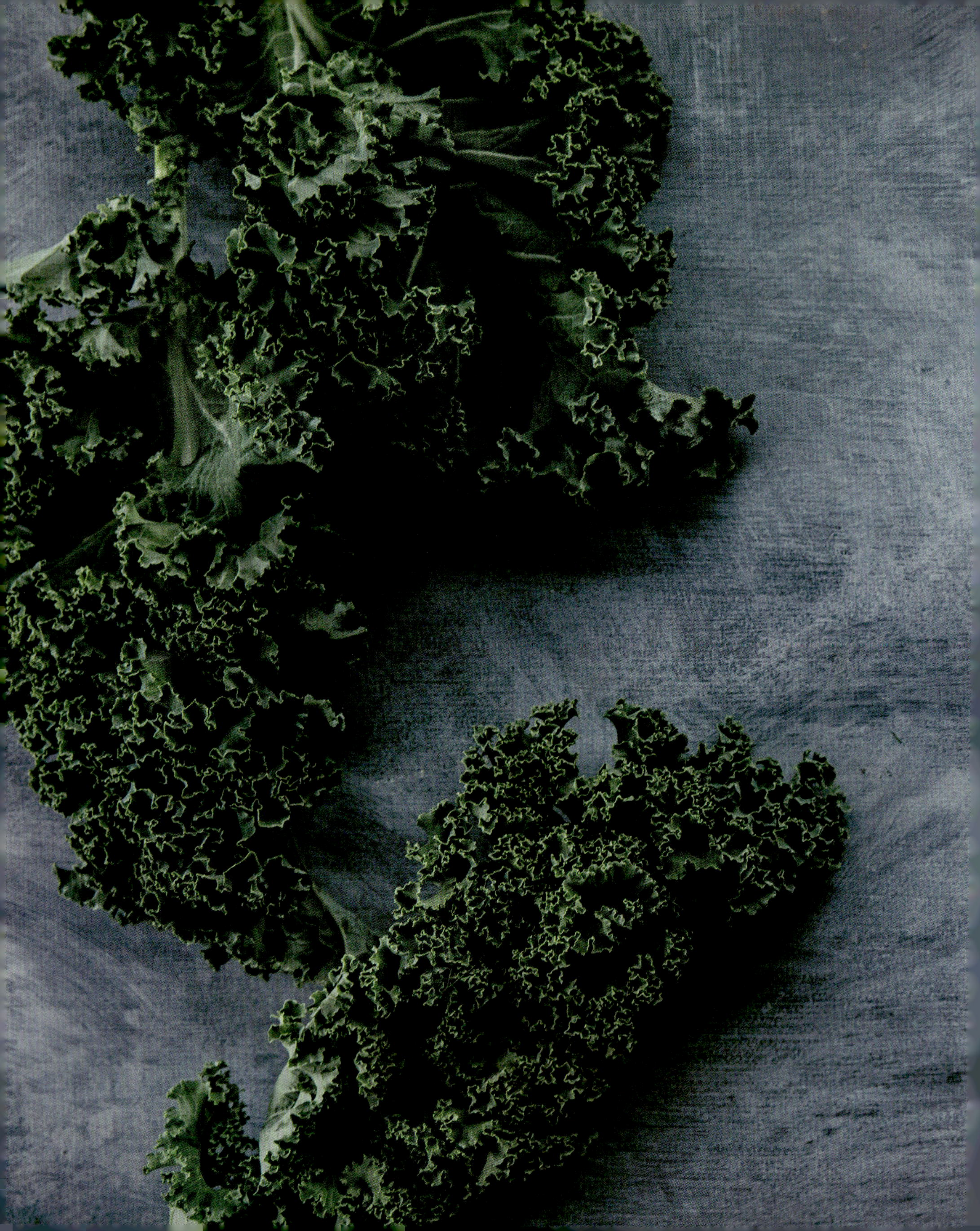

VEGETABLES AND GRAINS

Nutrition can be complex and confusing, but one thing is clear: we should all be eating more vegetables. This chapter is a good place to start. Simple recipes like Braised Kale and Apple Slaw (page 239), Caramelized Brussels Sprouts with Kimchi Sauce (page 235), and Roasted Cauliflower with Chermoula Sauce (page 236) can be served together to make a meal or served alongside almost any other savory dish in this book. These cruciferous vegetables support your health in numerous ways, from helping to lower cancer risk to reducing the chronic inflammation associated with various diseases.

Choose whatever vegetables are freshest in your market in any particular season. Eating with the seasons is a key concept of the Ayurvedic diet. Stick with dark leafy greens like kale and chard in the fall and winter and juicier "fruit-like" vegetables such as zucchini and eggplant in the summer. It can be difficult to recognize seasonal produce in modern American grocery stores, where you'll find summer foods like ears of sweet corn and fresh tomatoes even in the winter. To eat with the seasons, shop at a local farmer's market or check out the chart on page 18. Adjust the recipes here to enjoy the seasonal produce available in your area. For instance, if you can't find cauliflower for Roasted Cauliflower with Chermoula Sauce (page 236), use broccoli. Use whatever root vegetables you enjoy most for Turmeric Cider-Braised Root Vegetables (page 244).

Either way, you can't go wrong with eating seasonal vegetables and whole grains. Both of these food groups provide energy, moderate amounts of protein, and important nutrients that support a clear mind and a stable nervous system. If you are trying to eat less meat, start by having a filling grain and vegetable meal one night. On any given meatless Monday in the fall, enjoy a supper of Pineapple Purple Rice (page 240) and Warm Beets and Fennel with Orange Vinaigrette (page 243). Then notice how your body reacts. You may find that cutting back on meat in the evening helps you sleep better. Vegetables are much easier for our bodies to process in the evening, when our digestion naturally slows down. A meal made up entirely of vegetables and grains may sate your hunger while deepening the restorative sleep that your body needs to remain at peak health.

Roasted Asparagus with Watercress and Lemon Caper Dressing

↓V ↓P ↓K

ROASTING IS BY FAR the best way to cook asparagus. It delivers even heat all around the spears and lightly browns the vegetable, bringing out its sweetness. Olive oil, capers, and lemon balance out any grassy taste. You can serve this dish cold or hot.

Ayurvedic Insight: One of the best early spring vegetables, asparagus balances all three doshas. The brininess of capers and warming qualities of lemon zest also offset its coolness.

Serves 4

1 bunch white and/or green asparagus (about 1 pound), ends trimmed

1 tablespoon grapeseed oil or sunflower oil

1/4 cup plus 2 tablespoons extra-virgin olive oil

2 tablespoons rinsed and drained capers

2 tablespoons grated lemon zest

2 tablespoons fresh lemon juice

2 tablespoons chopped fresh basil, plus a few whole leaves for garnish

1/4 teaspoon fine sea salt

3 cups lightly packed watercress

1. Preheat the oven to 400°F.

2. Toss the asparagus and grapeseed oil on a sheet pan, shaking the pan to coat the spears. Arrange the asparagus in a single layer and roast until it is almost tender, 5 to 7 minutes. If you pick up a spear, it should bend slightly but not go completely limp. Remove from the oven and let cool to room temperature.

3. To make the dressing, combine the olive oil, capers, lemon zest, lemon juice, chopped basil, and salt in a small blender and puree until smooth and creamy with small flecks of basil.

4. Arrange a bed of watercress on a serving platter or 4 individual plates. Lay the asparagus on top and drizzle on the dressing. Garnish with the basil leaves.

OPTIONS

- Choose whatever thickness of asparagus you prefer. Young, early-spring asparagus is pencil thin and roasts in just 2 to 3 minutes. Late-spring asparagus is thicker and more flavorful but can have a woodier taste near the root end. Medium-thick is preferred here. To trim it, simply hold it horizontally in the air with two hands and bend. The stalk will naturally break where it becomes tender.

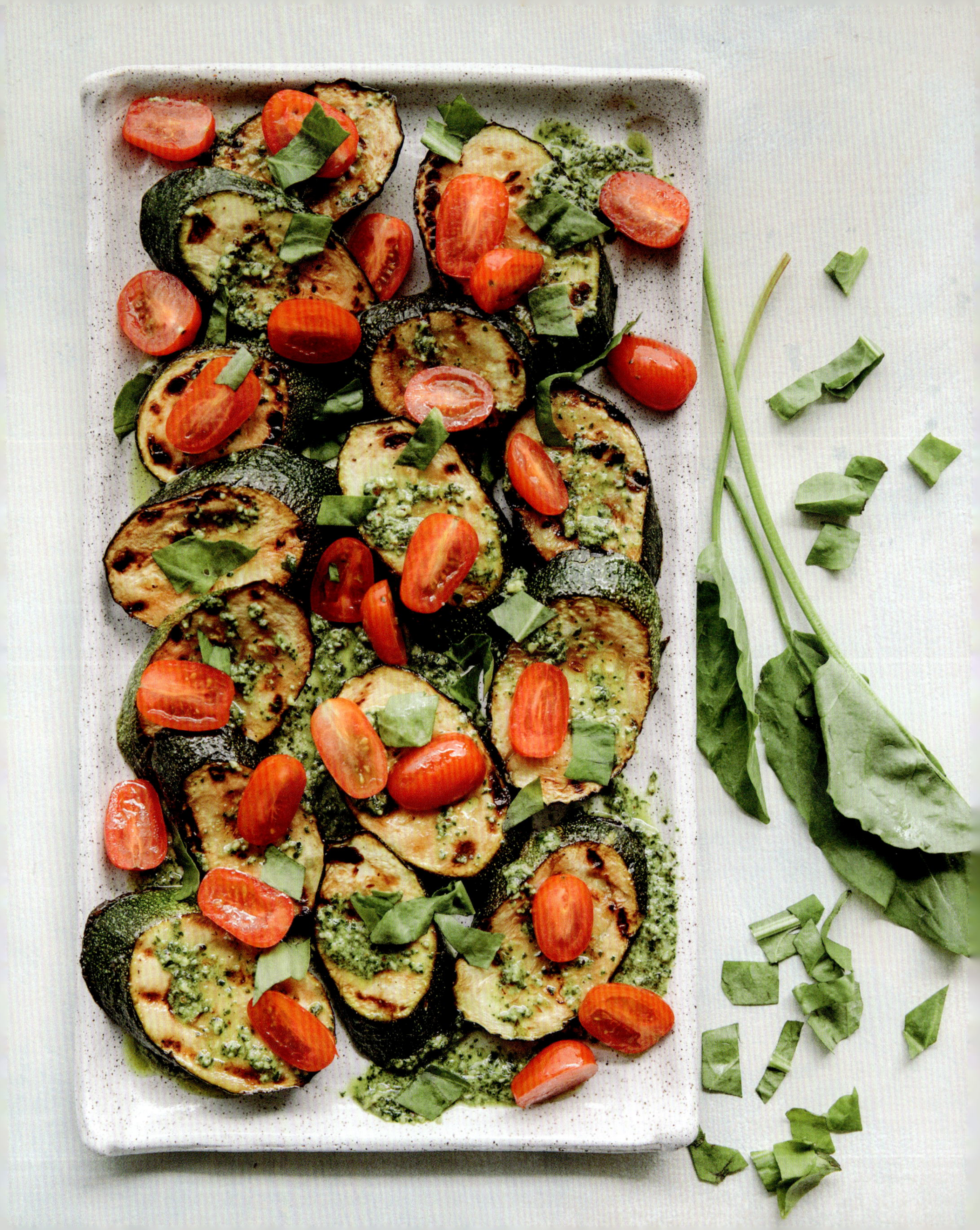

Grilled Zucchini with Cherry Tomatoes and Sorrel Puree

↓V
↓P
=K

GROWING UP IN Massachusetts, I remember running around in the summer and nibbling on wild greens like dandelion and sorrel. Plain old zucchini really gets a lift from the puckery taste of sorrel. Grilling the zucchini also gives it deeper, browned flavors. Just be sure to keep your grill heat moderate to avoid burning the zucchini, which is quite tender.

Ayurvedic Insight: Zucchini and tomatoes are very watery, making them perfect for dry vata and hot pitta types. Sorrel and watercress also balance out the wateriness so that kaphas can enjoy them from time to time.

Serves 4

SORREL PUREE

1½ cups packed sorrel leaves
½ cup packed watercress leaves
½ cup extra-virgin olive oil
¼ cup walnuts
3 garlic cloves
2 tablespoons chèvre (soft goat cheese) or ricotta (optional)
½ teaspoon fine sea salt
¼ teaspoon freshly ground black pepper

ZUCCHINI AND TOMATOES

2 medium zucchini, cut on an angle into ovals about 1 inch thick (2 to 3 inches long)
2 tablespoons grapeseed oil
1 tablespoon balsamic vinegar
½ teaspoon fine sea salt
Pinch of freshly ground black pepper
1 cup cherry tomatoes, halved

1. Preheat a grill for medium heat.

2. For the sorrel puree, put the sorrel, watercress, oil, walnuts, garlic, chèvre (if using), salt, and pepper in a food processor. Blend until pureed liked pesto, stopping periodically to scrape down the sides.

3. For the zucchini, toss the zucchini, oil, vinegar, salt, and pepper in a medium bowl.

4. Scrape the grill grate clean and lay the zucchini ovals on the grill. Cook just until they are golden brown on the bottom, 3 to 4 minutes. Flip with tongs and cook just until the zucchini is tender yet still a bit crunchy, 2 to 3 minutes more.

5. Arrange the zucchini on a serving platter or individual plates and spoon the sorrel puree over the top. Garnish with the halved cherry tomatoes and serve.

OPTIONS

- If grilling isn't an option, you could just roast the zucchini or sauté it.
- If you can't find sorrel, replace it with 1½ cups baby arugula, 1 tablespoon grated lemon zest, and 1 tablespoon lemon juice.

- For vegan sorrel puree, skip the chèvre or replace it with a vegan cream cheese such as Kite Hill.
- Use the sorrel puree on any cooked veggies, toss it with pasta, or use it as a sandwich spread.

Roasted Eggplant with Tomatoes, Raisins, and Mint

↑V
↑P
↓K

WHAT GROWS TOGETHER goes together: eggplant and tomatoes both thrive in the summer and marry happily in this light, clean-tasting preparation. The raisins and mint brighten up all the flavors here, so if you're not a fan of eggplant, give it another try. You can make this dish in the morning, let it marinate all day, then serve it later, either at room temperature or cold.

Ayurvedic Insight: Eggplant is heating and absorbs water. Its high fiber content also makes it a great replacement for grains if you're looking for a filling, grain-free meal.

Serves 4 to 6

6 cups 1½-inch cubes skin-on eggplant
½ teaspoon fine sea salt
2 tablespoons grapeseed oil or sunflower oil
1½ cups ½-inch diced ripe tomatoes (cherry, plum, heirloom)
¾ cup ½-inch diced red bell peppers
½ cup chopped fresh mint, plus a few sprigs for garnish
¼ cup golden raisins
2 tablespoons thinly sliced scallion greens
2 tablespoons extra-virgin olive oil
1 tablespoon fresh lemon juice
1 tablespoon red wine vinegar
2 teaspoons minced fresh garlic
¼ teaspoon freshly ground black pepper

1. Preheat the oven to 400°F.

2. Toss the eggplant, salt, and grapeseed oil on a sheet pan. Use your hands to evenly coat the eggplant, then arrange it in a single layer.

3. Roast until the eggplant is lightly browned on the bottom, 6 to 8 minutes. Use a metal spatula to loosen the pieces and flip them. Roast until they are fork-tender, 6 to 8 minutes more. The tips should be nicely browned.

4. Transfer the roasted eggplant to a serving bowl. Stir in the tomatoes, peppers, mint, raisins, scallions, olive oil, lemon juice, vinegar, garlic, and black pepper. Taste the mixture and add more salt, pepper, or lemon juice until it tastes good to you. Serve garnished with the mint sprigs.

OPTIONS

- For more protein, add some crumbled feta and scatter on a handful of toasted pine nuts.
- Serve the eggplant over cooked couscous or quinoa.

Sautéed Swiss Chard with Almonds and Currants

=V
↓P
↓K

I TEND TO GIVE main dishes bold flavor profiles but keep the accompaniments simple so they don't compete with the main course. This simple, sweet, and crunchy Swiss chard is a good example. It's perfectly at home alongside full-flavored dishes like Roasted Chicken with Sesame Cider Glaze (page 220) and Summer Vegetable Tian with Chèvre and Smoked Sea Salt (page 187).

Ayurvedic Insight: Dark, leafy greens are drying, astringent, and perfect for absorbing the excess oil of pitta and kapha. The salt and warming garlic and pepper here also make this dish suitable for vata types to enjoy in the summer.

Serves 4 to 6

2 bunches Swiss and/or rainbow chard (12 ounces each bunch)
1/4 cup extra-virgin olive oil
1/2 cup dried currants
1 teaspoon finely chopped garlic
1/4 teaspoon fine sea salt
2 pinches of freshly ground black pepper
1 cup almonds, toasted and chopped

1. Separate the chard leaves from the stems. Finely chop the stems and coarsely chop the leaves.

2. Heat a large sauté pan over medium heat for 1 minute. Swirl in the oil, then add the currants and chard. Cook until the chard is wilted, 3 to 4 minutes, tossing constantly. Stir in the garlic and cook for 30 seconds. Remove from the heat and season with the salt and pepper. Sprinkle on the almonds.

OPTIONS

- You can use this recipe as a template and substitute raisins or dried cranberries for the currants and hazelnuts or pistachios for the almonds.

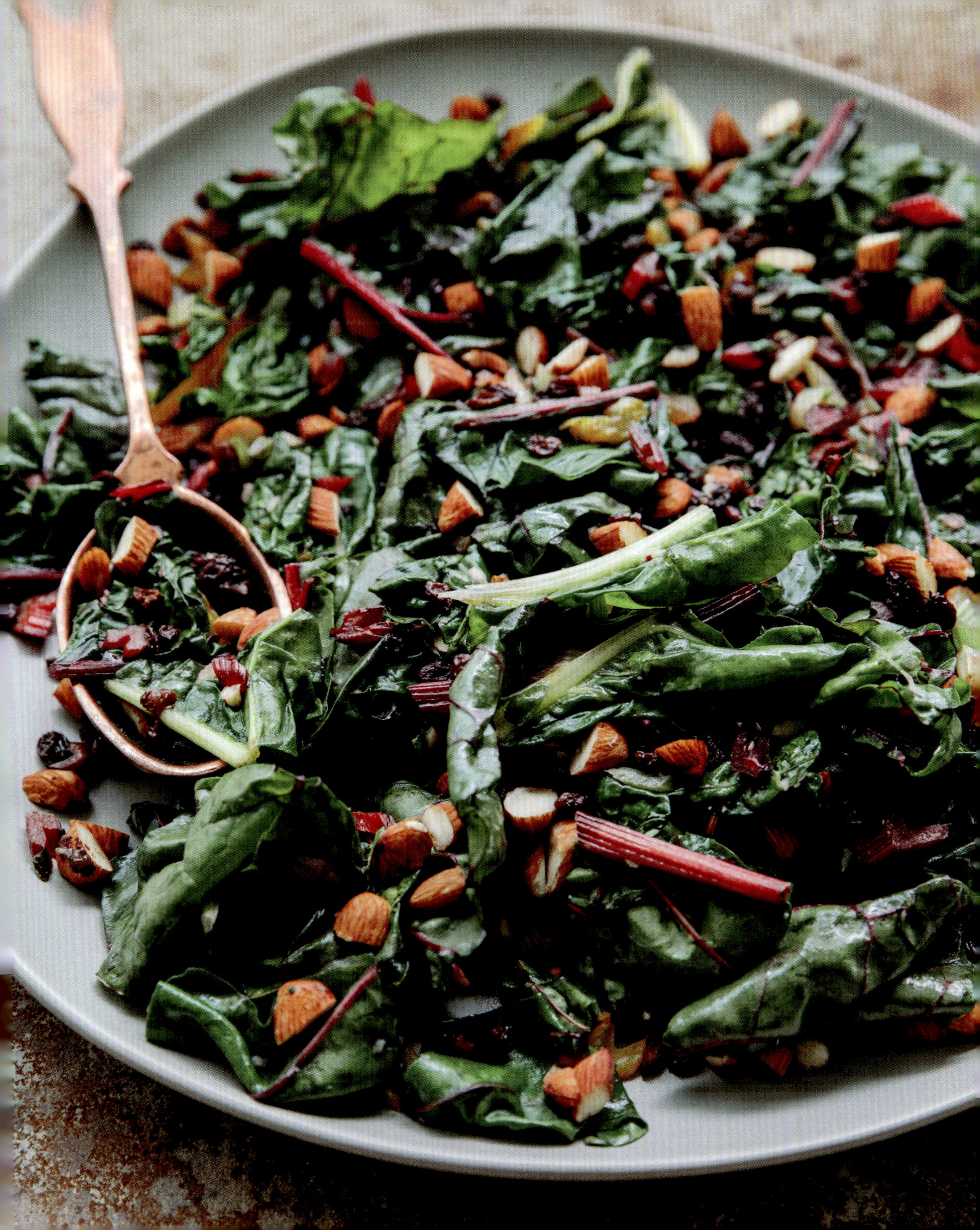

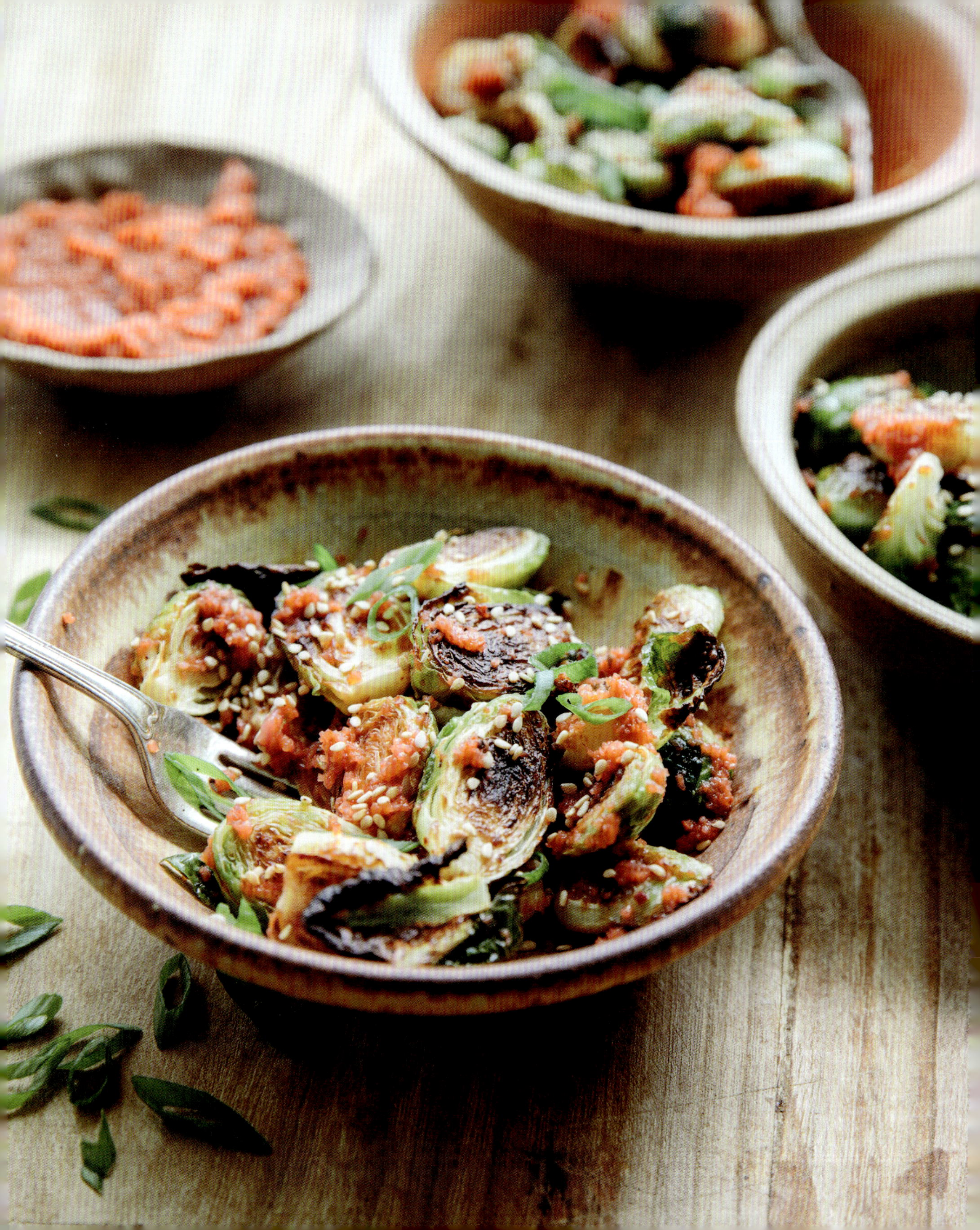

Caramelized Brussels Sprouts with Kimchi Sauce

↑V
=P
↓K

AS A FERMENTED FOOD, kimchi provides some fantastic prebiotics and probiotics to improve your digestive health. Just don't cook it or you'll kill all the good stuff. That's the idea behind kimchi sauce, a sort of vinaigrette made with finely chopped kimchi, maple syrup, and olive oil. It works perfectly with pan-seared Brussels sprouts.

Ayurvedic Insight: In the fall, the bitter and dry qualities of Brussels sprouts help to dry out excess heat buildup from the summer. The warmth of kimchi makes this dish best for kapha, yet pitta types can also enjoy it by using a little less of the sauce.

Serves 4 to 6

BRUSSELS SPROUTS

1½ pounds Brussels sprouts, trimmed and halved lengthwise

3 tablespoons toasted sesame oil

Sea salt and freshly ground black pepper

¼ cup minced shallots

2 tablespoons minced fresh ginger

KIMCHI SAUCE

1 cup drained and coarsely chopped kimchi

3 tablespoons extra-virgin olive oil

2 tablespoons pure maple syrup

2 tablespoons unsweetened brown rice vinegar

Pinch of crushed red pepper flakes

½ teaspoon toasted sesame seeds

1. Preheat the oven to 350°F.

2. For the Brussels sprouts, heat 2 large oven-proof sauté pans over medium-high heat. When hot, divide the sesame oil and Brussels sprouts between the pans, season the sprouts with salt and pepper, and toss to coat evenly. Use tongs or your hands to place the sprouts cut sides down, then cook until the sprouts are lightly browned on the bottoms, about 5 minutes. Place the pans in the hot oven and roast until the sprouts are golden brown on the bottoms, 5 to 8 minutes more.

3. Remove from the oven and stir in the shallots and ginger.

4. For the kimchi sauce, combine everything except the sesame seeds in a blender or food processor and blend or pulse until slightly chunky, 10 to 15 seconds. You should still see bits of cabbage in the mixture. Taste the sauce and season it with more salt if needed.

5. Pour the sauce over the bottom of a serving platter or 4 to 6 individual plates. Spoon the sprouts over the sauce and garnish with the sesame seeds.

OPTIONS

- We use pure maple syrup instead of white sugar because it's available locally here in Massachusetts, and it's delicious. You could use agave nectar or brown rice syrup.
- For a paleo version, replace the vinegar with lemon juice.
- For a vegan version, use vegan kimchi made without fish sauce.

Roasted Cauliflower with Chermoula Sauce

=V
↓P
↓K

CHERMOULA, A MIDDLE EASTERN HERB and spice condiment, pairs well with most fish and vegetable preparations. It's fantastic on roasted cauliflower, and this dish makes the ideal accompaniment to Braised Sumac Chicken and Lentils with Za'atar Yogurt Sauce (page 222).

Ayurvedic Insight: While cauliflower is generally best for pitta and kapha types, roasting it in oil makes it enjoyable for vatas as well.

Serves 4 to 6

1 head of cauliflower, cut into medium florets
2 tablespoons grapeseed oil
2 cups coarsely chopped fresh cilantro, plus more for garnish
1 cup coarsely chopped fresh parsley, plus more for garnish
2 garlic cloves, smashed
Grated zest and juice of 1 lemon, plus grated zest for garnish
1½ teaspoons ground cumin
1 teaspoon paprika
1 teaspoon fine sea salt
¼ cup extra-virgin olive oil

1. Preheat the oven to 400°F.

2. Toss the cauliflower and grapeseed oil on a sheet pan, using your hands to thoroughly rub the florets with oil. Roast until the cauliflower is golden brown and fork-tender, 10 to 15 minutes.

3. To make the chermoula sauce, place the remaining ingredients and ¼ cup water in a small food processor and puree until mostly smooth, periodically scraping down the sides of the bowl. The sauce should be thick yet pourable from a spoon. If it's too thick, blend in a bit more water.

4. To serve, spoon the sauce over the bottom of a serving platter or 4 to 6 individual plates. Top with the cauliflower and garnish with parsley, cilantro, and lemon zest.

OPTIONS

- Don't stress about picking all of the stems off the cilantro. Just get the thick ones off the bottom and leave the thinner ones.
- For a bit more flavor, mix ras el hanout or harissa spice mix with the grapeseed oil and toss it with the cauliflower before roasting.
- You can roast the whole head of cauliflower and serve it over the sauce family style. Coat the entire head with grapeseed oil, drizzling some into the inner crevices under and inside the head. Roast it in a cast-iron skillet until it is fork-tender in the center, basting the cauliflower with the oil periodically as it cooks.
- The chermoula sauce tastes wonderful on grilled vegetables, roasted winter squash, grilled fish, and roasted chicken.
- For those who hate cilantro, make the sauce entirely with parsley.

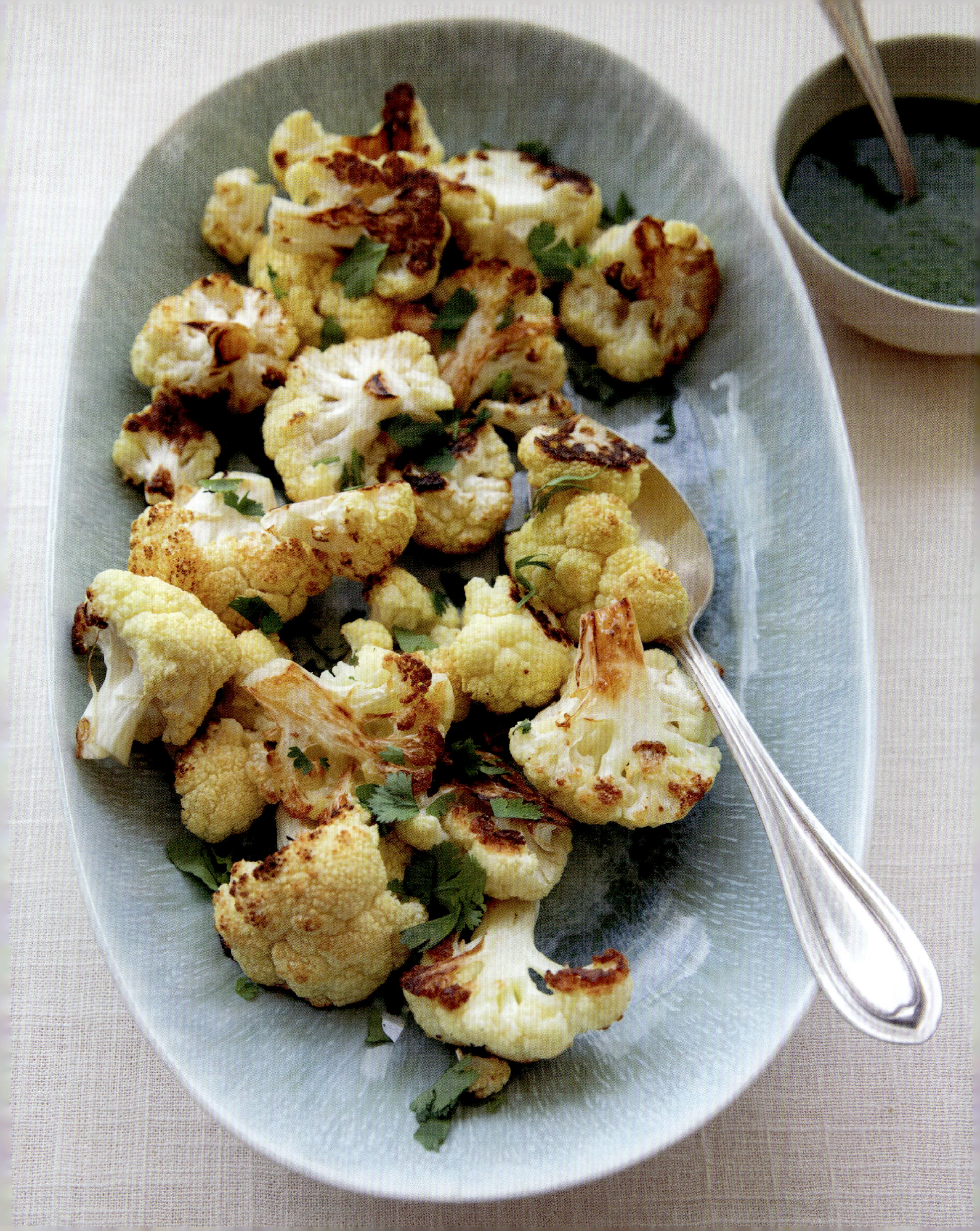

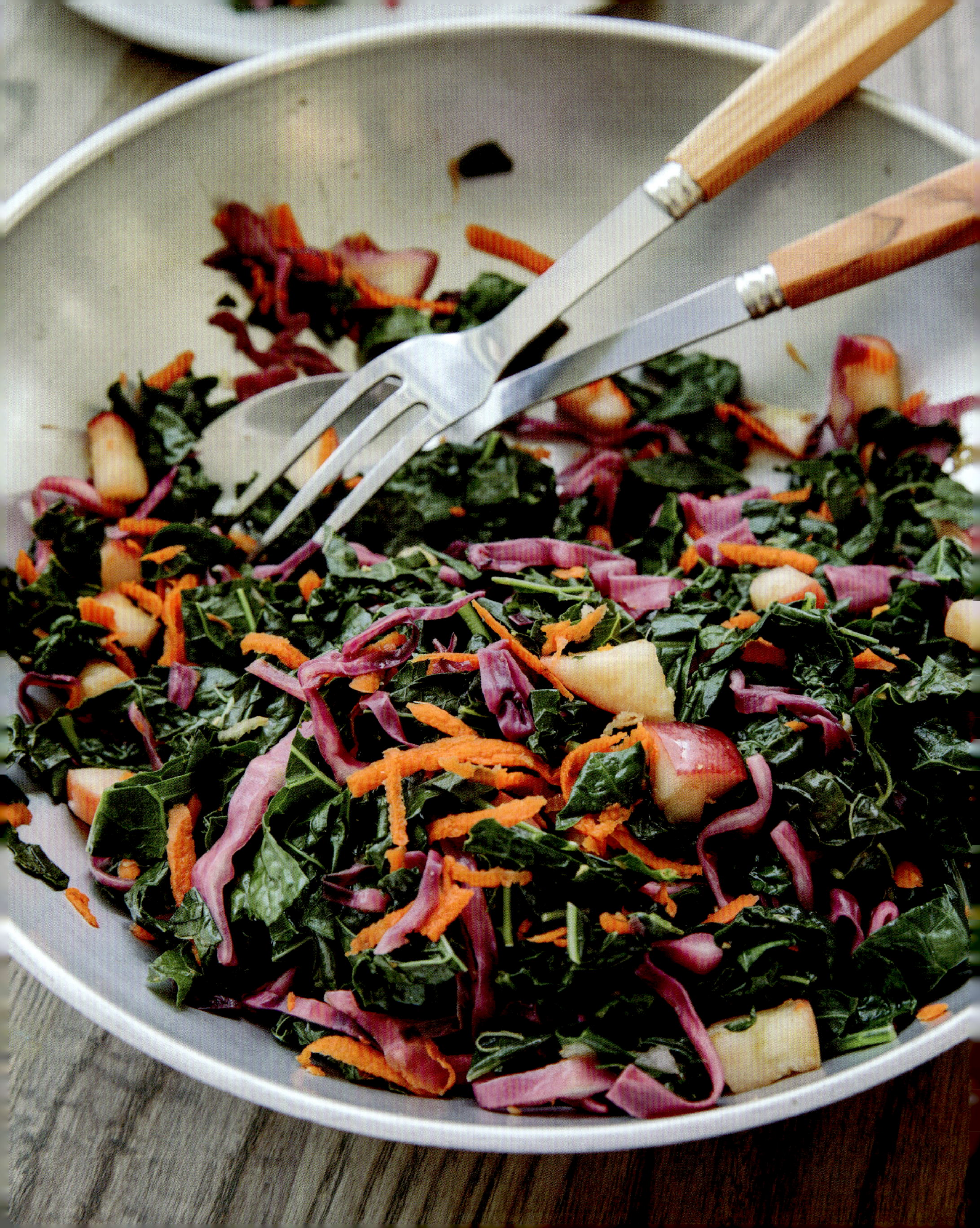

Braised Kale and Apple Slaw

WARM SLAW MAY seem odd to Americans, but it's a great way to eat your greens in the winter. Plus, according to Ayurveda, we should be eating cooked foods in cooler weather because our bodies run cold then too, and warm foods help to stoke our digestive fire. Here, the crunchy sweetness of carrots and apples balances the bitter astringency of cabbage and kale.

Ayurvedic Insight: Pitta and kapha types will enjoy the astringent qualities of this slaw, but it's a little too dry and cooling for vatas. Add a bit more ginger and oil to make it more vata friendly.

↑V ↓P ↓K

Serves 4 to 6

1 tablespoon extra-virgin olive oil

1 cup thinly sliced red cabbage

6 cups lightly packed shredded lacinato kale (8 ounces, about 1 bunch)

1/2 cup grated carrots

1/2 cup 1/4-inch diced red apples with skin

1 teaspoon minced fresh ginger

1 tablespoon cider vinegar

1/2 teaspoon fine sea salt

1/4 teaspoon freshly ground black pepper

1. Heat a large sauté pan over medium heat. When hot, put in the oil and cabbage, shaking the pan to coat the cabbage. Cook until a bit softened but not browned, 2 to 3 minutes. Stir in the kale and cook for 2 to 3 minutes, tossing now and then.

2. Stir in the carrots, apples, and ginger and cook until the carrots are still crisp-tender, about 1 minute. Stir in the cider vinegar and 1 tablespoon water and cook until most of the liquid evaporates. Season with salt and pepper and serve.

OPTIONS

- If you adhere to a raw diet, you could serve this slaw cold. Just mix everything together.
- For a paleo version, replace the vinegar with lemon juice.

Pineapple Purple Rice

↓V
↓P
↓K

PURPLE RICE, OR CHINESE BLACK RICE, is a medium-grain rice sometimes used in desserts. Its awesome purple color comes from anthocyanin, which has tons of health benefits, such as helping to fight inflammation and promoting healthy neural function. Toasting the rice in coconut oil gives it a tropical aroma, while red bell peppers, yellow pineapple chunks, and green scallions complement its dark purple color.

Ayurvedic Insight: Purple rice is loaded with digestion-improving fiber and various nutrients that make this dish balancing for all three doshas.

Serves 6

1½ cups purple rice (aka forbidden rice)
3 tablespoons coconut oil
1 cup ¼-inch diced pineapple
½ cup slivered almonds, toasted
½ cup thinly sliced scallion greens
¼ cup ¼-inch diced red bell peppers
1 teaspoon fine sea salt

1. Rinse the rice in a fine-mesh strainer under cool running water for 1 minute. Let drain.

2. Combine the rice and coconut oil in a medium saucepan, tossing to coat the rice. Over medium heat, cook the rice until it smells nutty and toasted, 3 to 5 minutes, stirring frequently. Add 3 cups water and bring the rice to a simmer. Cover, reduce the heat to low, and cook until the rice is tender, 20 to 25 minutes. When done, let the rice sit off the heat, covered, for 5 minutes.

3. Using a fork, gently fluff the rice to separate the grains. Gently fold in the pineapple, almonds, scallions, bell peppers, and salt. Serve hot. You can also serve the rice at room temperature or cold. It keeps for about a day in the refrigerator.

OPTION

- You can use other varieties of rice such as wehani. Cook it as directed on the package.

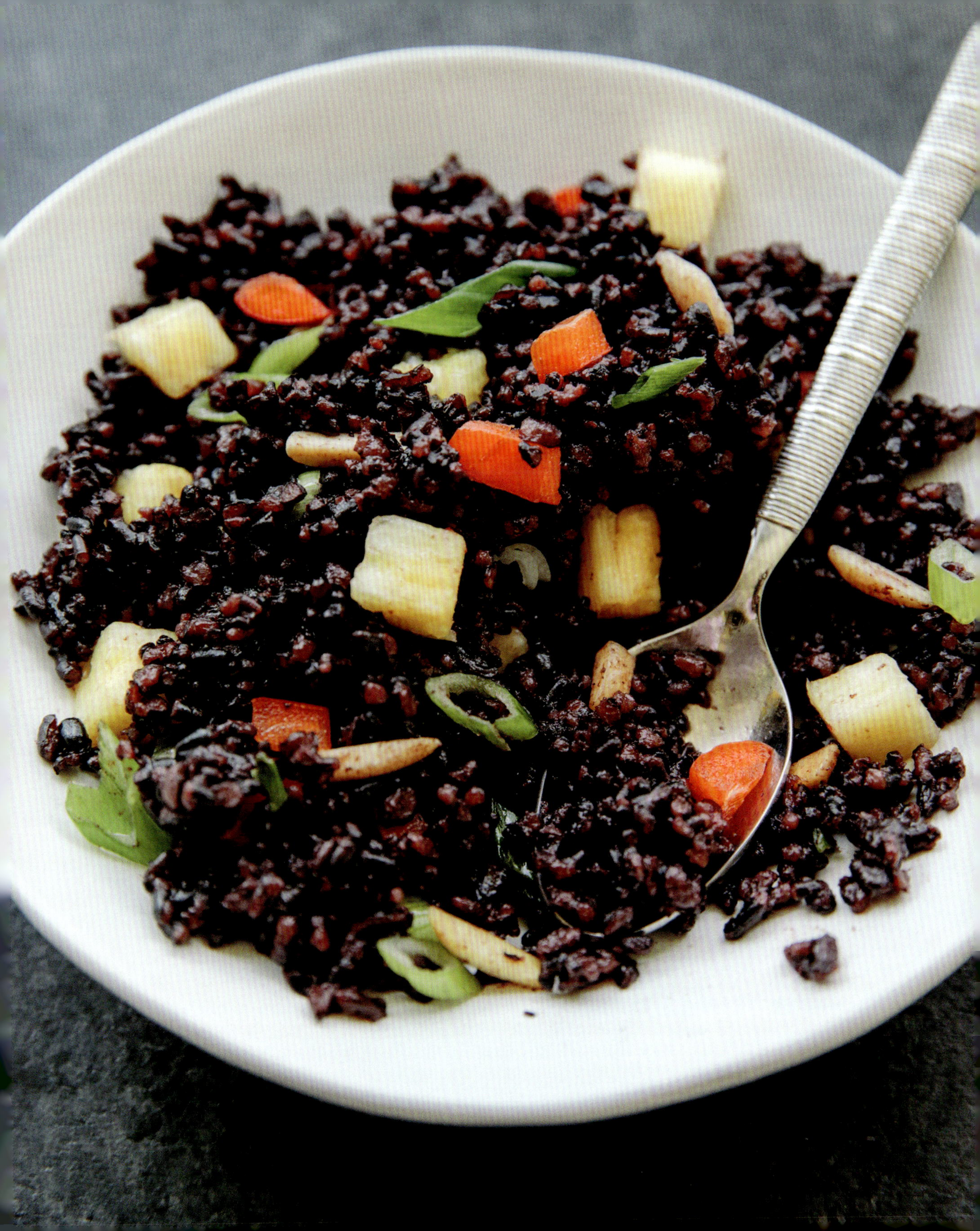

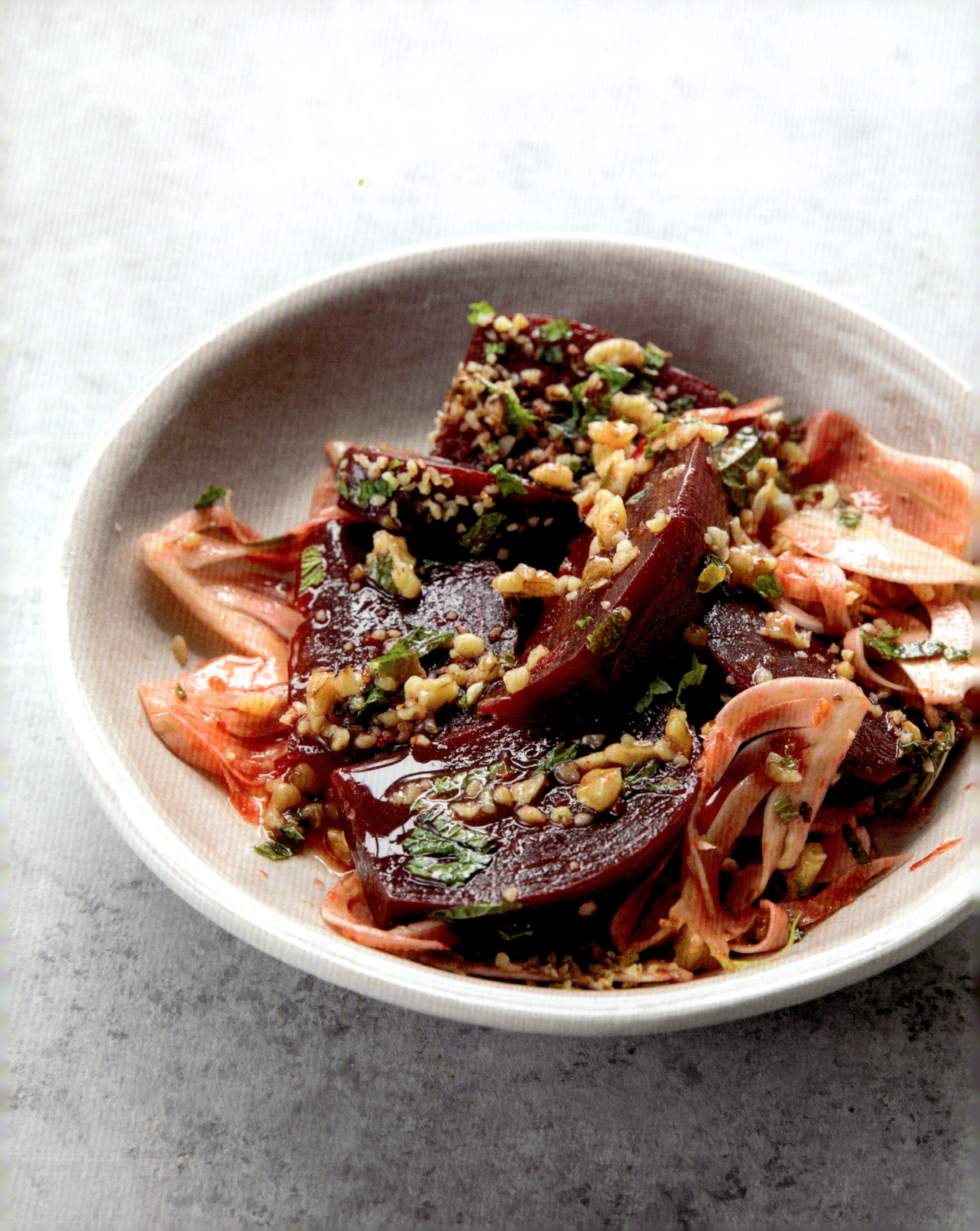

Warm Beets and Fennel with Orange Vinaigrette

↓V ↓P ↓K

HERE'S A TASTY, colorful way to serve beets. Simply simmer beet wedges to tenderness, then top them with a bright orange dressing infused with the flavor of fennel. Shaving the fennel paper thin releases its aromas while keeping it nice and crunchy. Toasted walnuts and mint round out the fall flavors and colors.

Ayurvedic Insight: When beets are in season, eat them with abandon, as they help to support healthy gall bladder and liver function.

Serves 4 to 6

1½ pounds beets (about 6 small), peeled and cut into eighths (about 4 cups)

1 seedless navel orange

1 tablespoon brown rice vinegar

½ teaspoon honey or agave nectar

2 tablespoons extra-virgin olive oil

½ cup shaved fresh fennel bulb (sliced paper thin on a mandoline)

¼ teaspoon fine sea salt

⅛ teaspoon freshly ground black pepper

2 tablespoons walnuts, toasted and chopped

1 tablespoon chopped fresh mint

1. Place the beets in a medium saucepan with just enough water to cover, about 3 cups. Cover and bring to a boil. Reduce the heat to low and simmer until the beets are fork-tender, 18 to 20 minutes.

2. While the beets cook, make the vinaigrette. Grate the zest from the orange into a small bowl. Squeeze in ¼ cup of the juice, then whisk in the vinegar, honey, and oil. Stir in the fennel and let the mixture stand at room temperature until the beets are ready.

3. Drain the cooked beets well and arrange them on a serving platter or on 4 to 6 individual plates. Season with the salt and pepper, then drizzle with the vinaigrette. Top with the walnuts and mint.

OPTIONS

- If you have leftover whole roasted beets, peel them and use them in place of the simmered beets here.
- For a paleo version, replace the vinegar with lemon juice.

Turmeric Cider-Braised Root Vegetables

↓V
↓P
↓K

WE ROAST A LOT of root vegetables at Kripalu. To keep them from drying out, I like to braise or "broast" them with a splash of water, or in this recipe, apple cider. When the cider cooks down, it leaves a shiny glaze on the roots. Turmeric gives the glaze a bright orange color and provides some anti-inflammatory and antioxidant benefits, thanks to a compound called *curcumin*.

Ayurvedic Insight: The oil and vinegar here balance out the earthiness of root vegetables, so this nourishing dish can be enjoyed by all three doshas.

Serves 4 to 6

2 tablespoons extra-virgin olive oil
2 tablespoons cider vinegar
3/4 cup apple cider
1/2 teaspoon ground cinnamon
1/2 teaspoon ground turmeric
1/4 teaspoon fine sea salt
1/8 teaspoon freshly ground black pepper
1 1/2 cups 3/4-inch diced rutabaga
1 1/2 cups 3/4-inch diced parsnips
1 1/2 cups 3/4-inch diced carrots
1 1/2 cups 3/4-inch diced turnips
2 teaspoons chopped fresh parsley

1. Preheat the oven to 350°F.

2. In a small bowl, whisk together the oil, vinegar, cider, cinnamon, turmeric, salt, and pepper.

3. Place the rutabaga, parsnips, carrots, and turnips in a 4-quart baking dish or roasting pan. Pour on the cider mixture and mix well. Cover the dish with foil and roast until the vegetables are barely fork-tender, about 30 minutes. Remove the foil, give everything a stir to coat the vegetables, and continue roasting until the liquid reduces, thickens slightly, and glazes the vegetables, 10 to 12 minutes more.

4. Toss with the parsley and serve.

OPTIONS

- Use any root vegetables you like here. If celeriac and kohlrabi are fresh at the market, use them. You can also use any fresh herb, such as thyme, parsley, or sage (go easy on sage because it is strong).

Kitchari

↓V ↓P ↓K

THE QUINTESSENTIAL AYURVEDIC healing food, kitchari is a simple rice and split mung bean dish flavored with various spices such as turmeric, cumin, and mustard seeds. It's like the chicken soup of Indian food. It's quick and easy to make, so you can enjoy it anytime you want a healthy reset. If you're feeling sick or you overindulged during the holidays, eat this for a day or two in a row. You can double the recipe and keep some kitchari in the fridge.

Ayurvedic Insight: A traditional part of the detoxing, purifying regimen called *panchakarma*, kitchari provides a full complement of beneficial amino acids in a complete meal that is easy to digest. All doshas can enjoy it freely.

Serves 4

1 tablespoon ghee or coconut oil
1 teaspoon brown mustard seeds
2 teaspoons ground cumin
1 teaspoon ground turmeric
Pinch of freshly ground black pepper
1/4 cup yellow split peas (moong dahl)
1/2 cup uncooked white basmati rice
2 tablespoons chopped fresh cilantro
1 teaspoon fresh lemon juice
1/2 teaspoon fine sea salt

1. Heat the ghee in a medium saucepan over medium-low heat. Stir in the mustard seeds and cook until they begin to pop, 2 to 3 minutes. Stir in the cumin, turmeric, and pepper and cook until fragrant, about 30 seconds. Stir in the split peas and rice and cook until the rice is lightly toasted, 2 to 3 minutes, stirring once or twice.

2. Add 4 cups water and bring to a simmer over high heat. Reduce the heat to low, cover, and cook until the rice and peas are tender and most of the liquid is absorbed, 10 to 15 minutes. The kitchari should be slightly wet, and the rice should be just moist enough to stick everything together. Turn off the heat and let the kitchari sit for 5 minutes with the lid on. If you like your kitchari soupy, or if it appears too thick, stir in up to 1 cup more water to thin it out. Once it has rested, remove the lid and stir in the cilantro, lemon juice, and salt. Serve hot.

OPTION

- Add your favorite vegetables after toasting the rice, and try different spices to find the blend that best suits your taste.

Vegetable Biryani

↓V
↓P
↓K

A CLASSIC KRIPALU RECIPE, this basic rice dish is a staple on Indian restaurant menus. It marries perfectly with Coconut Chana Saag (page 180). If you want the rice grains to remain separate and retain their long shape, look for basmati rice that has been aged for one to three years. Most of the rice sold in the United States is aged for only about six months and cooks up wetter and looser, but you can find aged rice at Indian markets and specialty food stores.

Ayurvedic Insight: Cooking basmati rice with pungent ingredients like onions, garlic, and turmeric mitigates its cooling properties. Even kids love this dish and generally don't mind the veggies.

Serves 4

1/4 cup minced yellow onions
1 tablespoon ghee or extra-virgin olive oil
1/2 cup 1/4-inch diced carrots
1/2 teaspoon ground turmeric
1 cup uncooked white basmati rice
2 teaspoons minced fresh ginger
1 teaspoon finely chopped garlic
1/4 cup dark raisins
1/2 cup fresh or frozen and thawed green peas
1/4 cup roasted cashew halves and pieces
1/4 teaspoon fine sea salt

1. Heat a medium saucepan over medium-low heat for 2 minutes. Put in the onions and ghee, shaking the pan to coat the onions. Cover and sweat over low heat until the onions are translucent, 3 to 5 minutes.

2. Stir in the carrots, turmeric, and rice. Cook over medium heat until the carrots are almost tender and the rice is colored orange with turmeric and smells lightly toasted, 2 to 3 minutes.

3. Stir in the ginger and garlic and cook until fragrant, about 30 seconds. Stir in the raisins and 1½ cups water. Cover and bring to a gentle simmer over high heat, then reduce the heat to low and cook until the liquid is absorbed and the rice is tender, 12 to 18 minutes. Remove from the heat and let rest, covered, for 5 minutes.

4. Using a fork, gently fluff the rice to separate the grains. Gently fold in the peas, cashews, and salt just until they are incorporated. Serve hot.

OPTION

- For a main dish to serve two, add 8 to 12 ounces cooked tofu cubes, shrimp, or chicken tossed with 1 teaspoon curry powder and 1 tablespoon ghee or olive oil.

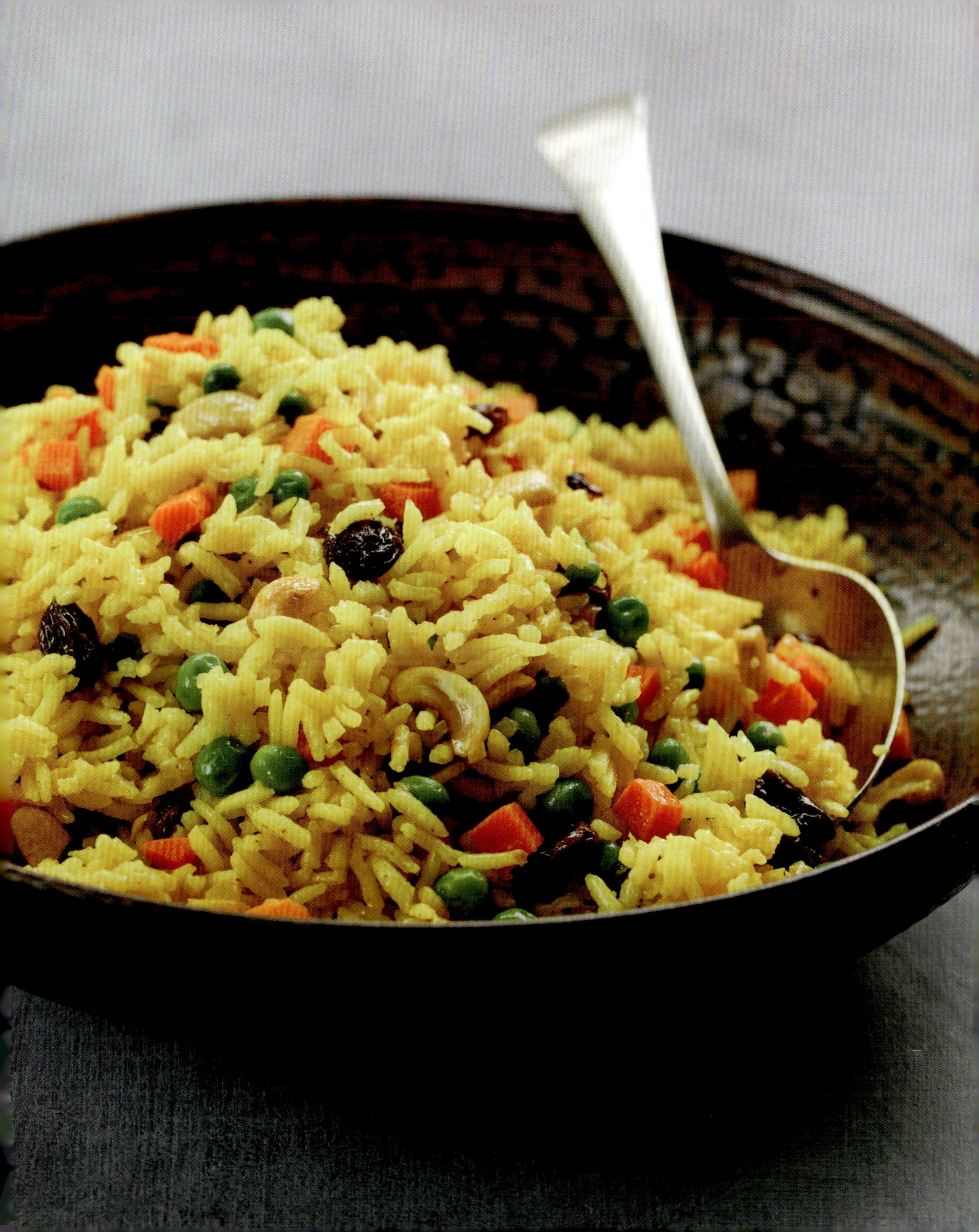

Cauliflower and Millet Mash

↑V
↓P
↓K

ONE OF THE SIMPLEST recipes in the book, this dish is always a sleeper hit in my cooking classes. It provides the creamy satisfaction of mashed potatoes without weighing you down. For a balanced three-part plate, pair it with almost any vegetable dish, such as Caramelized Brussels Sprouts with Kimchi Sauce (page 235), and any protein-based dish, such as Roasted Chicken with Sesame Cider Glaze (page 220).

Ayurvedic Insight: The light and dry qualities of cauliflower and millet help to evaporate excess mucus, which in turn supports healthy digestion. Try this dish if you are prone to allergies in the springtime.

Serves 4 to 6

1/2 cup millet

4 ounces chopped cauliflower florets (about 1 1/2 cups)

1/2 teaspoon fine sea salt

1 to 2 tablespoons ghee or extra-virgin olive oil

2 tablespoons chopped fresh parsley, for garnish

1. In a fine-mesh sieve, rinse the millet under cool running water, then let drain. Transfer the millet to a medium saucepan with a lid. Add 2½ cups water, the cauliflower, and salt. Bring to a boil over high heat, then reduce the heat to low, cover, and simmer gently for 35 minutes. After 30 minutes, give the mixture a stir. The millet should have broken apart and when you stir, it will thicken the liquid in the pot. When the mixture is very soft and thick, take it off the heat and let stand for 5 minutes.

2. Puree the mixture with an immersion blender or in an upright blender or small food processor. If using an upright blender or food processor, avoid a blowout by slightly cooling the mixture and partially removing the center lid of the machine. Puree the mixture until it is supersmooth. It will be thick. Blend in the ghee and serve the mash hot, garnished with the parsley.

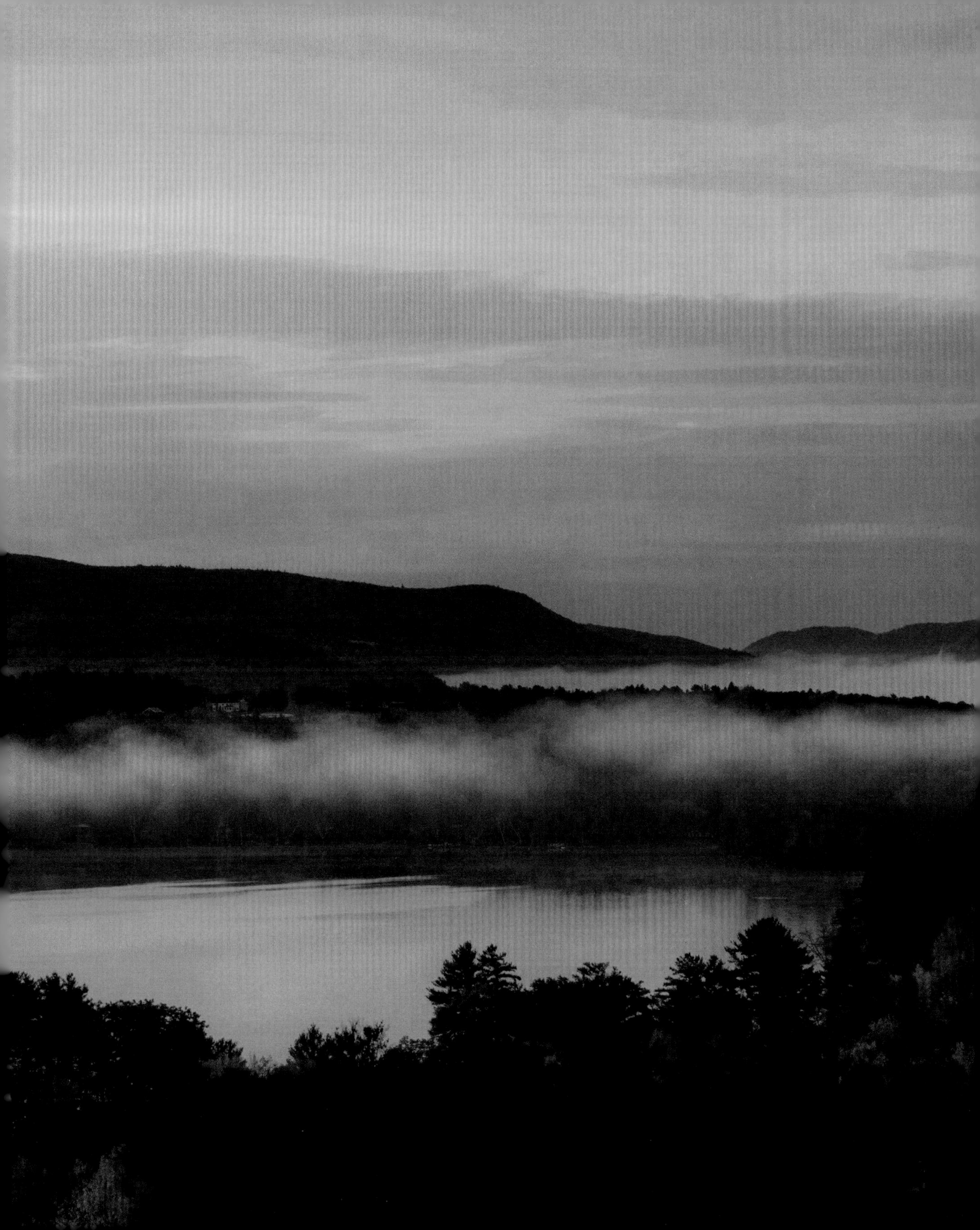

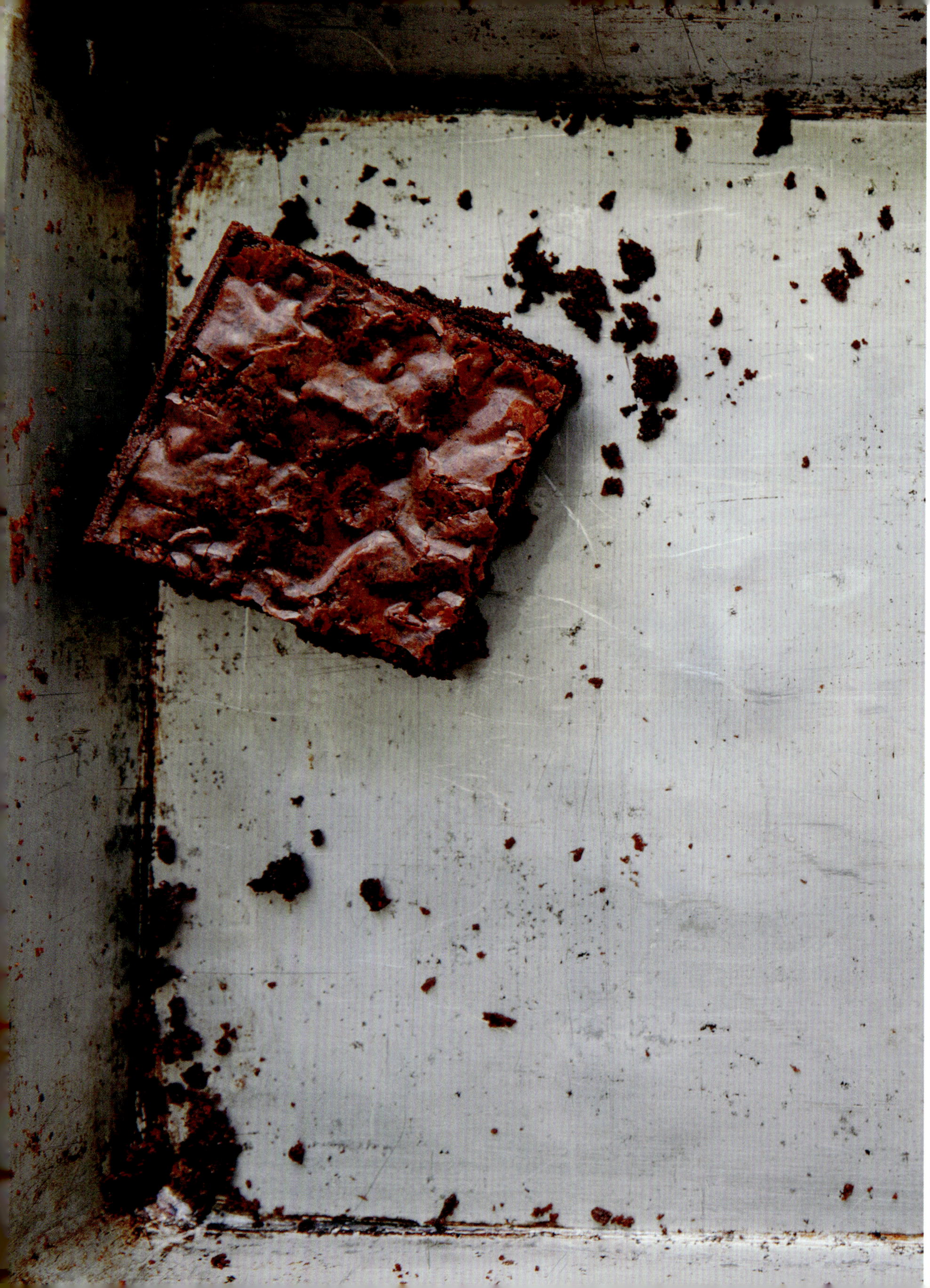

SOMETHING SWEET

Sweet is one of our most basic tastes. According to Ayurveda, it is best balanced by all the other tastes in a complete meal. At Kripalu, we help to satisfy the sweet tooth by providing small portions of familiar cakes, cookies, and other desserts at the end of a nourishing meal. Our emphasis is on whole grains and whole-food sources of sugar such as fruit and maple syrup.

Our Gluten-Free Salted Double Chocolate Chip Cookies (page 253) are a good example of an indulgence that won't put you in a sugar coma. They are chocolaty and decadent, yet full of fiber-rich oat flour. Likewise, Gluten-Free Whole-Grain Vegan Brownies (page 261) incorporate flax meal, oat flour, and buckwheat flour to make these rich, fudgy treats more nutritionally balanced.

Made with whole-grain flours, these sweets lower your overall glycemic load, which is a broad measurement of how quickly foods get metabolized by your body. Even though granulated sugar, maple syrup, and agave nectar are simple sugars with a high glycemic index (your body metabolizes them quickly), the fiber in whole grains like oat flour and in fruit as well as the fat in butter and vegetable oils have a low glycemic index, so they slow down the absorption of the simple sugars and lower the overall glycemic load. Simply put, using whole grains allows you to enjoy a little something sweet without a dramatic spike in your blood sugar. If you have a whole-grain cookie at the end of a meal loaded with fiber-rich, plant-based food, your overall glycemic load is reduced even further.

That said, moderation and mindfulness are key concepts when it comes to sweet treats. Before indulging in a brownie, cookie, or slice of cake, be sure you are seated and relaxed. Take the time to appreciate the sweet taste and fully enjoy every bite. Eating a single cookie can be an incredibly joyful experience, and savoring it mindfully with full satisfaction can reduce your desire to eat a whole batch in one sitting.

Ayurveda considers baked goods to be heavy and dense, so they are best enjoyed at lunchtime when digestion is strongest. That also gives you the advantage of time. You have all day to use this heavy, dense food for fuel and to burn it off. If the same baked goods were to be eaten after dinner or late at night, they might disturb your sleep and eventually cause weight gain.

Ayurveda also teaches us that like increases like and opposites bring balance. For that reason, favor cookies, cakes, and other baked goods in the cooler, drier months of fall and winter. Spring and summer are the seasons when damp, heavy weather prevails, and baked goods also produce dampness and heaviness. Plus, who wants to turn on the oven and heat up the kitchen during the sweltering days of summer?

Gluten-Free Salted Double Chocolate Chip Cookies

AT THE KRIPALU BAKERY, when anyone has an idea for a new baked good, we try it out and taste it. If it's good, we go with it. Our former bakery supervisor, Liz Lennon, came up with these nut-free cookies, and they manage to be chocolaty and sweet while somehow tasting remarkably light. Thanks, Liz!

Ayurvedic Insight: Cocoa powder is bitter, heating, and stimulating, making it most aggravating to vata and pitta types. However, Ayurveda recognizes that you are not eating just one ingredient; you are eating the marriage of all ingredients. Here, the coolness of coconut balances the heat of the cocoa, and the oiliness of butter mitigates the dryness of the flours. Enjoy in moderation.

Makes about twenty 3- to 4-inch cookies

1/2 cup sunflower seeds

2 1/3 cups (14 ounces) chopped bittersweet chocolate or chips

1 1/4 cups (7 ounces) chopped white chocolate or chips

2 cups gluten-free oat flour

1/2 cup natural (not Dutch or alkalized) cocoa powder

1 teaspoon baking powder

1 teaspoon baking soda

1 cup (2 sticks) unsalted butter, softened

3/4 cup organic cane sugar

1/2 cup packed light brown sugar

1 large egg

1 cup unsweetened dried shredded coconut

Flaky sea salt, such as Maldon

=V

=P

↑K

1. Preheat the oven to 350°F.

2. Spread the sunflower seeds on a baking sheet and toast in the oven until lightly browned and fragrant, 3 to 5 minutes. Remove from the pan and let cool. Line the baking sheet and another baking sheet with parchment paper and set aside.

3. Put 1¼ cups (8 ounces) of the bittersweet chocolate and ⅔ cup (4 ounces) of the white chocolate in a medium ovenproof bowl or saucepan. Place in the oven and heat until the chocolate begins to melt, 4 to 6 minutes. Watch it carefully and stir once or twice to make sure the chocolate doesn't scorch. When it is almost fully melted, remove from the oven and stir until the chocolate is smooth. Let cool slightly, stirring now and then to keep it smooth.

4. In a medium bowl, mix the oat flour, cocoa, baking powder, and baking soda.

5. Transfer the toasted sunflower seeds to a small food processor or clean spice mill along with 2 tablespoons of the mixed dry ingredients. Process just until the seeds are finely ground but do not turn to butter (the dry ingredients help prevent the seeds from becoming a paste). Set aside.

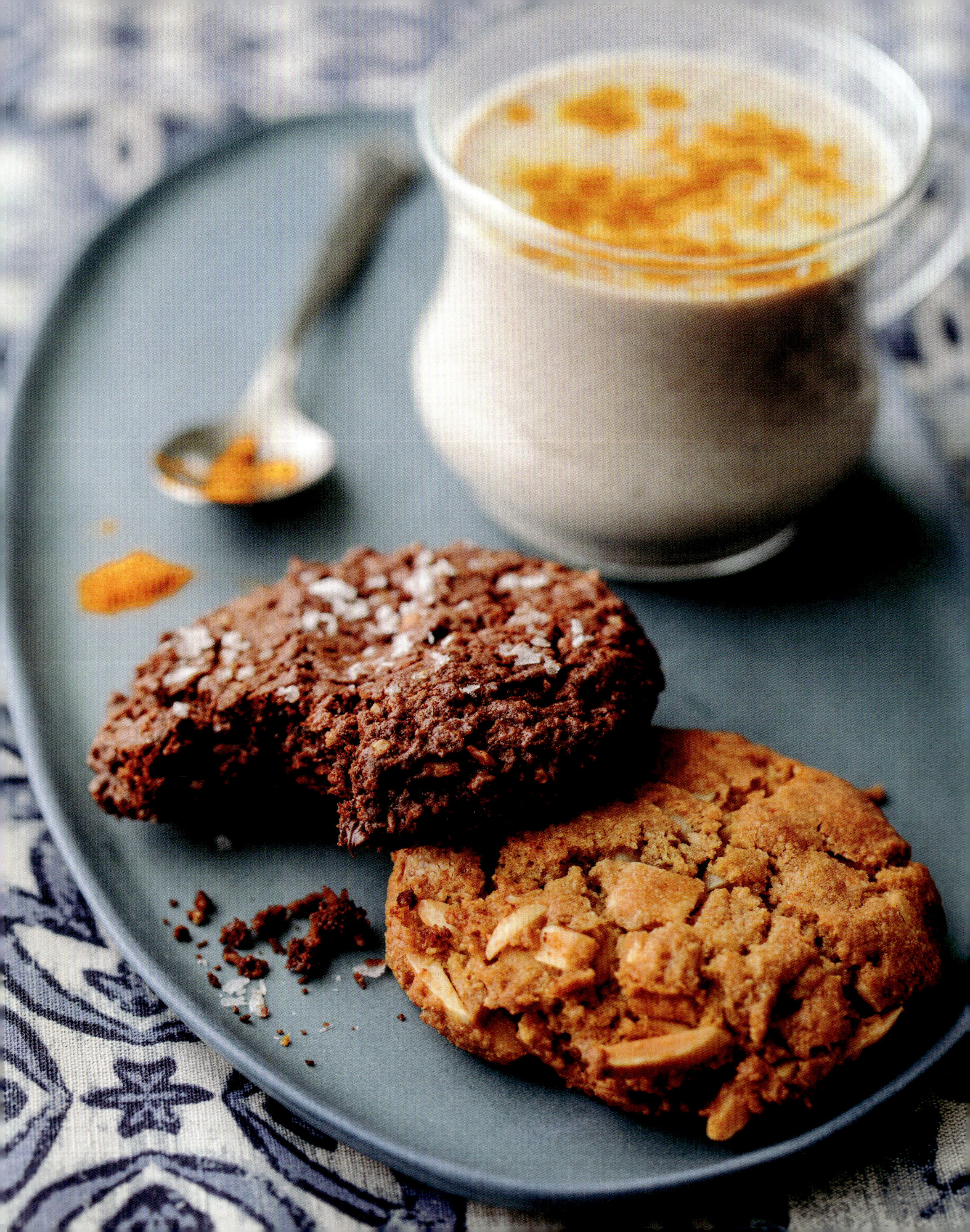

6. Put the butter, cane sugar, and brown sugar in the bowl of an electric mixer. Beat on medium speed until the mixture is light and fluffy. With the mixer running, add the egg and mix well. Scrape down the sides of the bowl, then return the mixer to medium speed and add the cooled melted chocolates. Turn the mixer to low speed and add the dry ingredients and the ground sunflower seeds, scraping down the bowl as needed. Fold in the coconut and remaining 1 cup (6 ounces) bittersweet chocolate and ½ cup (3 ounces) white chocolate.

7. Drop the dough in ¼-cup (2-ounce) portions onto the prepared baking sheets. You should have about 20 cookies. Gently press the cookies a bit to flatten them slightly and round them out. Sprinkle with the salt and bake until the cookies are set on the edges but still gooey in the middle, about 12 minutes total, rotating the pans midway through baking. Cool on the baking sheets for 15 minutes, then transfer to wire racks to cool completely.

Gluten-Free Rhapsody in Orange Cookies

=V

=P

↑K

DORA LEVINSON WAS a volunteer who worked in the Kripalu bakery. She had very little baking experience, but her ultimate goal was to create a signature cookie. Dora loved the taste of oranges and combined it with white chocolate in a cookie that tastes crispy, crunchy, and chewy all at once.

Ayurvedic Insight: If you were to enjoy a cookie in the springtime, this one would be ideal. It's gluten-free and kissed with orange, the perfect partner for a cup of tea.

Makes about twenty 3- to 4-inch cookies

1 3/4 cups almond flour
1 2/3 cups gluten-free oat flour
1 teaspoon baking soda
1 teaspoon fine sea salt
3/4 teaspoon xanthan gum
2/3 cup (11 tablespoons) unsalted butter, softened
1 1/2 tablespoons extra-virgin olive oil
3/4 cup packed light brown sugar
1/3 cup organic cane sugar
2 medium eggs (1 1/2 large eggs)
1 1/2 teaspoons vanilla extract
1/2 teaspoon orange extract
Grated zest of 1 1/2 oranges
1 1/2 cups (9 ounces) chopped white chocolate or chips
1 1/2 cups (5 3/4 ounces) slivered almonds

1. Preheat the oven to 350°F. Line 2 baking sheets with parchment paper and set aside.

2. In a medium bowl, mix the almond flour, oat flour, baking soda, salt, and xanthan gum. Set aside.

3. Put the butter, olive oil, brown sugar, and cane sugar in the bowl of an electric mixer. Beat on medium speed until the mixture is light and fluffy. With the mixer running, add the eggs, one at a time, scraping down the sides of the bowl between additions. Mix in the vanilla extract, orange extract, and orange zest. Turn the mixer to low speed and add the dry ingredients, scraping down the bowl as needed. Fold in the white chocolate and almonds.

4. Drop the dough in ¼-cup (2-ounce) portions onto the prepared baking sheets. You should have about 20 cookies. Gently press the cookies a bit to flatten them slightly and round them out. Bake until the cookies are golden on the edges and light gold on top, about 15 minutes total, rotating the pans midway through baking. Cool on the baking sheets for 15 minutes, then transfer to wire racks to cool completely.

Gluten-Free Graham Crackers

AT KRIPALU, WE BAKE our own graham crackers so we can use our local maple syrup and make the crackers gluten-free. These crackers are a bit thicker than store-bought versions but have a very similar taste.

Ayurvedic Insight: The various flours here make these gluten-free graham crackers suitable for all doshas in moderation. The spices also help to make them even easier to digest.

Makes twelve 5 x 2½-inch crackers (about 2½ cups crushed)

- 3 tablespoons unsalted butter, softened, plus more for greasing the sheet pans, if desired
- Oil spray for greasing the sheet pans, if desired
- 1 cup almond flour (almond meal)
- 3/4 cup gluten-free oat flour, plus more for dusting
- 1/2 cup buckwheat flour
- 1/3 cup arrowroot flour
- 1 1/2 tablespoons flax meal
- 2 tablespoons Sucanat or turbinado sugar
- 2 teaspoons ground cinnamon
- 1/2 teaspoon ground nutmeg
- 1/4 teaspoon ground ginger
- 1/2 teaspoon baking soda
- 1/2 teaspoon fine sea salt
- 1/3 cup maple syrup
- 2 tablespoons milk, any type

1. Preheat the oven to 325°F. Line 2 sheet pans (18 x 13 inches) with parchment paper or grease them with butter or oil spray.

2. You can mix these crackers with a machine or by hand. Either way, in a large bowl, mix the almond flour, oat flour, buckwheat flour, arrowroot flour, flax meal, Sucanat, cinnamon, nutmeg, ginger, baking soda, and salt. Gradually add the maple syrup, milk, and softened butter, mixing thoroughly. The dough will be firm yet pliable like pie dough.

3. Turn the dough out onto a lightly floured surface and roll it with a rolling pin into a large rectangle about ⅛ to ¼ inch thick. Cut the dough into 5 x 2½-rectangles. A wheeled pizza cutter works well for cutting. Re-roll the dough to cut as many rectangles as you can. You should have about 12. Use a spatula to transfer them to the prepared pans. Use a fork to prick the rectangles several times, which helps release steam and keep the crackers crisp. Bake until the crackers are light brown and look dry and crisp, 30 to 35 minutes. Let cool for 15 minutes in the pans. Transfer to wire racks to cool completely.

=V

=P

=K

Gluten-Free Chocolate Peanut Butter Bars

↑V
↑P
↑K

THE BAKERY STAFF KNOWS THAT, like many people, I love the combination of chocolate and peanut butter. They nailed it in this take on a popular treat. You really need only one because the layers of crushed graham crackers, sweetened peanut butter, and dark chocolate ganache taste so intense together. Just be sure to serve these bars cold. They start to melt when warm.

Ayurvedic Insight: Guests absolutely adore these chocolate peanut butter bars. They are very dense and rich, so are best enjoyed after the lunchtime meal. A sprinkle of powdered ginger over the top will help you digest them.

Makes 24

PEANUT BUTTER FILLING

- 1 2/3 cups (3 sticks plus 3 tablespoons) unsalted butter, melted, plus some for greasing the pan
- 2 1/2 cups peanut butter, creamy or crunchy
- 1/2 cup pure maple syrup
- 2 1/2 cups coarsely crushed Gluten-Free Graham Crackers (page 257) or store-bought crackers

GANACHE TOPPING

- 1/3 cup heavy cream
- 3 tablespoons pure maple syrup
- 7 ounces bittersweet or semisweet chocolate, finely chopped (or 1 cup chocolate chips)

1. For the peanut butter filling, lightly butter a 13 x 9-inch baking pan and set aside.

2. Put the peanut butter in a large mixing bowl. You can mix by hand or in a machine on medium-low speed. Mix the melted butter and maple syrup in a medium bowl, then gradually add the butter mixture to the peanut butter, stirring until everything is combined. Fold in the crushed graham crackers and pour the filling into the prepared pan, spreading it evenly to the edges. The filling will be somewhat loose.

3. Chill the filling until firm, about 1 ½ hours in the refrigerator or 45 minutes in the freezer.

4. For the ganache topping, combine the cream and maple syrup in a small saucepan and bring to a gentle simmer over medium heat. Remove from the heat and mix in the chopped chocolate, stirring until the chocolate is melted and the mixture is smooth. If the ganache appears a little grainy, stir in a little more cream until it is completely smooth and shiny.

5. Spread the ganache evenly over the chilled peanut butter filling all the way to the edges. Chill until firm, about 45 minutes in the refrigerator or 25 minutes in the freezer.

6. Cut into 24 pieces (2-inch squares). To cut cleanly, dip a sharp knife in very hot water until heated through, then dry thoroughly. Between cuts, dip the knife in hot water and wipe it dry. Serve immediately or cover and refrigerate for up to 2 days. Serve chilled, as the bars begin to melt at room temperature.

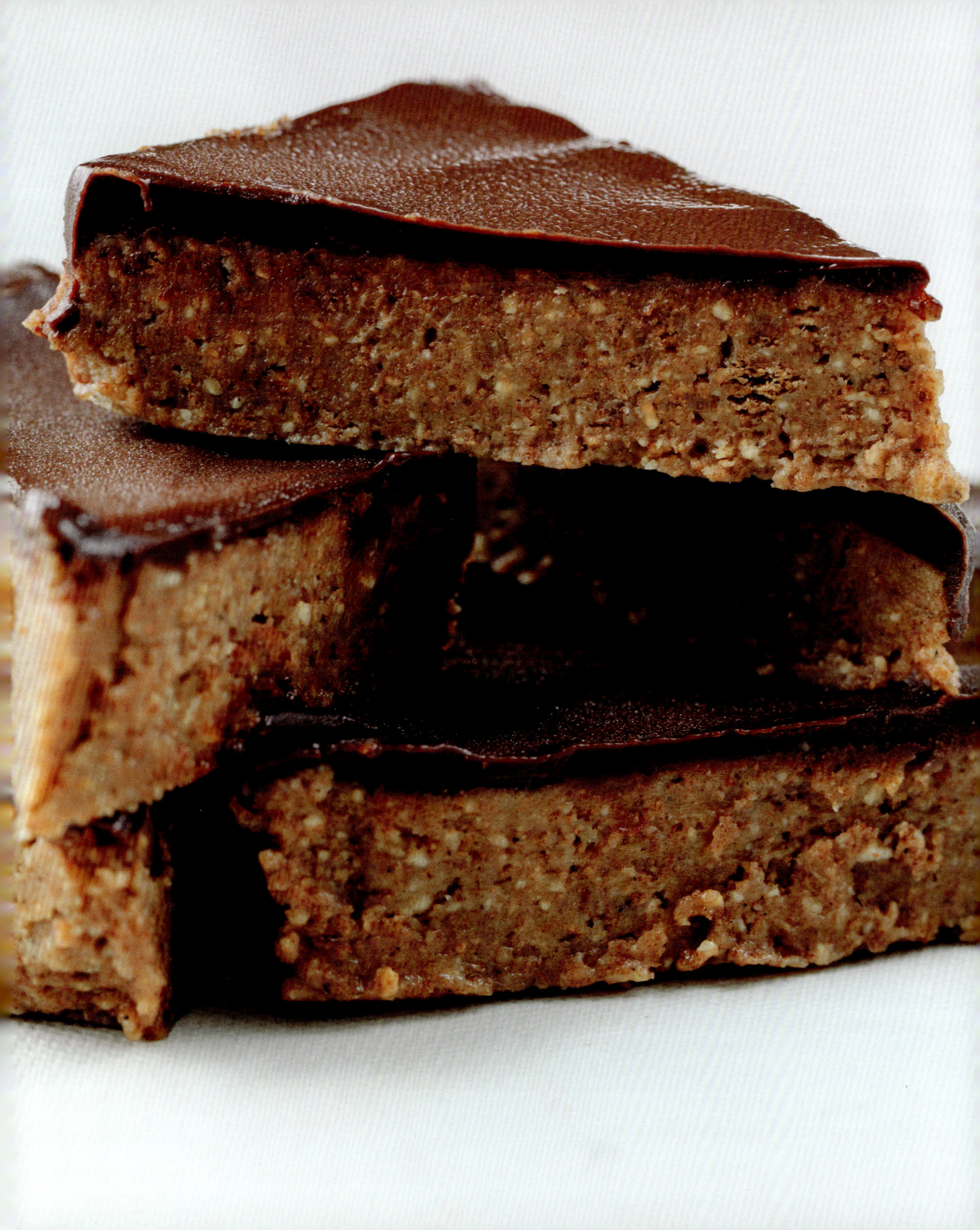

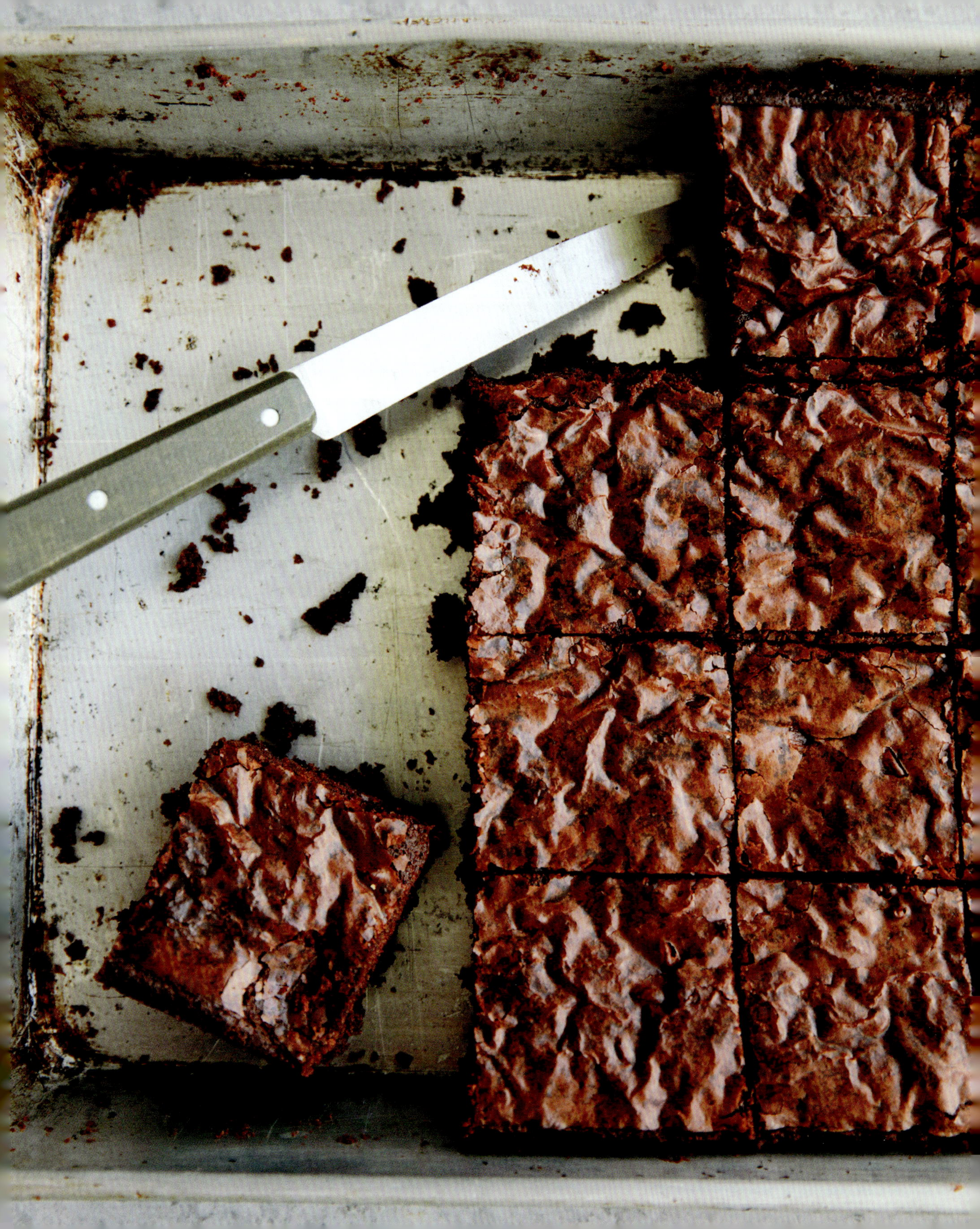

Gluten-Free Whole-Grain Vegan Brownies

↑V ↑P ↑K

BUCKWHEAT FLOUR GIVES these brownies a unique flavor reminiscent of cinnamon. The brownies get deliciously crisp on the edges while remaining rich and fudgy in the center. If you don't have Sucanat, you can replace it with turbinado sugar or coconut sugar.

Ayurvedic Insight: Cocoa powder and chocolate have some amazing health benefits, such as increasing circulation and reducing coughs. That said, these indulgent brownies are best enjoyed in small amounts and with full attention to savoring every bite.

Makes twelve 4-inch brownies

- 1 cup sunflower oil or other vegetable oil, plus more for greasing the pan
- 2 tablespoons flax meal
- 1/4 cup soy milk or other milk
- 1 cup Sucanat or turbinado sugar
- 3/4 cup plus 2 tablespoons maple syrup
- 2 teaspoons vanilla extract
- 1 1/2 cups gluten-free oat flour
- 1/2 cup buckwheat flour
- 1/2 cup natural cocoa powder
- 1 teaspoon baking powder
- 1/2 teaspoon fine sea salt
- 1 cup chocolate chips

1. Preheat the oven to 375°F. Grease a 13 x 9-inch baking dish with oil.

2. You can mix these by hand or with an electric mixer. Either way, in a large bowl, stir together the flax meal and milk. Let soak for at least 20 minutes and up to 1 hour.

3. Gently beat in the Sucanat on low speed until it starts to dissolve, about 5 minutes. Mix in the maple syrup and vanilla until incorporated. Then mix in the sunflower oil until incorporated.

4. In a medium bowl, combine the oat flour, buckwheat flour, cocoa powder, baking powder, and salt. Gradually stir the dry ingredients into the wet until well mixed. Fold in the chocolate chips and scrape the batter into the prepared pan.

5. Bake until the batter is just set yet still moist and fudgy in the center, 20 to 25 minutes. It will puff and fall on its own near the end of the baking time. It will also appear a little bubbly. Let cool before cutting.

OPTIONS

- These brownies are fudgy yet thin, about ¾ inch high. For thicker brownies, make 1½ times the recipe and bake them about 5 minutes longer.
- To add some dried fruit, soak 1 cup of chopped dried cherries, blueberries, or goji berries in 2 tablespoons warm water until the fruit plumps up, about 20 minutes. Fold the berries into the brownie batter along with the chocolate chips.

- Top each brownie with a dollop of Kripalu Whipped Cream (page 268) or Kripalu Cashew Cream (page 269).
- For easier cutting, line the entire brownie pan of brownies with a generous sheet of foil, oil the foil, and then, when cool, lift the entire brick of brownies from the pan.

Gluten-Free Vegan Peanut Butter Chocolate Banana Bread

↑V
=P
↑K

YEARS AGO, WHEN DEMAND for gluten-free foods started skyrocketing, we put this sweet bread on the menu. It has been popular ever since. With a good balance of chocolate and banana, you feel like you had dessert, but it's still relatively healthy.

Ayurvedic Insight: Ayurveda recommends against mixing raw fruit with other foods. However, when fruit is cooked, as in this dessert, it becomes another food entirely and is perfectly acceptable.

Makes one 9 x 5-inch loaf, about 10 slices

Oil spray
2 tablespoons flax meal
3/4 cup oat flour
1/2 cup buckwheat flour
1 1/4 teaspoons baking powder
1/2 teaspoon fine sea salt
1/2 cup creamy peanut butter
3 tablespoons unsweetened applesauce
2/3 cup organic cane sugar
3/4 cup mashed bananas
2 tablespoons soy milk
2/3 cup mini chocolate chips (about 4 ounces)

1. Preheat the oven to 325°F. Grease a 9 x 5-inch loaf pan with oil spray and set aside.

2. Put the flax meal in a small bowl and stir in ⅓ cup water. Let soak for at least 20 minutes and up to 1 hour.

3. In a medium bowl, mix the oat flour, buckwheat flour, baking powder, and salt. Set aside.

4. Meanwhile, put the peanut butter and applesauce in the bowl of an electric mixer. Using the paddle attachment on medium speed, mix until they are very well combined, 1 to 2 minutes. Scrape down the sides of the bowl and return the mixer to medium speed. Add the sugar and half the mashed bananas, mixing until the sugar is mostly dissolved, 1 to 2 minutes (the mixture shouldn't feel very granular when rubbed between your fingers). Scrape down the sides again, then add the dry ingredients in thirds, alternating with the milk and the soaked flax mixture. If necessary, stop and scrape down the sides during mixing to make sure everything is incorporated evenly. Turn the mixer speed to low, add the chocolate chips and remaining bananas, and mix just until the bananas are still a bit lumpy.

5. Scrape the batter into the prepared pan and bake just until the bread is firm to the touch and a toothpick inserted in the center comes out almost clean, 50 to 55 minutes.

OPTIONS

- Slices of this bread taste delicious griddled with a little butter. Or try making French toast with it.

Pumpkin Welcome Bread

=V

=P

↑K

WE SERVE "WELCOME" breads on Fridays and Mondays, our busiest days for guest check-in. They are not really desserts but are offered at the end of the first evening's meal for a taste of something sweet and comforting.

Ayurvedic Insight: Pureed pumpkin combined with the warmth of ginger, cinnamon, nutmeg, and cloves makes this bread best for cool fall mornings. A smear of softened butter is most welcome.

Makes one 9 x 5-inch loaf, about 10 slices

- 6 tablespoons unsalted butter, softened, plus more for greasing the pan
- 3/4 cup all-purpose flour
- 3/4 cup whole-wheat pastry flour
- 2/3 cup organic cane sugar
- 1 1/2 teaspoons ground cinnamon
- 1/2 teaspoon ground ginger
- 1/2 teaspoon ground nutmeg
- 1/4 teaspoon ground cloves
- 3/4 teaspoon baking powder
- 1/2 teaspoon baking soda
- 1 teaspoon fine sea salt
- 3/4 cup Sucanat or turbinado sugar
- 2 large eggs, at room temperature
- 1/3 cup milk, any kind
- 1/2 teaspoon vanilla extract
- 3/4 cup canned or pureed pumpkin

1. Preheat the oven to 350°F. Grease a 9 x 5-inch loaf pan with butter and set aside.

2. In a medium bowl, mix the all-purpose flour, whole-wheat pastry flour, sugar, cinnamon, ginger, nutmeg, cloves, baking powder, baking soda, and salt.

3. Put the butter and Sucanat in the bowl of an electric mixer. Using the paddle attachment on medium speed, cream the butter and Sucanat until the mixture is fluffy and lighter in color, about 5 minutes. Scrape down the sides of the bowl, then return the mixer to medium speed and add the eggs one at a time, beating thoroughly between each addition. Scrape down the sides again, then with the mixer on low speed, add the dry ingredients in thirds, alternating with the milk, vanilla, and pumpkin. As necessary, stop and scrape down the sides during mixing to make sure everything is evenly incorporated.

4. Scrape the batter into the prepared pan and bake until the top is well browned and a toothpick inserted in the center comes out clean, 55 to 65 minutes.

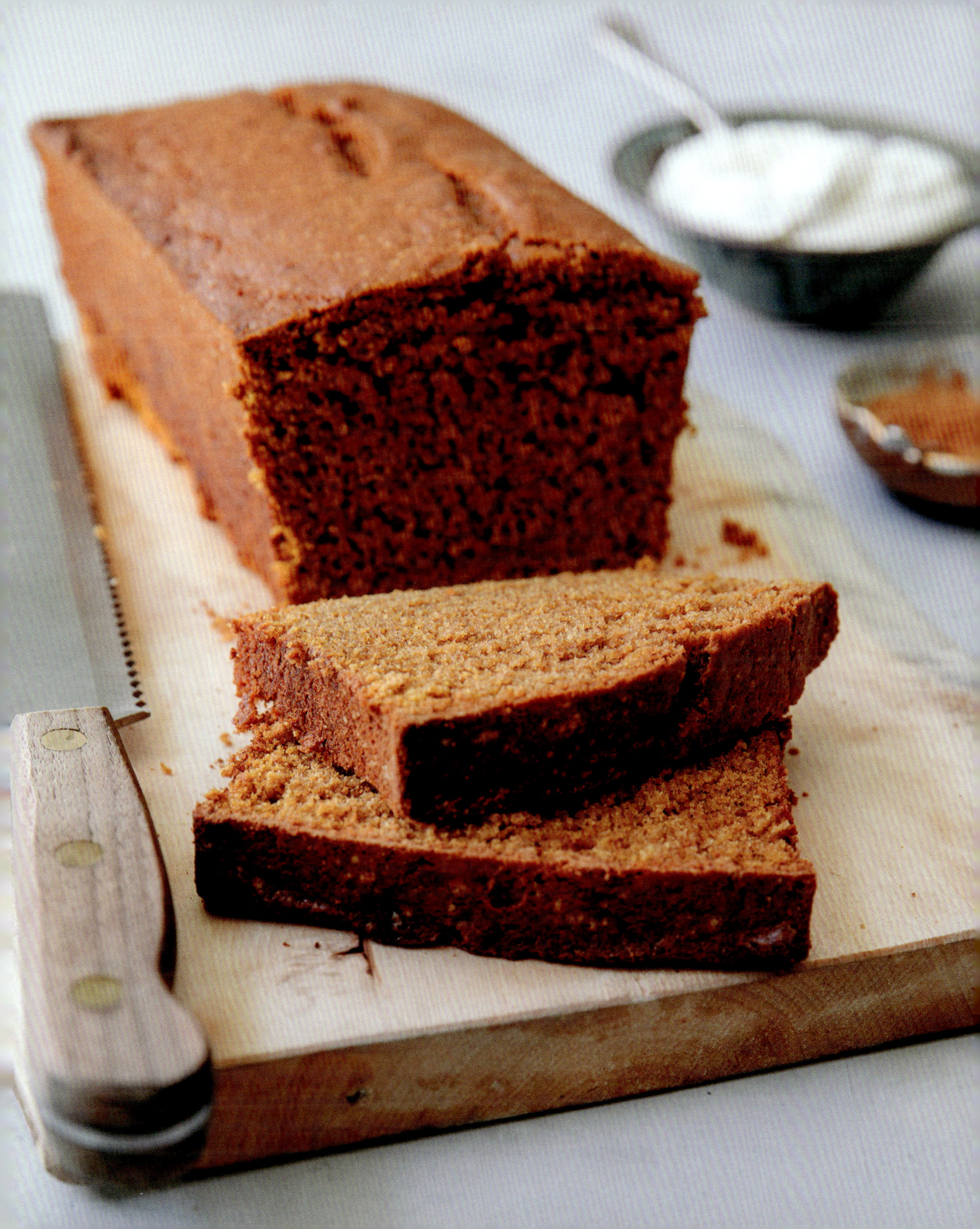

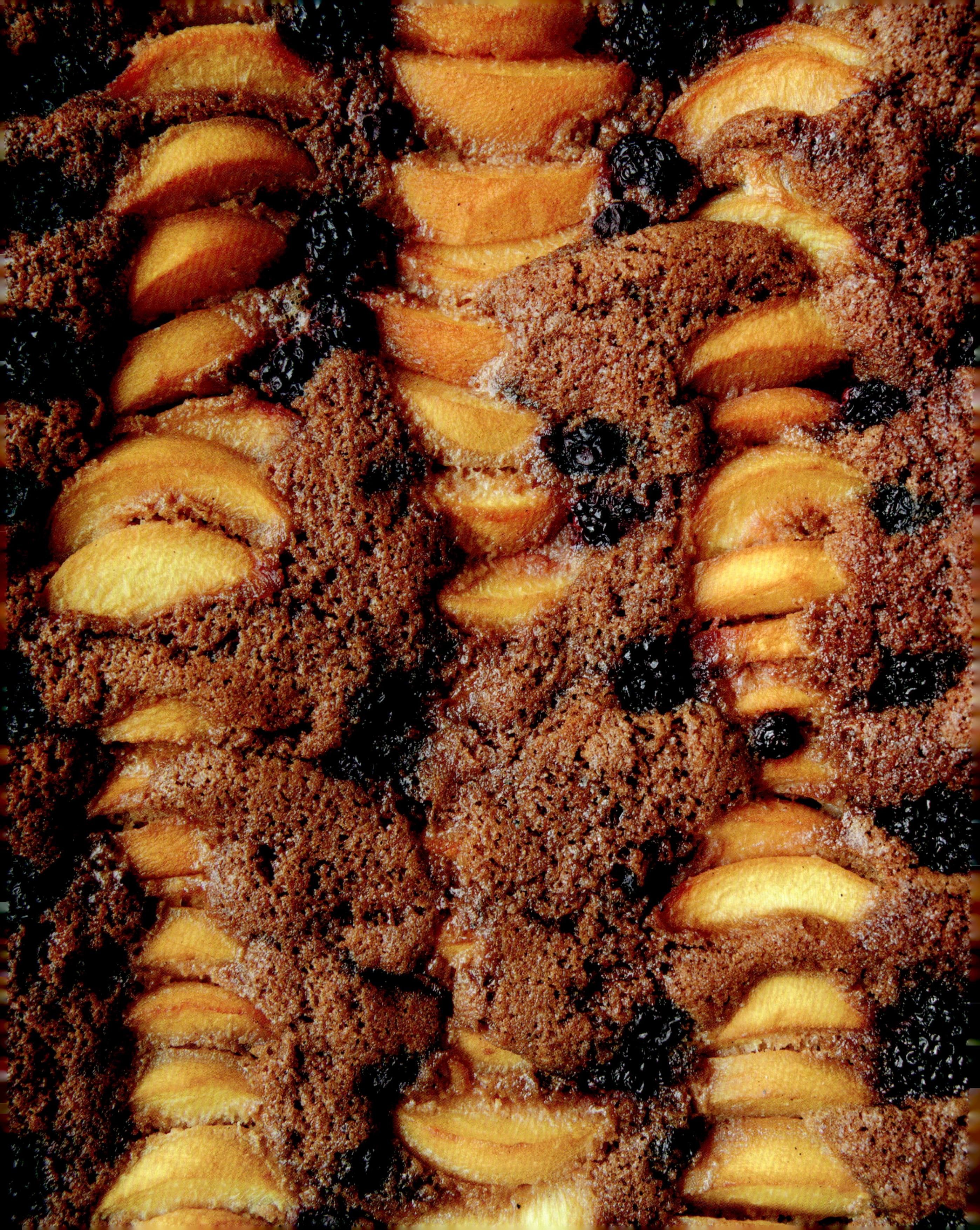

Peach Cake

HERE'S AN OLD-SCHOOL sheet cake that's as simple as it is delicious. Spelt flour makes the cake light and easily digestible while sliced fresh peaches sink into the top of the cake, creating wonderful hollows for dollops of softly whipped cream.

Ayurvedic Insight: The dry, heating, and astringent qualities of the ancient grain spelt make it less aggravating to kapha than modern varieties of wheat.

Makes one 13 x 9-inch cake (15 servings)

↑V
=P
=K

1 cup (2 sticks) unsalted butter, softened, plus more for greasing the pan

2 cups whole spelt flour, preferably sprouted

2 teaspoons baking powder

1 teaspoon baking soda

1⅓ cups coconut sugar, plus more for sprinkling

4 large eggs, at room temperature

2 teaspoons vanilla extract

1 pound (about 4 cups) thinly sliced pitted peaches

Kripalu Whipped Cream or Cashew Cream (recipes follow; optional)

1. Preheat the oven to 325°F. Grease a 13 x 9-inch baking pan with a little butter.

2. In a medium bowl, mix the flour, baking powder, and baking soda.

3. Put the butter and coconut sugar in the bowl of an electric mixer. Beat on medium speed until the mixture is light and fluffy. With the mixer running, add the eggs, one at a time. Scrape down the sides of the bowl, then return the mixer to medium speed and add the vanilla. Turn the mixer speed to low and gradually add the dry ingredients, scraping down the bowl to make sure everything is incorporated.

4. Spread the batter into the prepared pan, smoothing out the top. The batter will be somewhat thick. Arrange the peach slices evenly over the batter and sprinkle with coconut sugar.

5. Bake until the cake is golden brown and a toothpick inserted in the center comes out clean, 50 to 60 minutes. Let cool, then cut into 15 pieces. Serve with whipped cream, if desired.

OPTIONS

- In the summer, use fresh ripe peaches or even nectarines. In the off-season, frozen and thawed peach slices work fine.
- For more color and flavor, scatter ½ cup fresh blueberries over the peaches before sprinkling on the sugar.
- We like to use sprouted whole spelt flour in this cake. It gives the cake a tender texture, and many of our guests find sprouted spelt flour easier to digest than regular wheat flour. You could also use einkorn flour, another ancient wheat flour that many of our guests find even easier to digest.

KRIPALU WHIPPED CREAM

=V
↓P
↑K

COLD CREAM, A COLD BOWL, and cold beaters are the keys to making whipped cream quickly and easily. Sometimes we use honey here, but maple syrup is our favorite natural sweetener.

Ayurvedic Insight: Sweet cream and maple syrup make a great combination for balancing the hot aggravated qualities of pitta.

Makes about 2 cups

1 cup cold heavy cream

5 tablespoons pure maple syrup

1/2 teaspoon vanilla extract

1. Chill the bowl and beaters of an electric mixer.

2. Beat the cold cream on medium speed until it starts to thicken, 1 to 2 minutes. Add the maple syrup and vanilla, and beat just until the beaters leave soft peaks when lifted from the cream. Overbeating can cause the cream to become stiff and grainy. Serve immediately.

OPTION

- Whipped Coconut Cream: For a plant-based version, replace the heavy cream with a 14-ounce can of pure coconut cream and proceed with the recipe. If you can't find coconut cream, chill two 14-ounce cans of coconut milk, then open the cans and spoon off the white coconut cream from the top, leaving the clear coconut juice below. You can use the leftover coconut juice to flavor smoothies and soups, such as Chilled Mango Soup (page 100).

Kripalu Cashew Cream

THIS VEGAN CREAM doesn't get as light and fluffy as dairy whipped cream, but it's still a very rich and satisfying dessert topping.

Ayurvedic Insight: Magnesium is known as nature's chill pill. The high magnesium content of cashews helps this sweet treat to balance the nerves of those who feel stressed, agitated, or anxious.

↓V
=P
↑K

Makes about 2 cups

1⅔ cups cashew pieces
¼ cup honey
¼ teaspoon vanilla extract

1. Soak the cashews in water to cover for 8 hours or up to 24 hours.

2. Drain and rinse the cashews, then transfer them to a food processor or high-speed blender. Process until the nuts are very finely ground. With the machine running, gradually add the honey, processing until incorporated. Gradually add the vanilla, then just enough water, 3 to 4 tablespoons, to achieve a thick texture similar to sour cream. Process until very smooth, 2 to 4 minutes. Serve immediately or refrigerate for up to 2 days.

Gluten-Free Vegan Carrot Cake

=V
=P
=K

SOME VERSIONS OF CARROT CAKE are cloyingly sweet. Our take on this classic dessert is lightly sweet and moist, so you can actually taste the shredded carrots, walnuts, and currants.

Ayurvedic Insight: The warm and dry qualities of buckwheat make it balancing for damp kapha types.

Makes one 13 x 9-inch cake (15 SERVINGS)

1/2 cup sunflower oil, plus more for greasing the pan
1/4 cup flax meal
2/3 cup unsweetened applesauce
2 1/4 cups gluten-free oat flour
2/3 cup buckwheat flour
2 teaspoons ground cinnamon
2 teaspoons baking powder
1 teaspoon baking soda
1 teaspoon fine sea salt
3 1/4 cups (about 15 ounces) grated carrots
2/3 cup orange juice
3/4 cup plus 2 tablespoons organic cane sugar
6 ounces (about 1 1/2 cups) walnuts, chopped
6 ounces (about 1 cup) currants
2 cups Spiced Vegan Vanilla Frosting (recipe follows)

1. Preheat the oven to 325°F. Grease a 13 x 9-inch baking pan with oil.

2. In a small bowl, mix the flax meal and applesauce. Let soak for at least 20 minutes and up to 1 hour.

3. In the bowl of an electric mixer, combine the oat flour, buckwheat flour, cinnamon, baking powder, baking soda, and salt. Add the carrots and beat on medium speed until the carrots are coated with flour and the flour begins to appear moist, 2 to 3 minutes. With the mixer running, add the soaked flax meal and beat until well combined. Gradually add the orange juice, then the sunflower oil. Add the sugar and beat until the sugar is dissolved, 1 to 2 minutes. Mix in the walnuts and currants.

4. Scrape the batter into the prepared pan and bake until the cake is set and a toothpick inserted in the center comes out with just a few moist crumbs clinging to it, about 1 hour and 10 minutes. The cake will crack with small fissures on top. Cool the cake in the pan on a wire rack.

5. When completely cool, spread the frosting evenly over the surface. Then cut the cake into 15 servings.

OPTIONS

- This cake is about 1 inch high. For a thicker cake, make 1½ times the recipe and add 10 to 15 minutes to the baking time. When the cake cracks in tiny fissures, it is getting close to being done.
- If you like, replace the Spiced Vegan Vanilla Frosting with Kripalu Cream Cheese Frosting (page 272).

Spiced Vegan Vanilla Frosting

THE PERFECT TOPPING for carrot cake, this frosting is equally at home on Pumpkin Welcome Bread (page 264) or any spice cake. Transform it into a simple vanilla frosting for birthday cake by leaving out the ground spices and adding a bit more vanilla.

Ayurvedic Insight: Due to the butter, frosting is off the menu for most vegans. While processed oils make this frosting suitable for vegans, Ayurveda recommends avoiding heavily processed foods. Moderation is paramount here.

Makes about 2½ cups

3 cups confectioners' sugar

2 tablespoons pumpkin pie spice

2/3 cup 100% palm shortening, such as Spectrum

1/2 cup (1 stick) vegan butter sticks, softened (not whipped), such as Earth Balance

2 teaspoons vanilla extract

2 tablespoons soy milk or canned full-fat 100% coconut milk

1. Sift the confectioners' sugar and pumpkin pie spice into a bowl. Set aside.

2. Put the palm shortening in the bowl of an electric mixer and beat on medium speed until smooth, 1 to 2 minutes. Add the softened vegan butter and beat until well combined.

3. Turn the mixer speed to low and add the sugar mixture, scraping down the bowl as necessary to prevent lumps. Add the vanilla and mix until smooth. Finally, mix in the soy milk, beating just until the frosting is smooth and spreadable. Use immediately.

=V

↑P

↑K

OPTIONS

- If you don't have pumpkin pie spice, mix 1½ teaspoons ground cinnamon, ½ teaspoon ground nutmeg, ½ teaspoon ground ginger, and ½ teaspoon ground cloves.
- *Vegan Vanilla Frosting:* To spread this frosting on Gluten-Free Vegan Swami Kripalu Birthday Cake (page 273), omit the pumpkin pie spice and increase the vanilla to 1 tablespoon.

Kripalu Cream Cheese Frosting

=V

=P

↑K

HERE'S A MORE TRADITIONAL frosting for carrot cake, minus the confectioners' sugar. Honey gives it a unique floral aroma that complements the carrots and walnuts in the cake.

Ayurvedic Insight: Un-aged soft cheese such as cream cheese is favorable for pitta types who get aggravated by salty aged cheeses.

Makes about 1½ cups

1 cup (8 ounces) cream cheese, at room temperature

3 tablespoons honey

1/2 teaspoon vanilla extract

Put the cream cheese in the bowl of an electric mixer and beat on medium speed until smooth, 1 to 2 minutes. Scrape down the sides of the bowl, then beat in the honey and vanilla, scraping down the bowl as necessary to incorporate all of the ingredients. Use immediately.

Gluten-Free Vegan Swami Kripalu Birthday Cake

IN 2015 OUR HEAD BAKER, Cathy Ligenza, was asked to create a celebration cake for the one hundredth birthday of Swami Kripalu, the namesake of the Kripalu Center for Yoga & Health. Cathy developed this simple gluten-free, vegan white cake redolent with the perfume of coconut and vanilla. It is extremely easy to make, and we still serve it for staff celebrations to this day.

Ayurvedic Insight: According to Swami Kripalu, "The highest spiritual practice is self-observation without judgment." Enjoy a modest slice of this birthday cake just as he would: with full abandon.

Makes one 13 x 9-inch cake (15 servings)

- 1/4 cup sunflower oil, plus more for greasing the pan
- 1 cup brown rice flour
- 1 cup tapioca flour
- 3/4 cup coconut flour
- 1 1/4 cups organic cane sugar or coconut sugar
- 1 1/4 teaspoons baking powder
- 1 1/4 teaspoons baking soda
- 1 1/4 teaspoons fine sea salt
- 1 teaspoon xanthan gum
- 1/3 cup unsweetened applesauce
- 2/3 cup canned full-fat 100% coconut milk
- 1 tablespoon plus 1 teaspoon vanilla extract
- 1 teaspoon fresh lemon juice
- 2 1/2 cups Vegan Vanilla Frosting (page 271)

=V
=P
=K

1. Preheat the oven to 375°F. Grease a 13 x 9-inch baking pan with oil.

2. In a large bowl, sift together the brown rice flour, tapioca flour, coconut flour, sugar, baking powder, baking soda, salt, and xanthan gum.

3. In the bowl of an electric mixer, beat the applesauce, coconut milk, oil, vanilla, and lemon juice on medium speed until combined, 1 to 2 minutes. Turn the mixer to low and gradually add the dry ingredients in several additions, scraping down the sides of the bowl between additions. Mix until the batter is thick and smooth, 2 to 3 minutes. Gradually add 1 1/4 cups warm water, scraping down the bowl to make sure all the ingredients are incorporated. Increase the speed to medium-low and beat until the batter is very smooth, 1 to 2 minutes more.

4. Scrape the batter into the prepared pan and bake until the cake is deep golden brown, springs back when pressed, and a toothpick inserted in the center comes out completely clean, about 30 minutes. Cool the cake in the pan on a wire rack.

5. When completely cool, spread the frosting evenly over the surface. Then cut the cake into 15 servings.

OPTIONS

- To make a round 2-layer birthday cake, grease two 9-inch round cake pans, then dust them with brown rice flour, tapping out the excess. Bake as directed. Double or triple the frosting recipe. Spread the frosting over the top of the first layer, add the second layer, and spread the frosting over the top and sides.
- Or, to make a 4-layer cake as shown in the photo (page 275), make two round layers as described above. Then, cut each layer in half horizontally to make four layers. Spread raspberry or strawberry jam on the first layer, frosting on the second layer, jam again on the third layer, and then spread frosting on the top and sides.

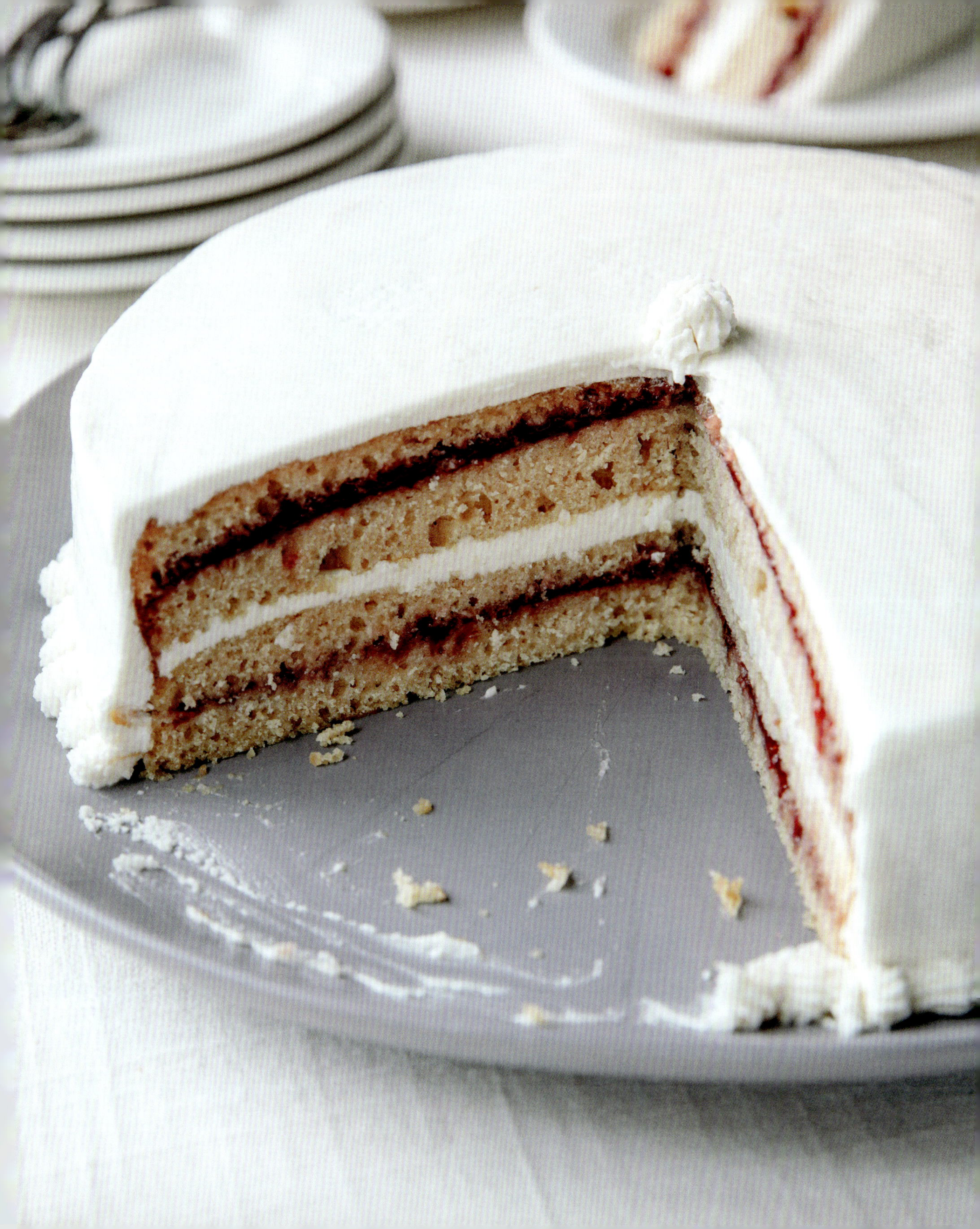

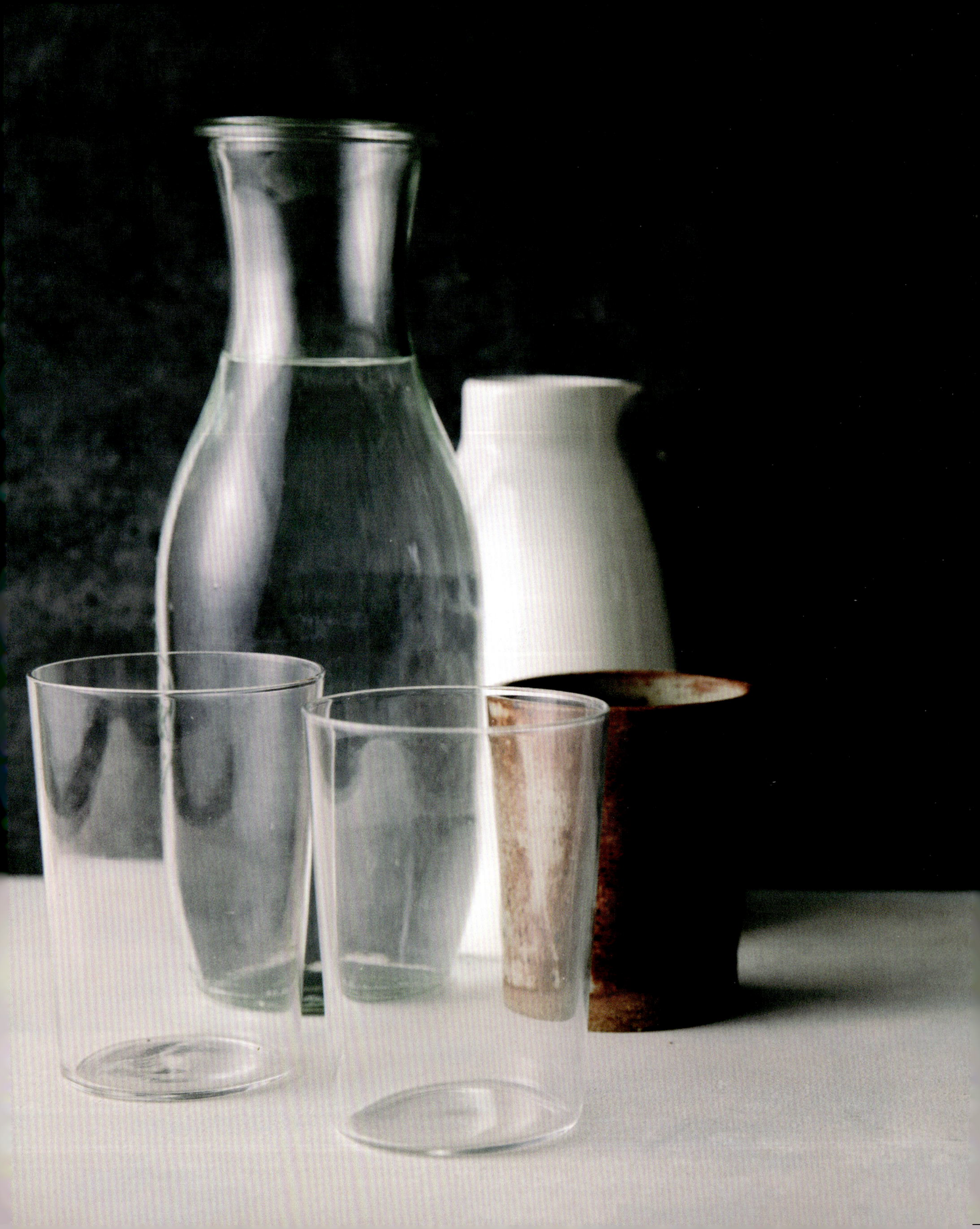

JUICES, TEAS, AND TONICS

Perhaps nowhere else can the power of self-healing be found so readily as in a cup of tea, juice, or healing broth. We encourage you to consume these preparations at all times of day for hydration, cleansing, detox, and refreshment.

At Kripalu, we make all of our beverages in-house, with the exception of local apple cider and our wide selection of hot teas. In the fall and winter months, we offer hot Kripalu Chai (page 282) and soothing Ojas Milk (page 285) to stoke your digestive fire. When summertime rolls around, guests love to cool off with Iced Lavender Black Tea (page 286), Thai Basil Lemonade (page 289), and the occasional Kripalu Switchel (page 291), a New England specialty made from pure maple syrup, cider vinegar, and fresh ginger.

Interestingly, one of the most beneficial qualities of beverages is their temperature. Water transfers temperature very effectively. In the winter or whenever you feel cold, consuming a hot beverage or broth will soothe and comfort your entire body simply by balancing its temperature with something warm. Likewise, in the summer or whenever you feel hot, iced beverages cool down your body temperature, making you feel refreshed and revitalized.

Another beautiful aspect of teas and beverages is that they extract other healthful components into the liquid. On a cold, damp morning, a cup of hot Kripalu Chai (page 282) brings not only warmth but also the anti-inflammatory and digestive benefits of ginger and cardamom along with the antibacterial and immune-boosting effects of cinnamon and cloves. In the warmer months, a glass of Cucumber, Kale, Ginger, and Apple Juice (page 292) will provide you with a veritable medicine chest of vitamins, minerals, and antioxidants in a refreshing beverage that's easy on the digestive system.

It's true that beans, lentils, whole grains, vegetables, and fruits are foundational components of a healthy diet. But hot and cold beverages can also increase your nutrient intake while improving your mood. Enjoy them often.

Morning Broth

WE OFFER THIS clean-tasting broth on the Buddha Bar every day. It falls somewhere between beverage and soup. In the morning hours, it is a very gentle way to break the fast. Plus, it's easy to make, and you can use whatever vegetables you like.

Ayurvedic Insight: On some mornings, your body may not be up for a full breakfast. If your digestion is feeling sluggish, this light soup will get you going without bogging you down.

Serves 4

5 cups Vegetable Stock (page 281) or water (to omit onions)

3/4 cup 1/4-inch diced peeled sweet potatoes

1/4 cup 1/4-inch diced carrots

1/4 cup 1/4-inch diced celery

1 small piece (about 1/2 inch) kombu

1/2 cup chopped kale, preferably lacinato

Fine sea salt or tamari

In a medium saucepan, combine the stock, sweet potatoes, carrots, celery, and kombu. Cover and bring to a simmer over medium heat. Reduce the heat to low and simmer gently, covered, until the sweet potatoes are fork-tender, about 15 minutes. Turn off the heat and stir in the kale. It should wilt and turn bright green in a minute or two. Taste the broth and season it with salt until it tastes good to you. Remove the kombu and serve warm.

OPTION

- Use any combination of firm and leafy vegetables you like here: turnips and daikon work, as do spinach and chard.

↓V
↓P
↓K

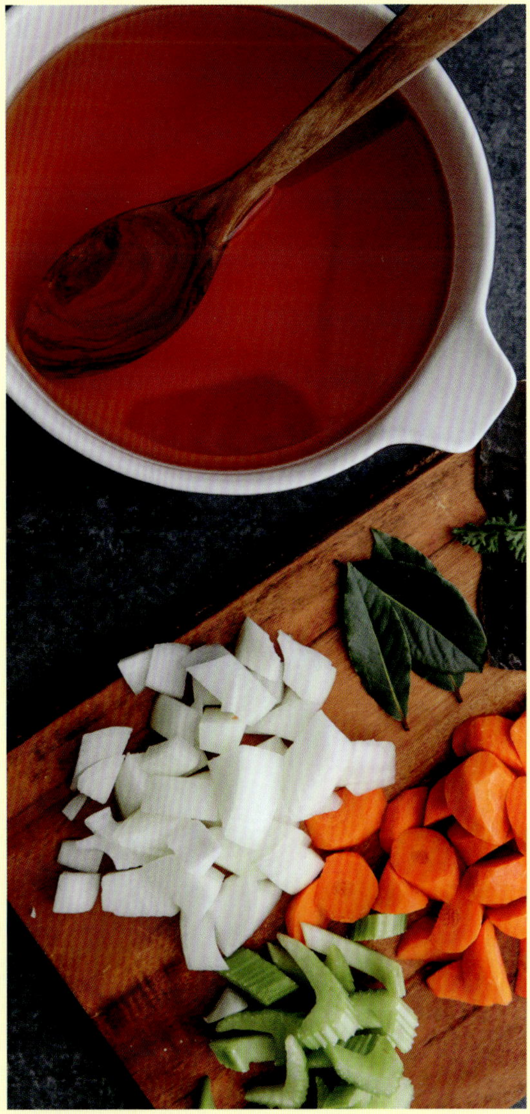

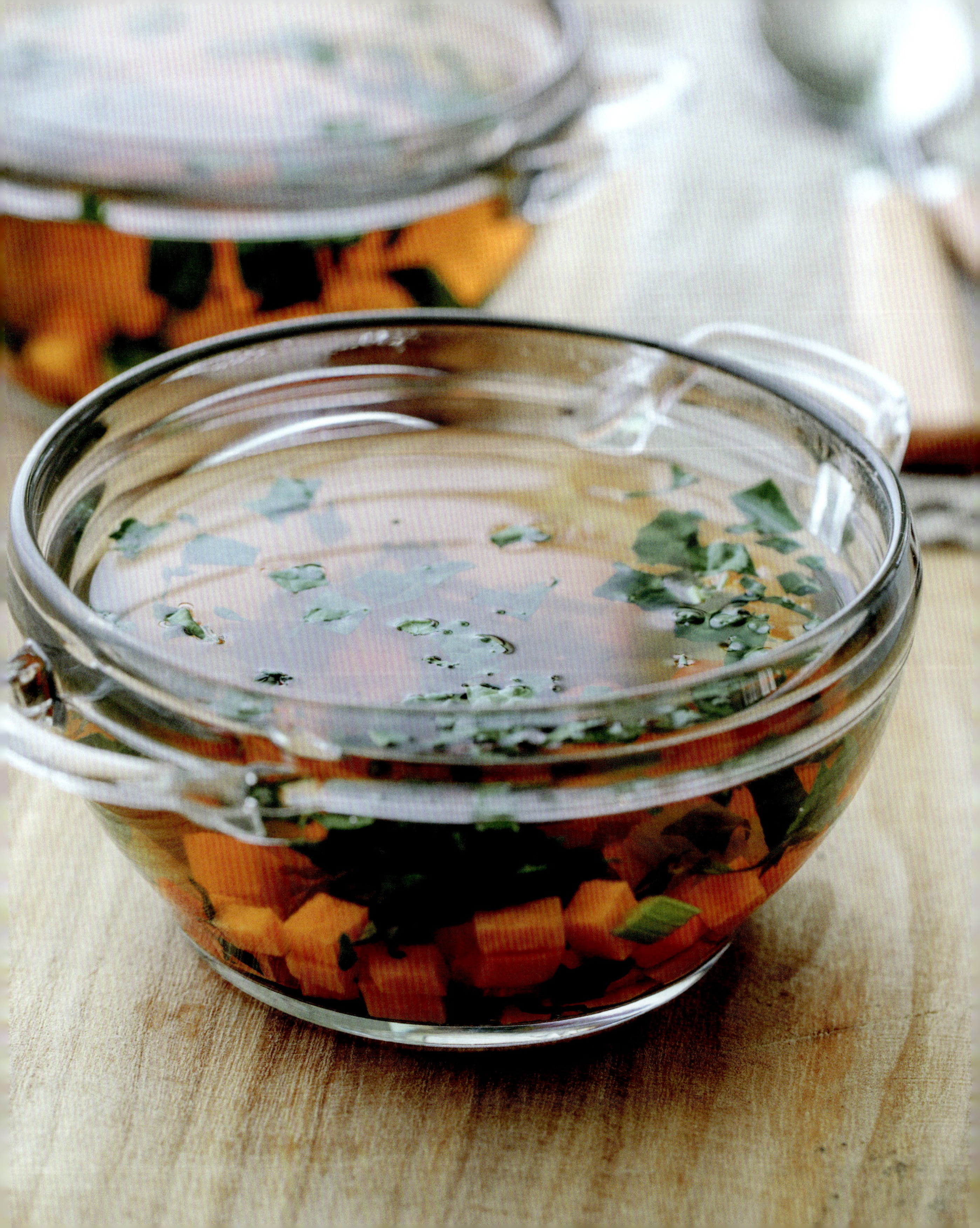

VEGETABLE STOCK

↓V ↓P ↓K

NEUTRAL-TASTING STOCK IS the foundation of Kripalu's healing hot beverage, Morning Broth (page 279). We also use it in dozens of dishes, from simmered breakfast grains such as Upma (page 70) to sauces like Gluten-Free Vegan Gravy (page 130) and main dishes like Braised Sumac Chicken and Lentils with Za'atar Yogurt Sauce (page 222). Keep some of this stock in the freezer and a restorative beverage or tasty meal will never be far away.

Ayurvedic Insight: Homemade vegetable stock will always be more flavorful and nutritious than store-bought stock. Just keep a bag of your fresh vegetable trimmings in the freezer, and when you have enough, simmer them into stock.

Makes 4 quarts

4 medium onions, chopped
2 pounds carrots, chopped
6 stalks celery, chopped
1 bunch of fresh parsley, chopped
2 bay leaves
3-inch piece of kombu

1. Combine everything in a large stockpot and add 6 quarts water. Bring to a boil over high heat, then reduce the heat to medium-low and simmer gently, uncovered, for 30 minutes. Turn off the heat and let sit for 30 minutes.

2. Strain the stock through a fine sieve. Use immediately, refrigerate for up to 1 week, or freeze for up to 1 month.

OPTIONS

- Include some of the brown onion skins for darker color in the broth.
- For deeper flavor, simmer the broth for up to 2 hours.

Kripalu Chai

↑V
=P
↓K

WE SUGGEST CHAI as an alternative to hot coffee. Ginger, cinnamon, cardamom, cloves, star anise, and black peppercorns make it nourishing, flavorful, soothing, and stimulating all at once.

Ayurvedic Insight: On cold, damp days, caffeine jump-starts your system. However, it is a little too heating for summer weather. It is generally too heating for pitta and vata types as well, but they may enjoy this chai prepared without the tea and only the spices. If you use almond milk in place of dairy milk, this beverage can be balancing for kapha types as well.

Serves 4

2 tablespoons whole cardamom pods
2 teaspoons whole cloves
2 cinnamon sticks
1 piece of star anise
1/2 teaspoon black peppercorns
1 tablespoon thinly sliced fresh ginger
2 cups milk, any type
4 black tea bags
1 to 3 tablespoons rapadura, packed dark brown sugar, or other sweetener of choice

1. Cover the cardamom, cloves, cinnamon, star anise, and peppercorns with cheesecloth on a sturdy work surface. Use a rolling pin or a cast-iron skillet to gently crush the spices and help release their aromas. Wrap the crushed spices and the fresh ginger in the cheesecloth or put them in a large tea ball.

2. Combine the milk, 2 cups water, and spice bundle in a medium saucepan and bring to a boil over high heat. Reduce the heat to medium-low and simmer gently for 15 minutes.

3. Return the mixture to a boil over high heat, then turn off the heat and immediately add the tea bags. Let steep for 5 minutes, then strain.

4. Stir in your sweetener of choice, stirring to dissolve it. Serve warm.

OPTIONS

- For iced chai in warm weather, thoroughly chill the chai and serve it in tall glasses filled with ice.
- For a paleo version, omit the milk and increase the water to 3 cups. Or for a vegan version, use almond milk.

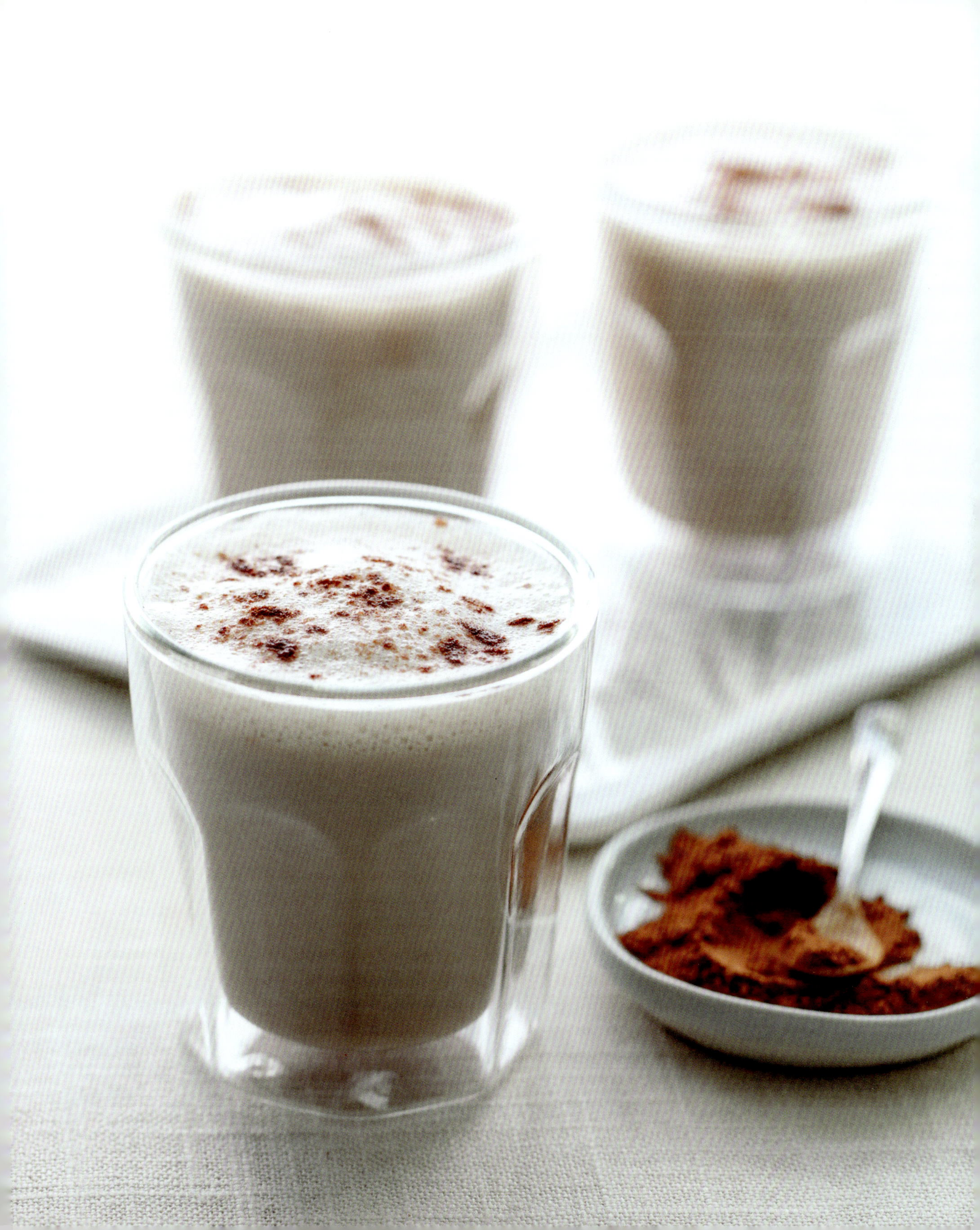

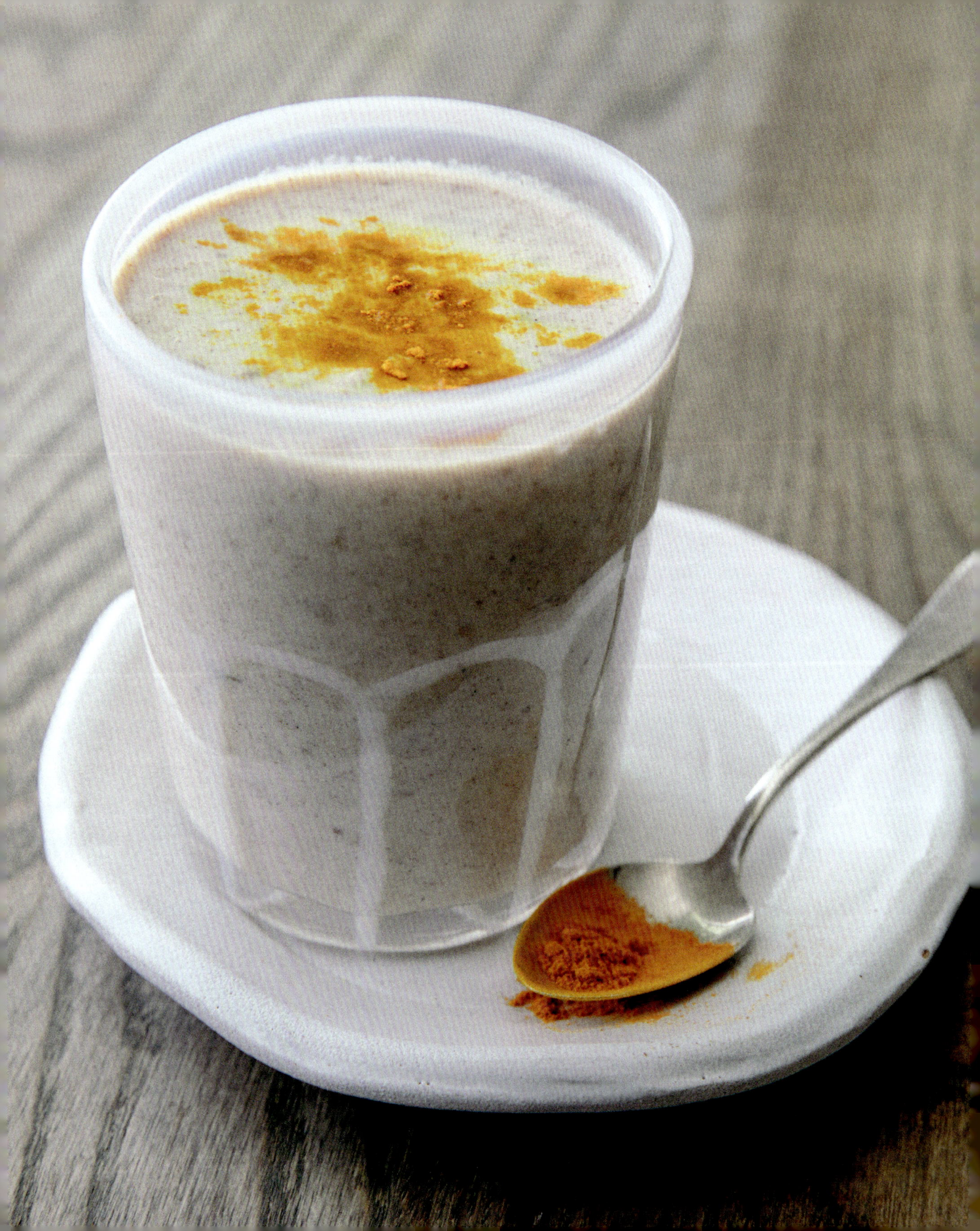

Ojas Milk

WARM SPICED MILK may be just what the doctor ordered when kids and adults need a little extra comfort. It also makes the ideal partner for Gluten-Free Salted Double Chocolate Chip Cookies (page 253) and Gluten-Free Rhapsody in Orange Cookies (page 256).

Ayurvedic Insight: Ojas is the life-sustaining vitality that promotes immunity in the body and resilience in the mind. Ojas can help keep you healthy during flu season and keep you energized when you are putting in overtime at work. This warm beverage is best enjoyed when digestion is strong, and it is more suitable for kapha when made with almond milk or rice milk.

Serves 4

1/4 cup slivered almonds

4 cups whole dairy milk, rice milk, or almond milk

8 whole dates, pitted and finely chopped

1/2 teaspoon ground ginger

1/2 teaspoon ground cinnamon

1/2 teaspoon ground cardamom

↓V

↓P

=K

1. Soak the almonds overnight in water to cover.

2. Drain the almonds and transfer to a medium saucepan along with the milk, dates, ginger, cinnamon, and cardamom. Bring the mixture to a simmer over medium heat and simmer gently until the dates are soft, about 8 minutes.

3. Make ½-cup servings with some dates and almonds in each cup.

OPTIONS

- For a smooth and frothy warm beverage, simmer everything as directed, then puree with an immersion blender or upright blender until smooth.
- *Golden Milk:* Stir in some ground turmeric with the other spices for its gorgeous golden color and its anti-inflammatory properties.

Iced Lavender Black Tea

↑V
=P
↓K

HERE'S OUR VERSION of Southern sweet tea with an infusion of lavender. The lavender has a calming, soothing effect while also improving brain function.

Ayurvedic Insight: Lavender helps to reduce stress and anxiety, making it the ideal partner for the stimulating effects of caffeine.

Serves 4

6 English Breakfast tea bags
2 tablespoons dried lavender
2 tablespoons honey or agave nectar

1. Bring 1½ cups water to a boil in a medium saucepan. Stir in the tea bags and lavender and remove from the heat. Cover and let steep for 5 minutes.

2. Strain the tea through a fine sieve, then stir in the honey and 2¾ cups cold water. Serve immediately over ice. You can also chill it for up to 3 days before serving.

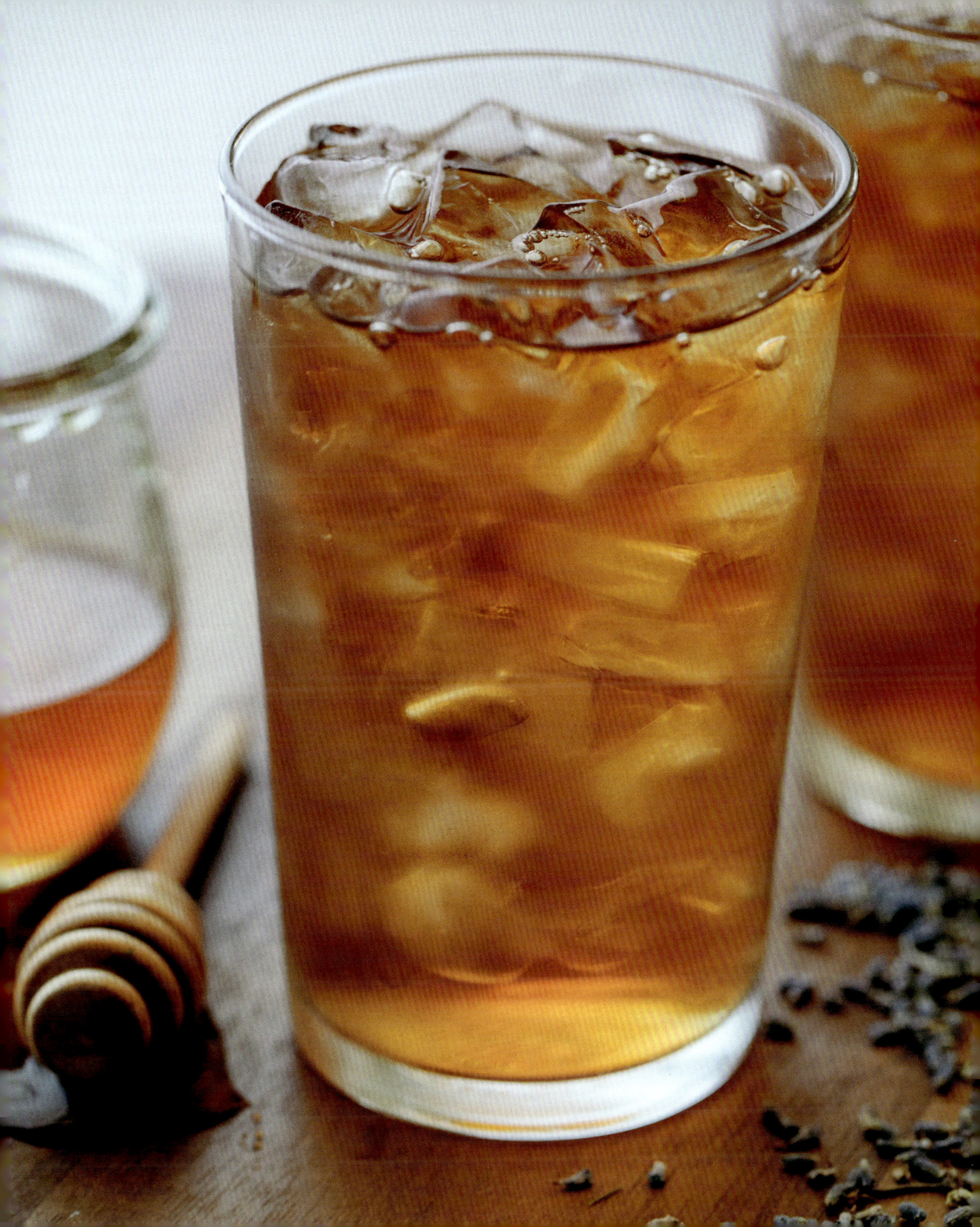

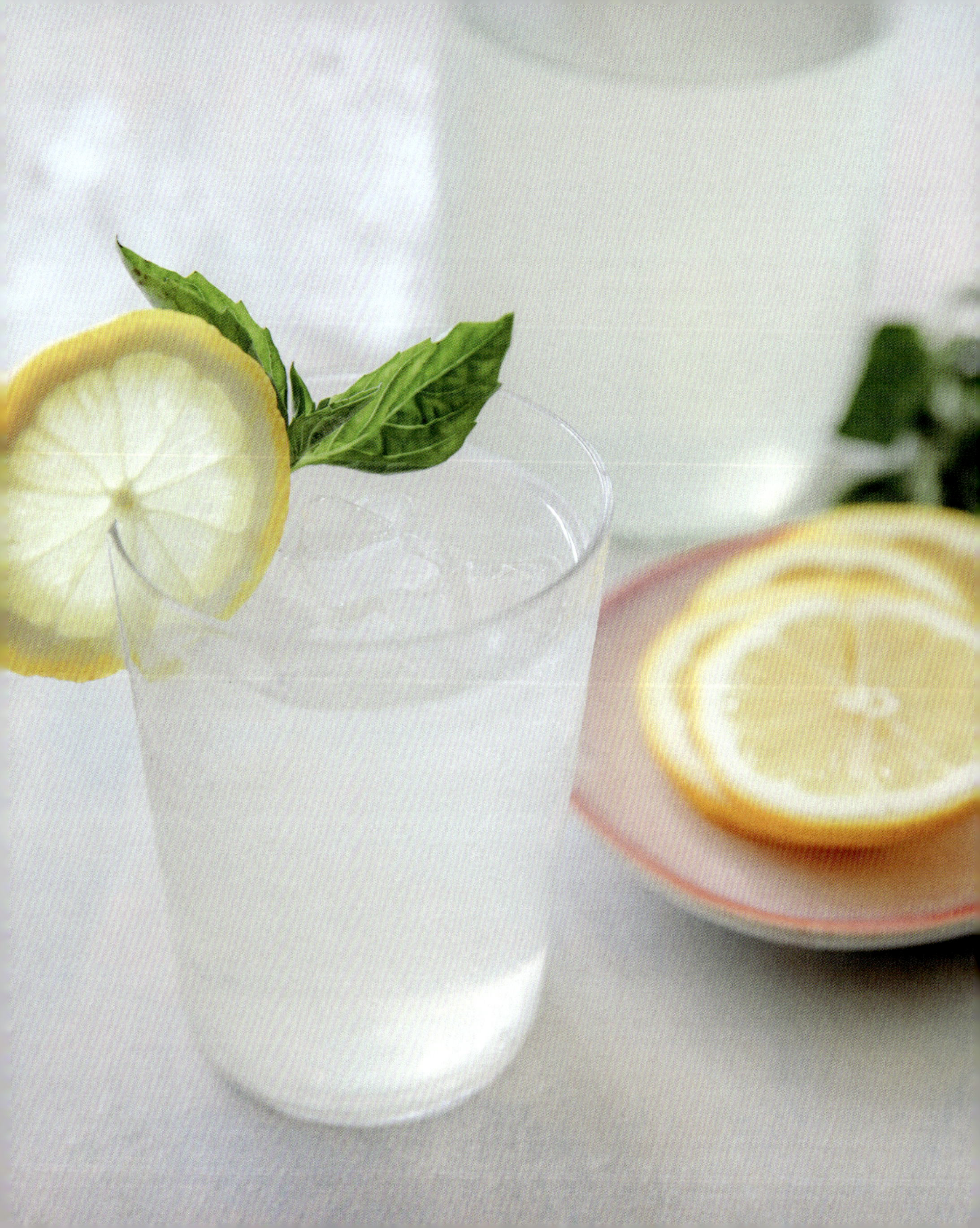

Thai Basil Lemonade

AT KRIPALU, THE AYURVEDIC HERB garden sits just above the main building. One hot summer, the herbs were growing like crazy and we infused them into various flavored syrups to make lemonade. This one is my favorite.

Ayurvedic Insight: In warmer months, the hot quality of alcohol coupled with the heat of the sun can cause inflammation that stifles digestion. This cold beverage is the perfect summer mocktail. Make it even more pitta friendly by swapping in lime for lemon.

Serves 4

1/2 cup packed Thai basil or basil leaves, plus more for garnish

1/2 cup organic cane sugar

Pinch of Himalayan salt

1/2 cup fresh lemon juice plus 4 lemon slices

4 cups seltzer or water

↓V

=P

=K

1. Combine the basil, sugar, salt, and ½ cup water in a small saucepan. Bring to a simmer over medium heat and simmer gently for 10 minutes. Remove from the heat and let cool. Chill this syrup mixture until it is cold, at least 1 hour and up to 5 days.

2. Remove the basil leaves and stir the lemon juice and seltzer into the syrup mixture. Serve in glasses over ice. Garnish each glass with a sprig of basil and a lemon ring on the rim.

OPTIONS

- Change the flavor by using rosemary or mint instead of basil in the syrup.

Moroccan Mint Iced Tea

↑V
↓P
↓K

THE SOOTHING COMBINATION of sweetened green tea and spearmint is a classic pairing throughout the Arab world. It is traditionally served hot, but we offer it over ice in the summer as an alternative to hot caffeinated beverages.

Ayurvedic Insight: Green tea contains less caffeine than coffee, making it more appropriate for pitta types. The cooling mint also helps improve digestion. If your digestion is feeling sluggish, enjoy it hot or at room temperature instead of iced.

Serves 4

3 green tea bags

1/4 cup packed fresh spearmint or peppermint leaves, plus a few for garnish

1 tablespoon honey or agave nectar

1. Bring 2½ cups water to a boil in a medium saucepan. Stir in the tea bags and mint, and remove from the heat. Cover and let steep for 7 minutes.

2. Strain the tea through a fine sieve, then stir in the honey and 2 cups cold water. Serve immediately over ice, garnished with a mint leaf. You can also chill it for up to 3 days before serving.

Kripalu Switchel

SWITCHELS ARE CLASSIC New England cold beverages made with maple syrup, cider vinegar, and ginger. Here's our version including turmeric, which gives it a beautiful golden color while helping to improve digestion.

Ayurvedic Insight: Sweet maple syrup, sour vinegar, pungent spices, and a touch of salt make this a very balanced beverage, perfect for warming up a sluggish digestive system.

Serves 4

2 tablespoons pure maple syrup

2 tablespoons raw cider vinegar, such as Bragg's

1 1/2 teaspoons minced fresh turmeric or 2/3 teaspoon turmeric powder

1 1/2 teaspoons minced fresh ginger

1/8 teaspoon fine sea salt

1. Combine the maple syrup, vinegar, turmeric, ginger, and salt in a half-pint jar. Cover and shake vigorously until combined, then refrigerate the mixture for 24 hours.

2. Strain the mixture through a fine strainer into a 1-quart jar, discarding the solids. Stir in 4 cups water and taste, adding a little maple syrup, vinegar, or water until it tastes good to you. Serve over ice.

↓V
↑P
=K

OPTIONS

- For a hot beverage in the cooler months, add 4 cups hot water to the switchel mixture instead of using cold water.
- For a paleo version, replace the vinegar with lemon juice.

Cucumber, Kale, Ginger, and Apple Juice

↑V
↓P
=K

HERE'S OUR BASIC KRIPALU green juice. It gives your digestive system a break while providing vital nutrients like vitamins A, C, and K, minerals like potassium and calcium, and the carotenoids *lutein* and *zeaxanthin*, which may help prevent macular degeneration and also have powerful antioxidant effects in the body.

Ayurvedic Insight: Favor juice when you want to lighten your digestive load. In the summer, this green juice offers nourishment as well as relief from a varied diet of proteins and fibrous vegetables.

Serves 4

4 cups lightly packed lacinato kale (stems are okay here)

2 English or hothouse cucumbers

2 apples, such as Pink Lady or Honeycrisp, cut into chunks

1/2 small fennel bulb, cut into chunks

1/4 cup packed cilantro leaves and small stems

1/2 lemon, peel removed

1 piece of fresh ginger, about 1/2 inch thick

Cut all the ingredients to fit your juicer and feed them in one by one, inserting the juiciest foods first. Extract the juice and divide among 4 glasses. If the juice is frothy, strain it through a fine-mesh sieve before serving.

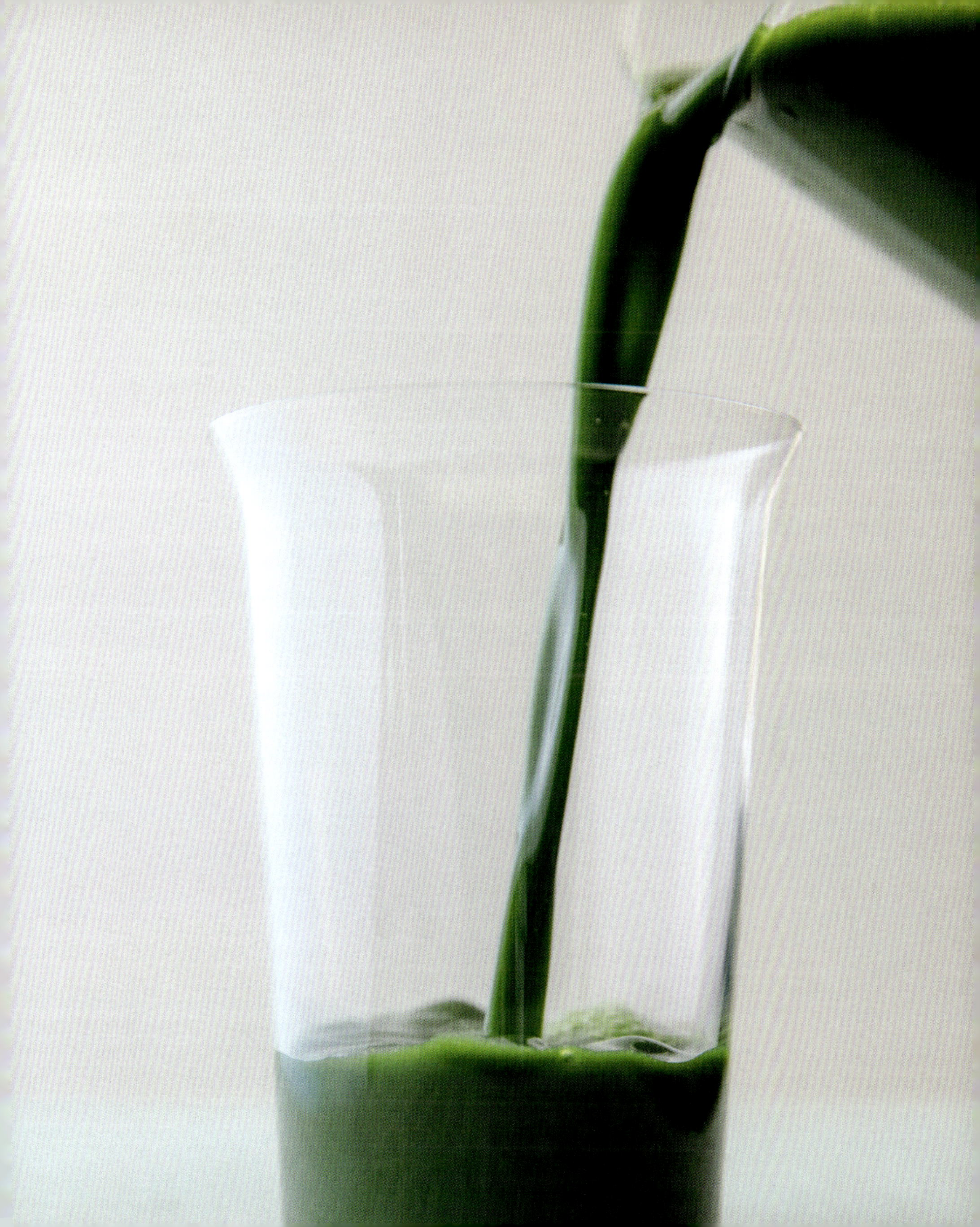

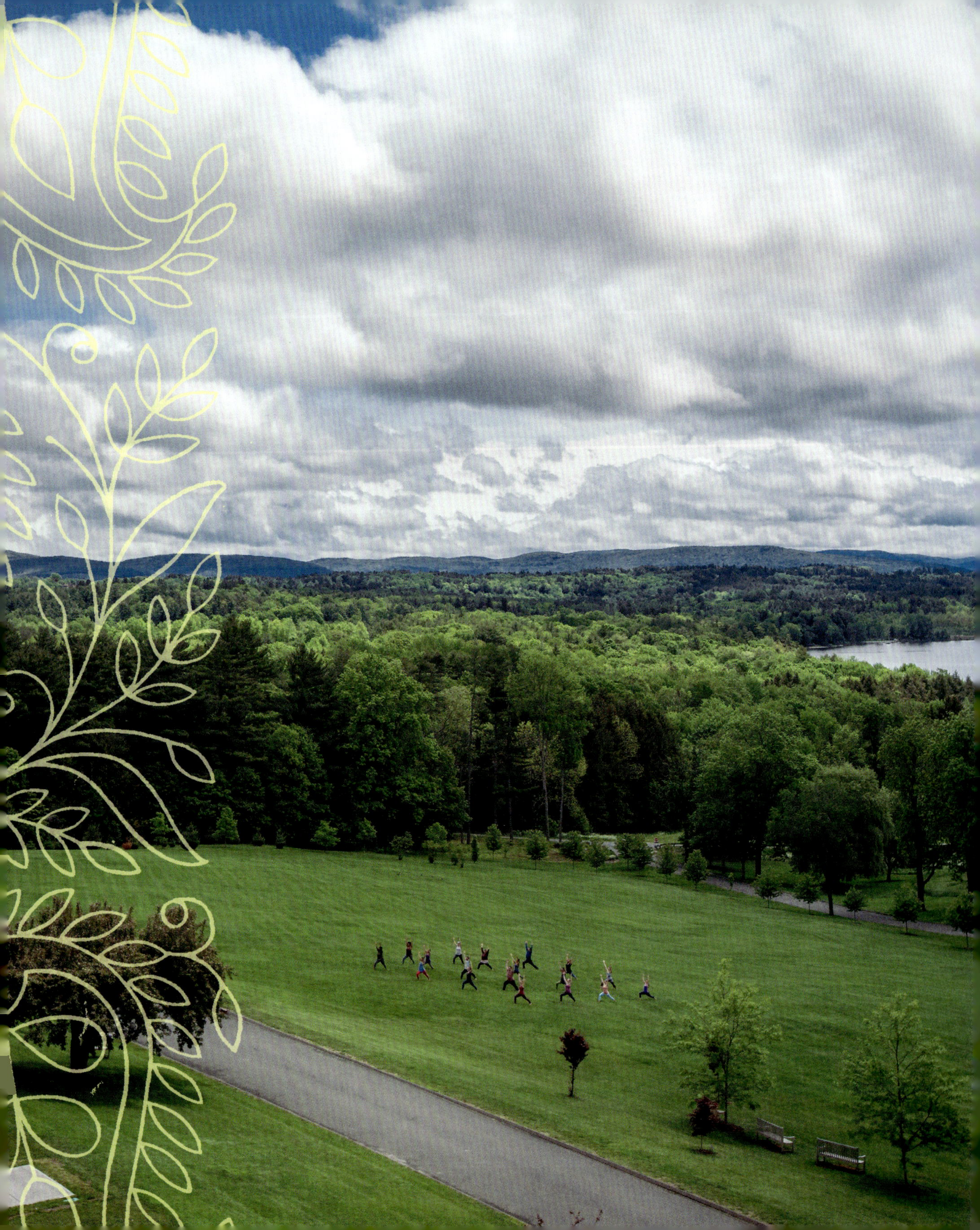

APPENDIX

SPECIAL-DIET RECIPES

All of our recipes are written with dietary restrictions and preferences in mind. Many are vegan or vegetarian, and most come with substitutes and options, so that the recipe can be made vegan, vegetarian, paleo, raw, sugar-free, dairy-free, gluten-free, or grain-free. Use the lists below to find the special-diet recipes you need. Recipes with an asterisk (*) will conform to the diet when following the variations or options listed in the recipe.

DAIRY-FREE RECIPES

GLUTEN-FREE RECIPES

GRAIN-FREE RECIPES

HEALTHY RESET (CLEANSE) RECIPES

PALEO RECIPES

RAW RECIPES

SUGAR-FREE RECIPES

VEGAN RECIPES

VEGETARIAN RECIPES

SIX-INGREDIENT RECIPES[†]

[†]Not counting salt, pepper, oil, and water

THIRTY-MINUTE RECIPES

GRATITUDE

I was blessed to inherit a unique and well-thought-out food service program at Kripalu. I want to honor and thank all of the cooks, volunteers, and chefs who came before me. They built the gastronomical foundation here and set the stage for our current chefs to successfully prepare the food that supports our guest experience to this very day.

A big shout-out to Erin Casperson, dean of the Kripalu School of Ayurveda, for all of her Ayurvedic insights throughout the book, for her sense of humor, and for keeping it real.

Thank you to our bakery manager, Cathy Ligenza, for her years of service, during which she developed the baking recipes in this book, and for her consistent effort in always looking for something new to bake.

To senior sous-chef Sinti Lin, for running our kitchen and for his support throughout the recipe testing.

To our operations manager, Steve Sherman, for his unending support in the department and for helping get the book photos done even when the right food didn't show up!

To my man, Dave Joachim, who managed to tease out all the information in this book from my crazy head and get it into print form. I haven't spent that much time on the phone with anyone since the '90s! Thank you for your expertise, patience, and laid-back approach to the work that you do. Thanks also to his wife, Christine Bucher, and sons, August and Maddox, for tasting all of the food during recipe testing—and raving about it!

To our agent, Sally Ekus, for helping to bring this project together for Kripalu as well as for bringing David on board. A big thank-you also to our editor, Marnie Cochran, for her levelheaded guidance throughout this book's development and to the rest of the staff at Ballantine for turning it into a success.

To Brian Samuels and Catrine Kelty, thank you for making the food leap off the page in these gorgeous photographs—and for the great food photography tips!

To executive sous-chef Shelby Drosehn, a born leader who has worked and laughed by my side since we both arrived here in 2010 and can be equally credited with any success the Kripalu Kitchen has had during my tenure.

Never-ending thanks to all the current cooks, sous-chefs, managers, servers, stewards, veggie preppers, bakers, those who purchase, those who put away, those who fix, and those who do all things clerical that make up the staff at Kripalu DFS (Dining and Food Service). You all collectively and consistently deliver the experience that those who visit us love so much . . . you are awesome!

To Terry Moore, my first boss and mentor, who took a chance and hired a shy fourteen-year-old kid with a Dutch boy haircut to be a bus boy in his restaurant and showed him what "service" was all about.

To Andrea Zahn and Ned Leavitt for all their work behind the scenes here at Kripula.

For my children, Hadyn, Jasmine, and Dessa, for always asking "Do you have work?" and being bummed out but understanding when I do. You inspire me every day to always do better.

Most important, to Amber Star for all you've done for our children and for your never-ending support while putting up with my craziness over the years, especially while writing this book. Thanks for listening when you'd heard the story a million times and being patient when I came up with a solution that you had already suggested.

Finally, to the thousands who walk through Kripalu's doors each year and give themselves and our food a shot: we are eternally grateful.

INDEX

Page references in *italics* refer to photographs.

ABOUT THE AUTHORS

JEREMY ROCK SMITH is the executive chef at Kripalu Center for Yoga & Health. A graduate of the Culinary Institute of America, Jeremy was trained in classical French cuisine and has cooked in fine-dining kitchens from Breckenridge, Colorado, to London, England. Jeremy and his team nourish Kripalu guests with approximately 1,200 healthy meals every day. In addition to overseeing all food service at Kripalu, Jeremy teaches guests about healthy food and cooking with weekly cooking demonstrations and frequent immersive programs on food and nutrition. Jeremy has also served as a faculty member of the Center for Mind-Body Medicine in Washington, DC. He lives with his family in the Berkshire Hills of Massachusetts.

jeremyrocksmith.com
Instagram: @jeremyrocksmith

DAVID JOACHIM has authored, edited, or collaborated on more than forty cookbooks, including several award winners and bestsellers, such as *The Food Substitutions Bible* and A Man, a Can, a Plan, a series of healthy cookbooks that has sold more than 1 million copies. His other cookbooks include *Cooking Light Global Kitchen* and *The Wicked Healthy Cookbook,* co-authored with chefs Chad Sarno and Derek Sarno. He lives near Allentown, Pennsylvania.

davejoachim.com

ABOUT THE TYPE

This book was set in Fournier, a typeface named for Pierre-Simon Fournier (1712–68), the youngest son of a French printing family. He started out engraving woodblocks and large capitals, then moved on to fonts of type. In 1736 he began his own foundry and made several important contributions in the field of type design; he is said to have cut 147 alphabets of his own creation. Fournier is probably best remembered as the designer of St. Augustine Ordinaire, a face that served as the model for the Monotype Corporation's Fournier, which was released in 1925.